OXFORD MEDICAL PUBLICATIONS

Colorectal Surgery

T0177745

Oxford Specialist handbooks published and forthcoming

Oxford Specialist Handbooks
in Surgery

Colorectal
Surgery

SECOND EDITION

EDITED BY

Richard G Molloy

Consultant Colorectal Surgeon
Queen Elizabeth University Hospital
Glasgow, UK

Graham J MacKay

Consultant Colorectal Surgeon
Glasgow Royal Infirmary
Honorary Professor
University of Glasgow
Glasgow, UK

Helen R Dorrance

Consultant Colorectal Surgeon
Queen Elizabeth University Hospital
Glasgow, UK

Patrick J O'Dwyer

Emeritus Professor of Surgery
University Department of Surgery
Queen Elizabeth University Hospital
Glasgow, UK

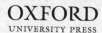

OXFORD
UNIVERSITY PRESS

OXFORD
UNIVERSITY PRESS

Great Clarendon Street, Oxford, OX2 6DP,
United Kingdom

Oxford University Press is a department of the University of Oxford.
It furthers the University's objective of excellence in research, scholarship,
and education by publishing worldwide. Oxford is a registered trade mark of
Oxford University Press in the UK and in certain other countries

First Edition published in 2010
Second Edition published in 2021

Impression: 1

Published in the United States of America by Oxford University Press
198 Madison Avenue, New York, NY 10016, United States of America

British Library Cataloguing in Publication Data
Data available

Library of Congress Control Number: 2020952851

ISBN 978–0–19–289624–7

DOI: 10.1093/med/9780192896247.001.0001

Printed in Great Britain by
Ashford Colour Press Ltd, Gosport, Hampshire

Preface

The primary focus of this book is as a revision tool for general surgical trainees preparing for the FRCS examination, and in particular those declaring colorectal surgery as an area of special interest. It has been written specifically to address the curriculum designed and approved by the Association of Coloproctology of Great Britain and Ireland and the Intercollegiate Surgical Curriculum Project.

The book is designed to provide easy access to relevant, up-to-date, and evidence-based information in a portable format which can be used at work or wherever time is available for study. While the handbook is not meant to replace the use of an in-depth reference text, it does aim to provide comprehensive coverage of the curriculum, including sections on related specialties and applied anatomy. Further sections address the presentation of colorectal disease in the outpatient clinic; a review of colorectal assessment tools; and detailed, practical information regarding the management of benign and malignant colonic and anorectal conditions.

The 2nd edition of the book has undergone extensive updating to reflect some of the recent innovations in surgical practice. The most significant updates have taken place in the oncology and inflammatory bowel disease chapters. Additional new sections include Robotic surgery, complete mesocolic excision, capsule colonoscopy and the role of qFIT in lower GI investigation. Management of benign colorectal disease has also been revised to reflect current approaches to rectal prolapse and haemorrhoidal disease including updated guidelines for functional bowel conditions.

The authors hope that this specialist handbook will be of interest to surgical trainees at all levels, including specialist nurses, general practitioners and allied healthcare professionals who may be involved in the management of this patient group.

Graham J MacKay
Richard G Molloy

Contents

Detailed contents

First edition contributors

Des Alcorn
Consultant Radiologist,
Gartnavel General Hospital,
Glasgow

John Anderson
Consultant Colorectal Surgeon,
Glasgow Royal Infirmary

Stuart Ballantyne
Consultant Radiologist,
Queen Elizabeth University
Hospital,
Glasgow

Pete Chong
Consultant Colorectal Surgeon,
Glasgow Royal Infirmary,

Helen R Dorrance
Consultant Colorectal Surgeon,
Queen Elizabeth University
Hospital,
Glasgow

Kate Fitzgerald
Consultant Breast and Oncoplastic
Surgeon
Griffith
Australia

Daniel Gaya
Consultant Gastroenterologist,
Glasgow Royal Infirmary

Vivienne Gough
Consultant Surgeon
Royal Alexandra Hospital
Paisley

Graham Haddock
Consultant in Paediatric Surgery,
Royal Hospital for Children,
Glasgow

David Hendry
Consultant Urological Surgeon,
Queen Elizabeth University
Hospital,
Glasgow

Angus Macdonald
Consultant Colorectal Surgeon,
Monklands Hospital,
Airdrie

Graham J MacKay
Consultant Surgeon
Glasgow Royal Infirmary

Alec McDonald
Consultant Oncologist,
Beatson West of Scotland
Oncology Centre,
Glasgow

Ruth McKee
Consultant Colorectal Surgeon
(retired),
Glasgow Royal Infirmary

Mathew McKernan
Consultant Gynaecologist
Letterkenny University Hospital
Ireland

Andrew McMahon
Consultant Surgeon,
Glasgow Royal Infirmary
Glasgow

Lindsay McNeil
Consultant in Palliative Care,
Royal Alexandra Hospital,
Paisley

Richard G Molloy
Consultant Colorectal Surgeon,
Queen Elizabeth University
Hospital,
Glasgow

Lisa Moyes
Consultant Surgeon
Queen Elizabeth University
Hospital,
Glasgow

Patrick J O'Dwyer
Emeritus Professor of Surgery,
Queen Elizabeth University
Hospital,
Glasgow

Christopher Payne
Consultant Colorectal Surgeon
Ninewells University Hospital
Dundee

Andrew Renwick
Consultant Colorectal Surgeon,
Royal Alexandra Hospital,
Paisley

Vlad Shumeyko
Consultant Transplant and
Hepatobiliary Surgeon,
Queen Elizabeth University
Hospital,
Glasgow

Graham Sunderland
Consultant Colorectal Surgeon
(retired),
Queen Elizabeth University
Hospital,
Glasgow

Michelle Thornton
Consultant Colorectal Surgeon,
Wishaw General Hospital,
Wishaw

Mark Vella
Consultant Colorectal Surgeon,
Royal Alexandra Hospital,
Paisley

Andy Winter
Consultant in GU Medicine and HIV,
Sandyford Initiative,
Glasgow

David Wright
Consultant Colorectal Surgeon,
Queen Elizabeth University
Hospital,
Glasgow

Second edition contributors

Kevin Burton
Consultant Gynaecological
Oncologist,
Glasgow Royal Infirmary,
Glasgow, UK

Daniel Gaya
Consultant Gastroenterologist,
Glasgow Royal Infirmary,
Glasgow, UK

Graham J MacKay
Consultant Colorectal Surgeon
Glasgow Royal Infirmary
Honorary Professor
University of Glasgow
Glasgow, UK

Nazia Mohammed
Consultant Oncologist,
Beatson West of Scotland
Oncology Centre,
Glasgow, UK

Richard G Molloy
Consultant Colorectal Surgeon
Queen Elizabeth University Hospital
Glasgow, UK

Second edition contributors

Symbols and abbreviations

➔	cross reference	bd	twice daily (bis die)
+ve	positive	BMI	body mass index
−ve	negative	BOPTA	benzyloxypropionictetra-acetate
~	approximately	BP	blood pressure
↑	increased	BSO	bilateral salpingo-oopherectomy
↓	decreased	CAD	circular anal dilator
→	leading to	cAMP	cyclic adenosine monophosphate
1°	primary	CBT	cognitive-behavioural therapy
2°	secondary	CCD	charge-coupled device
♀	female	CD	Crohn's disease
♂	male	CDAD	*Clostridium difficile*-associated diarrhoea
±	plus/minus	CDAI	Crohn's Disease Activity iIndex
AAD	antibiotic-associated diarrhoea	CEA	carcinoembryonic antigen
ACE	antegrade colonic enema	CF	cystic fibrosis
ACPO	acute colonic pseudo-obstruction	cfu	colony-forming unit
AFAP	attenuated familial adenomatous polyposis	CHRPE	congenital hypertrophy of the pigmented retinal epithelium
AFI	autofluorescence imaging	CIN	cervical intraepithelial neoplasia
AFP	alpha fetoprotein	CMI	chronic mesenteric ischaemia
AIDS	acquired immune deficiency syndrome	CMV	cytomegalovirus
AIN	anal intraepithelial neoplasia	CNS	central nervous system
AJCC	American Joint Committee on Cancer	CO_2	carbon dioxide
AMI	acute mesenteric ischaemia	COC	combined oral contraceptive
AP	anteroposterior	COPD	chronic obstructive pulmonary disease
APC	argon plasma coagulation	COX	cyclo-oxygenase
APER	abdominoperineal resection of the rectum	CRC	colorectal cancer
AS	ankylosing spondylitis	CRM	circumferential resection margin
5-ASA	5-amino-salicylic acid	CRP	C-reactive protein
ASA	American Society of Anesthesiologists	CsA	ciclosporin A
ASCA	anti-*Saccharomyces cerevisiae* antibody	CSCI	continuous subcutaneous infusion
ASCRS	American Society of Colon and Rectal Surgeons	CSM	component separation method
AST	aspartate transaminase	CT	computed tomography
AT	anti-thrombin	CTA	computed tomography angiography
ATLS	advanced trauma life support	CVP	central venous pressure
ATZ	anal transition zone	CXR	chest x-ray
AVM	arteriovenous malformation		
AXR	abdominal x-ray		
BCC	basal cell carcinoma		

DALM	dysplasia-associated lesion or mass
DEXA	dual energy x-ray absorptiometry
DFI	disease-free interval
DIC	disseminated intravascular coagulation
DIP	distal interphalangeal
DJ	duodenojejunal
DM	diabetes mellitus
DNA	deoxyribonucleic acid
DPAM	diffuse peritoneal adenomucinosis
DRE	digital rectal examination
DTPA	diethylene triamine pentaacetic acid
DVT	deep venous thrombosis
EA	epidural analgesia
EAS	external anal sphincter
EAUS	endoanal ultrasound
ECG	electrocardiography
ED	erectile dysfunction
EGFR	epidermal growth factor receptor
EHEC	enterohaemorrhagic *Escherichia coli*
EIA	enzyme immunoassay
EIEC	enteroinvasive *Escherichia coli*
EIM	extraintestinal manifestation
ELISA	enzyme-linked immunosorbent assay
EMG	electromyography
EMR	endoscopic mucosal resection
EOB	ethoxybenzyl
EPA	eicosapentanoic acid
EPEC	enteropathogenic *Escherichia coli*
ERCP	Endoscopic Retrograde Cholangiopancreatography
ERUS	endorectal ultrasound
ESD	endoscopic submucosal dissection
ESR	erythrocyte sedimentation rate
ETEC	enterotoxigenic *Escherichia coli*
EUA	examination under anaesthetic
FA	folinic acid
FAP	familial adenomatous polyposis
FB	foreign body
FBC	full blood count
FDG	fluorodeoxyglucose
FEV	forced expiratory volume

FI	faecal incontinence
FIT	faecal immunological testing
FNA	fine needle aspiration
FOB	faecal occult blood
FOBT	faecal occult blood testing
FRC	functional residual capacity
5-FU	5-fluorouracil
FVC	forced vital capacity
GA	general anaesthetic
GAVE	gastric antral vascular ectasia
GC	gonococcus
GCS	graduated compression stocking
G-CSF	granulocyte colony-stimulating factor
Gd	gadolinium
GI	gastrointestinal
GIP	gastric inhibitory polypeptide
GIST	gastrointestinal stromal tumour
GnRH	gonadotropin-releasing hormone
GP	general practitioner
GTN	glyceryl trinitrate
GUM	genitourinary medicine
HAART	highly active anti-retroviral therapy
HAPC	high amplitude propagated contractions
Hb	haemoglobin
hCG	human chorionic gonadotropin
Hct	haematocrit
HGM	hypertrophic gastric mucosa
HIAA	hydroxyindoleacetic acid
HIT	heparin-induced thrombocytopenia
HIV	human immunodeficiency virus
HLA	human leucocyte antigen
HMPAO	hexamethyl propylene amine oxime
HNPCC	hereditary non-polyposis colon cancer
HP	hyperplastic polyposis
HPB	hepato pancreatico biliary
HPN	home parenteral nutrition
HPV	human papilloma virus
HRT	hormone replacement therapy
HSV	herpes simplex virus
5-HT	hydroxytryptamine
HUS	haemolytic–uraemic syndrome
IAS	internal anal sphincter

IBD	inflammatory bowel disease	MS	multiple sclerosis
IBS	irritable bowel syndrome	MSI	microsatellite instability
IC	indeterminate colitis	MSM	men who have sex with men
ICA	ileocolic artery	MSSU	midstream specimen of urine
IFN	interferon	NA	noradrenaline
IFX	infliximab	NAAT	nucleic acid amplification test
IGAP	inferior gluteal artery perforator	NADH	nicotinamide adenine dinucleotide
IL	interleukin	NBI	narrow-band imaging
IM	intramuscular	NG	nasogastric
IMA	inferior mesenteric artery	NICE	National Institute for Health and Clinical Excellence
INR	international normalized ratio	NMDA	N-methyl-D-aspartic acid
IORT	intraoperative radiotherapy	NO	nitric oxide
IPAA	ileal pouch–anal anastomosis	NOD	nucleotide-binding oligomerization domain
IRA	ileorectal anastomosis	NOTES	natural orifice transluminal endoscopic surgery
IS	injection sclerotherapy		
IV	intravenous	NSAID	non-steroidal anti-inflammatory drug
IVC	inferior vena cava		
IVF	*in vitro* fertilization	N+V	nausea and vomiting
IVSR	intravenous steroid resistant	od	once daily (omni die)
IVU	intravenous urogram	OOS	outlet obstruction syndrome
JPS	juvenile polyposis syndrome	PAN	polyarteritis nodosa
LA	local anaesthetic	P-ANCA	perinuclear anti-neutrophil cytoplasmic antibody
LBO	large bowel obstruction		
LFT	liver function test	PCA	patient-controlled analgesia
LGV	lymphogranuloma venereum	PCOS	polycystic ovarian syndrome
LIF	left iliac fossa	PCR	polymerase chain reaction
LMWH	low molecular weight heparin	PDAI	Pouch Disease Activity Index
LN	lymph node	PDS	polydioxanone
LR	local recurrence	PDT	photodynamic therapy
LUQ	left upper quadrant	PE	pulmonary embolism
MALT	mucosa-associated lymphoid tissue	PEG	percutaneous endoscopic gastrostomy
MBP	mechanical bowel preparation	PET	positron emission tomography
MD	Meckel's diverticulum	PICC	peripheral inserted central catheter
MDT	multidisciplinary team		
MI	myocardial infarction	PID	pelvic inflammatory disease
min	minutes	PJS	Peutz–Jehgers syndrome
MMC	migrating myoelectric complex	PMB	post-menopausal bleeding
MMR	mismatch repair	PMCA	peritoneal mucinous carcinomatosis
MODS	multiorgan dysfunction syndrome		
6-MP	6-mercaptopurine	PMP	pseudomyxoma peritonei
MRCP	Magnetic Resonance Cholangiopancreatography	PN	parenteral nutrition
		PNE	peripheral nerve evaluation
MPSRUS	mucosal prolapse solitary rectal ulcer syndrome	PNTML	pudendal nerve terminal motor latency
MRI	magnetic resonance imaging	PO	orally (per os)
MRSA	methicillin-resistant *Staphylococcus aureus*	PPH	procedure for prolapse and haemorrhoids

PPI	proton pump inhibitor	SRUS	solitary rectal ulcer syndrome
PR	per rectum	SSI	surgical site infection
PRC	packed red cell	SSRI	selective serotonin reuptake inhibitor
PRN	as required (pro re nata)		
PS	performance status	STARR	stapled transanal rectal resection
PV	portal venous		
PPI	proton pump inhibitor	STI	sexually transmitted infection
qid	four times daily (quarter in die)	TAH	total abdominal hysterectomy
qFIT	quantitative feacal immunological test	TAP	transversus abdominus plane
		TB	tuberculosis
RA	rheumatoid arthritis	Tc	technetium
RAIR	rectoanal inhibitory reflex	TEM	transanal endoscopic microsurgery
RAP	resting anal pressure		
RBC	red blood cell	TENS	transcutaneous electrical nerve stimulation
RBL	rubber band ligation		
RCDAD	recurrent Clostridium difficile-associated diarrhoea	TFT	thyroid function tests
		THD	transarterial haemorrhoidal dearterialization
RCT	randomized controlled trial		
RFA	radiofrequency ablation	TI	terminal ileum
RIF	right iliac fossa	tid	three times daily (ter die sumendus)
RMI	risk of malignancy index		
RPC	restorative proctocolectomy	TIPS	transjugular intrahepatic portosystemic shunt
RPR	rapid plasma reagin		
RT	radiotherapy	TME	total mesorectal excision
RTA	road traffic accident	TNF	tumour necrosis factor
RUQ	right upper quadrant	TNM	tumour nodes metastases
s	seconds	tPA	tissue plasminogen activator
SBO	small bowel obstruction	TPMT	thiopurine methyltransferase
SC	subcutaneous	TPN	total parenteral nutrition
SCC	squamous cell carcinoma	TPPA	Treponema pallidum particle agglutination
SCFA	short chain fatty acids		
SCPRT	short course pre-operative radiotherapy	TS	thymidylate synthase
		TVS	transvaginal ultrasonography
SBRT	stereotactic body radiation therapy		
		U	units
SEMS	self-expanding metal stents	UC	ulcerative colitis
SIGN	Scottish Intercollegiate Guideline Network	UFT	tegafur–uracil
		UGIE	upper gastrointestinal endoscopy
SIRS	systemic inflammatory response syndrome		
		US	ultrasound
SLE	systemic lupus erythematosus	UTI	urinary tract infection
SMA	superior mesenteric artery	U&E	urea & electrolytes
SMV	superior mesenteric vein	VDRL	venereal disease research laboratory
SNS	sacral nerve stimulation		
SP	squeeze pressure	VEGF	vascular endothelial growth factor
SPIO	superparamagnetic iron oxide		
SRA	superior rectal artery	VIP	vasoactive intestinal polypeptide
SRC	signet ring cell carcinoma		
SRS	somatostatin receptor scintigraphy	VTE	venous thromboembolism
		WCC	white cell count
		WHO	World Health Organization

Chapter 1

Basic science

The anterior abdominal wall

An understanding of the anatomy of the abdominal wall is important for the colorectal surgeon to facilitate appropriate incisions optimizing patient recovery and producing a well-healed cosmetic scar. Vertical incisions crossing Langer's lines are often unsightly.

The anterior abdominal wall consists of skin, subcutaneous fat, areolar tissue, fascia, muscles, pre-peritoneal fat and peritoneum. The fascial layer (Scarpa's fascia) is well developed in the lower abdomen and particularly evident during inguinal hernia repair.

Superficial nerves

- Segmental cutaneous nerves run between the transversus abdominus and internal oblique with lateral and anterior branches (Fig. 1.1)
- Iliohypogastric and ilioinguinal nerves arise from the 1st lumbar nerve and are the most caudal superficial nerves
- Ilioinguinal nerve is absent in 10% of individuals
- The genitofemoral nerve arises from the 1st and 2nd lumbar nerves and supplies the upper, inner thigh and genital region
- Knowledge of the position of these nerves is of value in inguinal hernia repair and post-operative pain relief using local anaesthetic (LA).

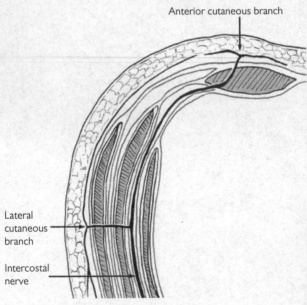

Anterior cutaneous branch

Lateral cutaneous branch

Intercostal nerve

Fig. 1.1 Superficial nerves of the anterior abdominal wall.

THE ANTERIOR ABDOMINAL WALL 3

Superficial blood vessels

- The lower intercostals, musculophrenic and epigastric arteries supply the abdominal wall cephalad to the umbilicus
- Caudal to the umbilicus, the superior epigastric artery is continuous with the inferior epigastric artery which lies deep to the rectus muscle
- The inferior epigastric artery arises from the external iliac artery just proximal to the inguinal ligament
- Superficial epigastric, superficial circumflex iliac and superficial external pudendal arteries are encountered in hernia repair and arise from the femoral artery. The associated veins drain to the saphenous vein.

Abdominal wall muscles

External oblique

- Arises from digitations on the external surfaces of the lower eight ribs
- Fibres pass down and forwards inserting into iliac crest (Fig. 1.2)
- Medially it forms the external oblique aponeurosis, becoming the inguinal ligament along its lower margin
- Merges into the anterior rectus sheath and linea alba in the midline.

Internal oblique

- Arises from anterior 2/3 iliac crest and lateral 1/2 of inguinal ligament
- Fibres pass up and medially, inserting into lower four ribs and linea alba
- Lower fibres originating from inguinal ligament arch down and medially, merge with fibres of transversus abdominus to insert at the pubic crest and iliopectineal line
- Medially the aponeurosis of the internal oblique splits, fusing with the external oblique to form the anterior rectus sheath and with transversus abdominus to form the posterior rectus sheath.

Transversus abdominus

- Arises from the iliopsoas fascia and inserts into the linea alba
- Fibres mostly run transversely, curving down and medially to form an arch over the inguinal canal
- Contributes to posterior rectus sheath with the aponeurosis of internal oblique to a point midway between umbilicus and symphysis pubis (arcuate line)
- Below this it fuses with internal and external oblique to form anterior rectus sheath.

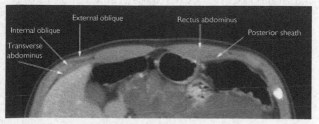

Fig. 1.2 CT of anterior abdominal wall musculature.

Linea alba, rectus sheath and rectus abdominus muscles
- The linea alba is a dense fibrous band extending from the xiphoid process to the pubic symphysis
- Formed by the decussation of fibres from the aponeurosis of external and internal oblique and transversus abdominus muscles
- At the umbilicus there is a single layer of fused fibrous tissue as a result of the space occupied by the umbilical cord at childbirth
- Fibres of anterior and posterior rectus sheaths cross the midline forming a triple layer crisscross pattern
- Rectus muscle is flat and strap-like, arising from the crest of the pubis
- Inserts into 5th–7th costal cartilages and the xiphoid
- Three tendinous intersections at xiphoid, umbilicus and midway between the two are all adherent to the anterior rectus sheath
- The pyramidal muscle is triangular in shape, arises from the symphysis pubis and inserts into the linea alba.

Fascia transversalis
- Lies deep to the transversus abdominus muscle and extends from side to side and from the rib cage above to the pelvis inferiorly
- In the lower abdomen it has specialized bands and folds and forms the posterior wall of the inguinal canal
- The fascia transversalis invests the cord structures as they pass through it forming a U-shaped sling. Thought to be an important part of the shutter mechanism closing the internal ring during episodes of increased intra-abdominal pressure.

Inguinal canal and spermatic cord
- The inguinal canal is covered by the external oblique aponeurosis
- The conjoint tendon is a variable structure, absent in ~20% of subjects and is formed by the fused aponeurosis of the internal oblique and transversus muscles (Fig. 1.3)
- Medially it arches posterior to the spermatic cord inserting into the iliopectineal line deep to the inguinal and lacunar ligaments. It forms the posterior wall of the inguinal canal with transversalis fascia
- The inguinal ligament is attached medially like a fan to the pectineal line and pubic tubercle forms the inferior part of the canal
- Spermatic cord receives fascial investments as it emerges from the deep ring from fascia transversalis (internal spermatic fascia), internal oblique (cremaster muscle) and external oblique (external spermatic fascia)
- The cord is composed of the vas deferens, testicular artery and vein (pampiniform plexus), lymphatics, artery to vas deferens, cremasteric artery and the genital branch of the genitofemoral nerve.

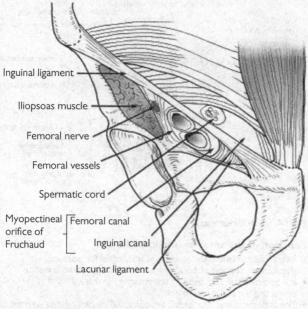

Fig. 1.3 The inguinal and femoral canals.

Pre-peritoneal space and peritoneum

- In the lower abdomen the fascia transversalis has two distinct layers: an anterior layer covers the internal aspect of the transversus muscle; the deep layer lies anterior to the pre-peritoneal fat and peritoneum
- The space between the layers is avascular and opened to enter the pre-peritoneal space of Bogros during totally extraperitoneal hernia repair (Fig. 1.4)
- In the midline the pre-vesical space of Retzius contains loose connective tissue and fat
- The myopectineal orifice of Fruchaud (Fig. 1.3), divided in two parts by the inguinal ligaments, represents a potentially weak part of the abdominal wall through which inguinal and femoral hernias occur.

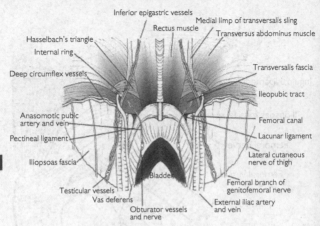

Fig. 1.4 Pre-peritoneal space.

Function of the anterior abdominal wall

- Intact function of the abdominal wall is essential for postural stabilization, support of breathing and for defecation and urination
- It is also necessary for bending and rotating the trunk as well as protecting the abdominal cavity
- The abdominal wall is an elastic structure and elasticity varies with age and sex
- Elasticity is greater in the vertical than the horizontal or oblique directions. This elasticity is one of the reasons why very severe blunt trauma is required to disrupt the abdominal wall and thus hernias secondary to trauma are rare.

Development of the GI tract

Foregut

Midgut

Development of the GI tract

The primitive gastrointestinal (GI) tract extending from the buccopharyngeal to the cloacal membrane begins to form during the second and third week of gestation. Cephalocaudal and lateral folding of the embryo incorporates an endoderm-lined cavity from the wall of the yolk sac which becomes the primitive gut.

Foregut

- Extends from just caudal to pharyngeal tube to the liver outgrowth
- Around week 4 the tracheobronchial diverticulum develops. It gradually separates to form the respiratory primordium and oesophagus
- The stomach appears as a fusiform dilatation around the 4th week. During subsequent development its appearance and position change due to longitudinal/anteroposterior (AP) axis rotation and differential rates of growth
- The duodenum is formed from the terminal part of foregut and cephalic part of midgut. As the stomach rotates the duodenum takes on its 'C' shape and becomes retroperitoneal.

Liver and pancreas

- The liver primordium appears in middle of week 3 as a diverticulum at the distal end of the foregut with rapidly developing strands of cells penetrating the septum transversum. As a result of rapid growth, the liver protrudes into the abdominal cavity. The mesoderm of the septum transversum becomes stretched, forming the falciform ligament
- The pancreas is formed from two buds originating in the endodermal lining of the duodenum.

Midgut

- At week 4, the midgut is suspended from posterior abdominal wall by a short mesentery. It communicates with yolk sac via the vitelline duct
- In adults, the midgut begins immediately distal to the ampulla of Vater. It extends to the junction of middle/distal third of transverse colon
- Its whole length is supplied by the superior mesenteric artery (SMA)
- Development of the midgut is characterized by rapid elongation of the gut and its mesentery, forming the primary intestinal loop. At the apex of the loop is an open communication with yolk sac, the vitelline duct
- The upper part develops into distal duodenum, jejunum and upper part of ileum. The lower part develops into ileum, caecum, appendix, ascending colon and proximal 2/3 of transverse colon.

Physiological herniation of the midgut

- There is rapid elongation of the primary intestinal loop, particularly the cephalad limb. Combined with rapid expansion of the liver this means that the abdominal cavity is temporarily too small. The intestinal loops herniate into the base of the umbilical cord during the 6th week of development (Fig. 1.5a)
- In addition, the intestinal loop rotates on the axis formed by the SMA
- Viewed from the front there is a 270° counter-clockwise rotation (Fig. 1.5b)

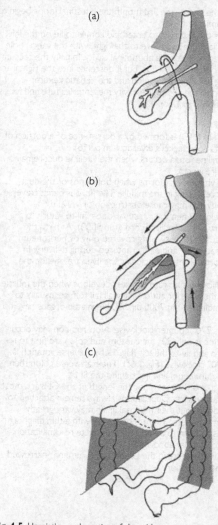

Fig. 1.5 Herniation and rotation of the midgut.

- At approximately the end of the 3rd month the intestinal loops begin to return to the abdominal cavity
- Proximal jejunum is the first part to enter and comes to lie on the left
- Subsequent loops lie more and more to the right, with the caecal pole being the last part to re-enter the abdominal cavity. Initially the caecum is in the right upper quadrant (RUQ), but it descends into the right iliac fossa (RIF) forming the ascending colon and the hepatic flexure
- As the loops return to the abdominal cavity mesenteries fuse and loops are fixed into position (Fig. 1.5c).

Midgut variations

- Meckel's diverticulum (MD) is formed by a persistence of a portion of the vitelline duct (◑ see Meckel's diverticulum p.416)
- An umbilical or vitelline fistula occurs when the vitelline duct remains patent over its entire length
- Enterocystoma or vitelline cyst forms when both ends of the duct fibrose with a cyst remaining in the middle. The fibrous bands traverse the abdominal cavity and may cause obstruction or volvulus
- Omphalocele develops when the intestinal loops fail to return to the abdominal cavity from the umbilical cord (1 in 5000). At birth the herniated loops cause a large swelling covered only by peritoneum and amnion. The sac is thin and easily ruptured during delivery. In the most severe form, all viscera including the liver are outside the abdominal cavity
- A congenital umbilical hernia (gastroschisis) develops when the muscle layers and skin of the anterior abdominal wall fail to fuse, usually to the right of the umbilicus (1 in 7000 births). Herniated organs have no covering layer
- Normal rotation is 270° counter-clockwise. Non-rotation may occur (Fig. 1.6a). If rotation is only 90° the caecum and colon are first to re-enter the abdomen and lie to the left (Fig. 1.6b). Reverse rotation is possible, usually 90° clockwise (Fig. 1.6c). The transverse colon then passes behind the duodenum and lies behind the SMA
- Duplication can occur anywhere along the length of the GI tract, most commonly in the ileal region. Duplications always remain attached to their segment of origin, but their mucosal lining may vary greatly
- Atresia may occur anywhere. There is no lumen with a thin diaphragm across the gut. It is thought to be due to incomplete re-canalization. It may also be due to vascular abnormalities
- Stenosis may occur anywhere in the GI tract. The lumen is narrowed often with proximal distension.

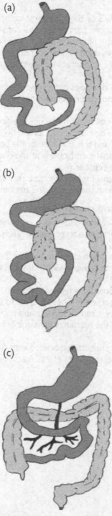

Fig. 1.6 Malrotation of the digestive system. Non-rotation (a) incomplete rotation (b) and reversed rotation (c).

Hindgut

- This forms the distal 1/3 of the transverse colon, descending colon, sigmoid, rectum and upper part of the anal canal
- The terminal part of the hindgut enters into the cloaca. This is an endoderm-lined cavity which is in direct contact with the surface ectoderm. At the point of contact between endo- and ectoderm is the cloacal membrane
- The urorectal septum develops and grows caudally. This divides the cloaca into the anterior urogenital sinus and the posterior anorectal canal
- By 7 weeks the urorectal septum reaches the cloacal membrane. This forms the perineum. The cloacal membrane divides into the urogenital membrane anteriorly and the anal membrane posteriorly
- By the 8th week the anal membrane is at the bottom of the anal pit, a depression within the ectoderm
- By the 9th week the anal membrane ruptures forming an open communication between the rectum and the outside (Fig. 1.7).

Imperforate anus and rectal atresia

- This is a range of clinical conditions and appearances from the anal canal ending at the anal membrane to complete failure of development of the rectum and anal canal
- A low lesion will have colon close to the skin. There may be anal stenosis or the anus may have failed to develop with the rectum ending in a blind end
- A high lesion has colon ending higher in the pelvis. Rectal fistulae are often observed in association. These may be found between rectum, vagina, urinary bladder, urethra and perineal surface
- In a persistent cloaca the rectum, vagina and urinary tract enter into a common channel
- Imperforate anus is frequently associated with other birth defects, commonly spinal defects, heart defects, tracheo-oesophageal fistula and oesophageal atresia.

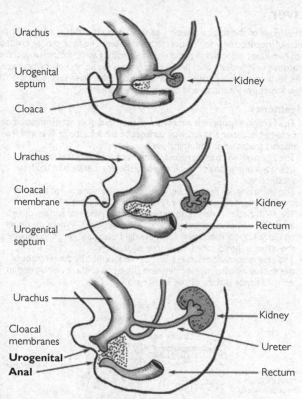

Fig. 1.7 Development of the hindgut.

Liver

Knowledge of the surgical anatomy of the liver is essential for safe performance of hepatectomy for colorectal metastases. The liver can be divided
into two lobes (right and left) and eight segments. Each segment is a discrete
anatomic unit with its own blood supply and venous and biliary drainage.
The technique of liver resection is based on these liver segments due to
their structural autonomy and constant arrangement.

Ligaments

- The falciform ligament is a crescent-shaped fold of peritoneum attached
  between superior and anterior surfaces of the left lobe of liver and the
  diaphragm/anterior abdominal wall
- The ligamentum teres or round ligament of the liver located in the
  free edge of the falciform is formed by the degeneration of the fetal
  umbilical vein
- The left triangular ligament between superior surface of left lobe and
  the diaphragm arises from the left leaf of the falciform
- The V-shaped coronary ligament attaches the posterior surface of right
  lobe to the diaphragm and posterior abdominal wall. Where the upper
  and lower layers meet, they form the right triangular ligament. Between
  the layers is the so-called 'bare area' of the liver
- The ligamentum venosum is a fibrous cord formed by the remnant of
  the ductus venosus running between the layers of the lesser omentum
  on the inferior surface of the liver (Fig. 1.8).

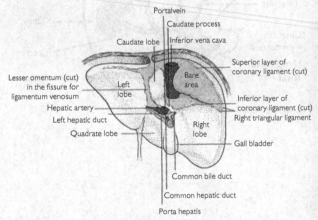

Fig. 1.8 Posterior view of the liver.

Reproduced from Rogers AW. (Eds.) (1992). *Textbook of anatomy*. London, UK: Churchill
Livingstone, Elsevier.

Lobar anatomy

- The left lobe consists of segments 1–4 nourished by the left hepatic artery and the left portal vein (Fig. 1.9)
- The right lobe consists of segments 5–8 and is nourished by the right hepatic artery and the right portal vein
- The anatomical division between right and left lobe is a plane through the medial margin of the gallbladder to the left side of the inferior vena cava (IVC) not through the falciform/teres ligament and umbilical fissure.

Venous drainage

- Venous drainage is through three major hepatic veins (right, middle and left) and multiple, small veins draining directly from the back of the right and caudate lobe to the IVC
- The major hepatic veins occupy three planes (scissurae), dividing the liver into 4 sectors, each of which is supplied by a portal pedicle
- Branching of the pedicles subdivides 4 sectors into 8 segments
- Often the left and middle hepatic veins form a confluence before entering the IVC
- Occasionally, a large inferior right hepatic vein is present that may provide adequate drainage of the right lobe
- Numerous short veins drain the caudate lobe directly into the IVC
- IVC lies in a groove on the posterior surface of the liver just to the right of the midline.

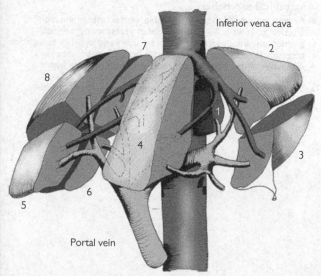

Fig. 1.9 The Couinaud classification of liver anatomy.

Portal and arterial supply

- Hepatic blood inflow represents about 1/4 of the cardiac output, demonstrating its central role in the body's metabolism
- The portal vein contributes 75% and the hepatic artery 25% to hepatic blood flow
- Portal pressure is normally 6–10mmHg
- Unlike the hepatic veins which run between segments, portal venous, hepatic arterial and ductal branches run centrally within segments
- Portal vein and hepatic artery divide into left and right branches before entering the hilum
- Usually right hepatic artery, portal vein and duct enter the liver substance almost immediately after branching, making pedicle dissection on the right more difficult than on the left
- The left branch of the portal vein and the hepatic duct take a long extrahepatic course at the base of segment 4 before joining the left hepatic artery to form a triad and entering the liver at the base of the umbilical fissure.

Biliary anatomy

- ~1500ml of bile is produced by the liver daily and excreted into the duodenum via the biliary tree. The importance of preservation of adequate biliary drainage post-hepatectomy cannot be underestimated
- Intrahepatic biliary anatomy is similar to the anatomy of the hepatic artery.

Anatomical anomalies

- Arterial anatomy of the liver is variable, with accessory and replaced arteries common. In 10–20% replaced or accessory right hepatic arteries arise from superior mesenteric artery and in 7–18% replaced or accessory left hepatic arteries originate from left gastric artery
- Anomalies of the hepatic ductal confluence are common, with the normal anatomy present in only ~2/3 of cases
- Identification of anatomical anomalies is important for favourable outcome at hepatectomy.

Small bowel

Anatomy

Anatomically small bowel includes duodenum, jejunum and ileum. Clinically the small intestine is often considered to be from duodenojejunal (DJ) flexure to ileocaecal valve. The DJ flexure can be identified at the insertion of the ligament of Treitz (fibromuscular band derived from the diaphragm near the oesophageal opening).

Jejunum and ileum

The small bowel is 5–7m in length with the first 2/5 jejunum and the last 3/5 ileum. There is no clear distinction between the two; however, jejunal mucosa is palpably thicker with longer villi and a wider calibre. The jejunal mesentery is thinner with fewer arterial arcades.

Small bowel is attached to posterior abdominal wall by mesentery fixed obliquely from right of L3 to left of L1 (15cm) and formed by a fold of peritoneum containing the blood supply, lymphatics and adipose tissue.

Aggregations of lymphoid tissue (Peyer's patches) become more numerous in the ileum along the anti-mesenteric border and are vital to the gut-mediated immune response.

Blood supply

- The SMA is an anterior branch from the aorta passing under the neck of pancreas, over 3rd part of duodenum and through root of mesentery
- Branches from left side of SMA (12–20) form vascular arcades (Fig. 1.10)
- Venous drainage follows arterial supply to superior mesenteric vein (SMV) and then portal vein.

Lymph drainage

- Follows arterial supply draining to the cistern chyli and thoracic duct.

Nerve supply

- Sympathetic supply from T9/10 is vasoconstricting and anti-peristaltic
- Parasympathetic supply is from vagus and ↑ peristalsis and secretion.

Wall layers

- Mucosa consists of a single layer columnar epithelium arranged in crypts and villous projections
- Villous architecture leads to a large surface area for absorption
- The crypts of Lieberkühn play a part in cell turnover and secretion
- Epithelial cells include enterocytes (absorptive), goblet (mucus-producing), enteroendocrine and Paneth cells
- Beneath the epithelial layer the lamina propria contains supporting connective tissue, a rich blood and nerve supply, lymphatics, lymphocytes, plasma cells, macrophages and mast cells
- The muscularis mucosa is the final layer of the mucosal lining
- Submucosa contains ganglion cells of Meissner's submucosal plexus
- Outside the submucosa there is an inner circular and outer longitudinal muscle. Between the muscle layers lies Auerbach's myenteric plexus which contributes to the control of motility
- The wall is completed by a well developed serosa, part of the visceral peritoneum.

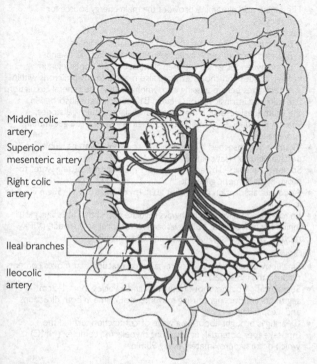

Fig. 1.10 Anatomy of the superior mesenteric artery.

Small bowel physiology

The primary role of the small bowel is the digestion and absorption of carbohydrates, proteins, fat, water, electrolytes, vitamins and minerals. Other functions include secretion and transportation.

Absorption

- 9 litres of fluid enters the small bowel daily (ingested fluid, saliva, gastric, pancreatic juice and bile) with only 1 litre passing to the colon
- Pancreatic bicarbonate neutralizes acidic chyme from the stomach
- Carbohydrate digestion begins with salivary and pancreatic amylase and is completed by disaccharidases in the duodenum and proximal jejunum. This results in monosaccharides which are absorbed by active transport and facilitated diffusion
- Protein breakdown begins with pepsin in the stomach but is predominantly in the duodenum by pancreatic peptidases including trypsin, chymotrypsin and lipase. Enzymes are activated by small bowel enterokinase and activated trypsin

- The amino acid glutamine provides the main energy source for enterocytes
- Fat digestion
  - Begins with lipolysis of triglycerides mediated by lipase
  - Bile salts form mixed micelles resulting in free fatty acids and monoglycerides which are then absorbed in the upper jejunum
  - Triglycerides and cholesterol are also made into chylomicrons within enterocytes before passing into lymphatics and the general circulation
- Bile salts and intrinsic factor/vitamin B12 complex are absorbed in the ileum (ileal resection may cause fat malabsorption, gallstones, vitamin B12 deficiency/macrocytic anaemia and reduced gut immune surveillance)
- Vitamins are absorbed by either active transport (water-soluble) or passive diffusion (fat-soluble: A, D, E, K)
- Sodium is absorbed by active transport mechanisms causing water to move by its osmotic gradient
- Adequate absorption requires at least 1m of small bowel (50cm if colon in circuit)
- Endocrine and paracrine pathways regulate absorption including gastric inhibitory polypeptide (GIP), vasoactive intestinal polypeptide (VIP), motilin, enteroglucagon, secretin and substance P.

Peristalsis
- Small bowel peristalsis is a coordinated contraction that moves contents through the intestine
- Segmentation occurs more frequently and involves short 1–2cm segments contracting, causing movement of chime in both directions and aids mixing
- Clearing is brought about by a wave of contraction termed the 'housekeeper potential' or migrating myoelectric complex (MMC) which occurs approximately every 90min.

Colon

Anatomy

The colon is variable in length, averaging 1.5m. It gradually reduces in calibre from 7–8cm in the caecum to 2.5cm in the sigmoid colon.

Characteristics of the large intestine include:

Taeniae coli

Consist of three condensations of outer longitudinal muscle which form bands beginning at the base of the appendix and eventually converging at the rectosigmoid junction. They are named after their relationship to the transverse colon: anterior (taenia libera), posteromedial (taenia mesocolica) and posterolateral (taenia omentalis).

Haustra

Sacculations occurring between the taeniae thought to be caused by the taeniae being relatively shorter than the length of the colon. Plicae semilunares are the folds between haustrae which can be seen at endoscopy or on radiological examinations.

Appendices epiploicae

Fat-filled pouches which hang from the serosal border of the colon. Care should be taken when dissecting as these may contain diverticulae at the points where supplying blood vessels pierce the bowel wall.

Caecum

Blind-ending pouch projecting below the ileocaecal valve usually situated in the right iliac fossa and covered by peritoneum. The ileocaecal valve is a transverse opening resembling a pair of lips with a sphincter created by thickening of the muscular layer of the terminal ileum (TI). The valve controls the flow of material into the colon and may prevent reflux. The caecum is at risk of rupture when the diameter reaches 12cm, usually due to distal obstruction.

Appendix

The appendix is found on the posteromedial aspect of the caecum at the confluence of the 3 taeniae. The average length is 8–10cm with a 5mm diameter. The appendix may lie in a variety of positions (pre-/retroileal, retrocaecal, pelvic).

Ascending colon

Laying in a retroperitoneal position on the iliac and lumbar fascia it is ~15cm in length from the ileocaecal valve to the hepatic flexure. Lateral to the bowel is the paracolic gutter with the infracolic compartment medially. The hepatic flexure is supported by a nephrocolic ligament with the lower pole of right kidney and duodenal loop inferiorly.

Transverse colon

The transverse colon loops down on mesentery from fixed points at the hepatic and splenic flexures. The mesentery extends between the lower renal poles across duodenum and pancreas.

The gastrocolic omentum connects it to the greater curvature of the stomach while the greater omentum is suspended from its anterior surface. The more acute splenic flexure lies high in the left upper quadrant (LUQ) inferior to the tip of the spleen and fixed by the phrenicocolic ligament.

Descending colon

The descending colon (30cm) from splenic flexure to pelvic brim is covered by peritoneum lying on left kidney as well as iliac and lumber fascia.

Sigmoid colon

The mobile sigmoid is variable in length, forming a Ω-loop from pelvic brim to sacral promontory. It is suspended on its own mesentery which forms a V-shaped attachment across the pelvic side wall. The left ureter and gonadal vessels and inferior mesenteric artery (IMA) lie at the base and should be clearly identified before ligation of the blood supply. The sigmoid colon may cross to the right side of the pelvis depending on length.

Blood supply

- Branches from the right side of SMA supply to the distal third of transverse colon and anastomose to form a marginal artery which is continuous with left colon blood supply from the IMA (Fig. 1.11)
- The middle colic is the first branch at the inferior border of pancreas supplying transverse colon and the splenic flexure in a third of patients
- The right branch, like the middle colic, is variable and supplies the ascending colon
- The ileocolic artery is a more constant terminal branch supplying caecum, appendix and ileum

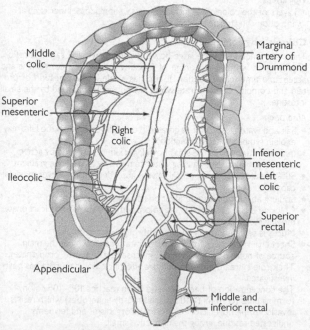

Fig. 1.11 Blood supply to the colon.

- The IMA comes directly off the left side of the aorta 4cm above the bifurcation and supplies from distal third of transverse to upper rectum
- The left colic gives an ascending and descending branch supplying splenic flexure and descending colon. The ascending branch contributes to the marginal artery of Drummond ('watershed zone').
- An arcade lower in the mesentery between middle and left colic called the 'meandering mesenteric artery' is sometimes found in arterial occlusive disease
- A number of sigmoid branches supply the sigmoid colon
- The terminal branch is called the superior rectal artery after it crosses the left common iliac artery
- Venous drainage follows the arterial supply draining to portal vein.

Lymph drainage
- Lymph drainage follows the arterial supply
- Epiploic (next to bowel wall), paracolic (around marginal supply) and then following the named mesenteric vessels
- Drainage is to the cisterna chyli via the para-aortic nodes.

Nerve supply
- Sympathetic supply from T6–L2/3. Important for epidural placement
- Parasympathetic supply from vagus and pelvic splanchnic nerves.

Wall layers
- Layers of the colonic wall include mucosa, submucosa, inner circular and outer longitudinal muscle and serosa.

Colonic physiology

The main functions of the large bowel include water and salt absorption, solidifying of waste and storage of faecal matter until a convenient and acceptable time for evacuation. It also has a role in the digestion of protein and complex carbohydrate which has not been absorbed by the small intestine.

Absorption
- Salt and water absorption is greater in the right colon than the left (may explain symptoms after resection)
- In a similar fashion to the small bowel, sodium is absorbed by active transport mechanisms causing water to move by its osmotic gradient
- 90% of fluid through ileocaecal valve is absorbed with 5–6litres maximal capacity
- Sodium absorption is dependent on its luminal concentration
- Chloride is also absorbed in the colon, with potassium and bicarbonate moving the other way
- Mucus is secreted from goblet cells throughout the colon
- Short chain fatty acids from carbohydrate breakdown are the main source of nutrition for the colonic mucosa (e.g. butyrate, propionate). Their role in treatment of conditions affecting colonic mucosa has been investigated.
- The concentration of bacteria in the colon reaches 10^{10}–10^{12} colony-forming units (cfu)/ml (>400 species mostly anaerobes) which resists invasion by pathogenic or opportunistic organisms and ferments undigested residue, giving the distinctive smell.

Peristalsis

- Colonic function is under the control of a complex, poorly understood endocrine and paracrine system with a variety of mediators involved (e.g. acetylcholine, opioids, noradrenaline (NA), 5-hydroxytryptamine (5-HT), somatostatin, cholecystokinin, substance P, VIP, nitric oxide NO))
- Motor innervation to the colon is via Auerbach's myenteric (sympathetic and parasympathetic for smooth muscle function) and Meissner's submucosal plexus (parasympathetic for absorptive functions)
- Segmentation as previously described in the small intestine allows mixing and absorption of water
- High amplitude propagated contractions responsible for onward movement of colonic content ('mass movement') occur ~5 times/day
- Colonic pressure activity is increased on wakening and after meals, reducing at night
- On average colonic transit time is 34h.

The rectum and pelvis

The rectum can be divided into thirds. The upper third is intraperitoneal and is covered anteriorly and laterally by peritoneum. The middle third is covered anteriorly by peritoneum whereas the lower rectum is entirely extraperitoneal. Anteriorly, the fascia of Denonvilliers separates the rectum from the bladder, prostate and seminal vesicles in males and the posterior vaginal wall in women. Posteriorly, Waldeyer's rectosacral fascia lies between the mesorectum and the sacrum.

The rectum differs from the colon in having a mesorectum rather than a mesentery. The mesorectum contains fat, blood vessels, nerves and lymph nodes enveloped by the fascia propria of the rectum. At the rectosigmoid junction, the taeniae diffuse out to provide a complete outer longitudinal muscle layer which also means that the rectum has no appendices epiploicae.

Rectum

- The rectum is 15–18cm length. Anatomically, the rectum extends from the third sacral vertebra to the dentate line
- From a surgical perspective, the upper limit is the sacral promontory, where the sigmoid mesentery ends and the appendices epiploicae disappear; the lower limit is the anorectal ring
- The rectum has three curves which correspond to the rectal valves of Houston. The middle valve (convex to left) lies at 9–10cm and corresponds to the anterior peritoneal reflexion.
- The upper third is covered by peritoneum anteriorly and to the sides, the middle third is only covered anteriorly and the lower third is entirely extraperitoneal.

Fascial attachments of the rectum

- The rectum and mesorectum is enveloped by the fascia propria. This condenses anteriorly to form the rectovesical fascia of Denonvilliers and is continuous inferiorly with the pelvic fascia over the levator ani
- Posteriorly, the lower part of the rectum is attached to the sacrum by Waldeyer's fascia, which blends into the rectal longitudinal muscle at the level of the puborectalis (Fig. 1.13)
- The lateral ligament of the rectum is a condensation of the perirectal tissue and is continuous with the fascia propria of the rectum. The ligament contains nerves which branch from the pelvic nerve plexus to enter the rectum. In 10% of individuals the lateral ligament may contain a middle rectal artery (Fig. 1.12).

Blood supply and lymphatics

- The IMA becomes the superior rectal artery (SRA) as it crosses the left common iliac artery and supplies the rectum
- The SRA subdivides into the superior haemorrhoidal arteries
- The inferior haemorrhoidal arteries from the internal iliac and occasionally (25% of cases) the middle rectal artery also contribute blood to the rectum
- Venous return follows the arteries

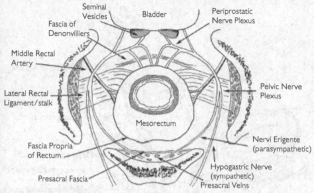

Fig. 1.12 Surgical anatomy of the rectum.

- Lymph from the upper 2/3 of the rectum drains to the inferior mesenteric nodes and then the para-aortic nodes. The lower rectum lymph drainage is variable both proximally and laterally along the middle rectal vessels.

Nerve supply

- The rectum receives a sympathetic supply from L1–3 via lumbar sympathetics, the pre-aortic plexus and post-ganglionic fibres which travel with the IMA and SRA
- The hypogastric nerve plexus supplies the lower rectum
- Parasympathetic supply is via the nervi erigentes (S2–4) which emerge from the sacral foramena and join the hypogastric nerves to form the pelvic plexus, which lies on the side wall of pelvis
- The autonomic nerves can be damaged during high ligation of the IMA, rectal mobilization at the pelvic promontory or pre-sacral region. The pelvic plexus may be damaged due to forceful rectal traction or division of the lateral stalks. Dissection anterior to fascia of Denonvilliers will damage the periprostatic plexus.

Anorectal spaces

- **Ischiorectal fossa** which communicates posteriorly with the **postanal space** (deep and superficial components)
- **Intersphincteric space** which communicates with the **perianal space**
- **Supralevator space** which lies between the peritoneum and the levators
- **Retrorectal space** lies between the fascia propria of the rectum and the presacral fascia (Fig. 1.13).

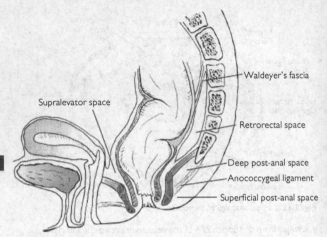

Fig. 1.13 The anorectal spaces. Sagittal view.

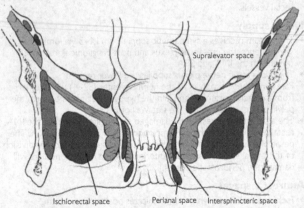

Fig. 1.14 The anorectal spaces. Frontal view.

The anal canal and sphincters

Anus

- The 'surgical' or functional anus extends from the anal margin or intersphincteric groove to the anorectal ring and measures 3–5cm
- The anatomical or embryological anus is shorter (2cm) and extends from the anal margin to the dentate line (Fig. 1.15).

Lining of the anal canal

- The proximal anal canal has 12–15 longitudinal mucosal folds (columns of Morgagni), which extend proximally to the anal valves located at the dentate line
- The 12–15 anal glands lie within the submucosa although some also penetrate the internal sphincter to lie in the intersphincteric plane. They secrete mucus via the anal ducts which empty into the anal crypts, which lie just above anal valve
- The lining of the anal canal can be broken into 3 distinct zones
  - Below dentate line it is lined by stratified squamous epithelium. This area is known as the anoderm or pectin
  - For a distance of 1–2cm above dentate line the lining is modified columnar epithelium which contains endocrine cells from above and melanin-containing cells from below the dentate line. This area is known as the anal transition zone (ATZ). This zone plays a critical role in the sensory function of the anal canal
  - The lining above the ATZ is rectal columnar mucosa
- The distal anal canal has 3 prominent folds at the 4, 7 and 11 o'clock positions
- These folds or vascular cushions play an important role in continence and contribute up to 15% of resting anal pressure. Abdominal straining cuts off venous return, leading to swelling of the anal cushions which acts as an effective seal to gas and liquid (Fig. 6.3). If the mucocutaneous junction descends distally to lie outside the high-pressure zone of the anal canal (e.g. prolapsing haemorrhoids), this barrier function may fail, giving rise to mucous and faecal staining.

Blood supply and innervation

- The anal canal receives its arterial supply and drainage, sympathetic and parasympathetic innervation and lymphatic drainage from the inferior mesenteric and superior rectal vessels and associated hypogastric nerve plexus
- For 1–2cm above the dentate, the anal canal lining is highly innervated and consists of several layers of cuboidal cells. This is known as the transition zone
- Below the dentate line, the anal canal has a squamous lining which has a somatic nerve supply. It also receives its blood supply and drains via the inferior haemorrhoidal system
- 10–12 anal glands (located in the internal anal sphincter (IAS) and intersphincteric plane) drain into the anal crypts at the level of the dentate line.

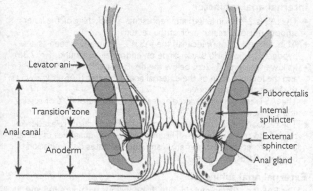

Fig. 1.15 Anatomy of the anal canal.

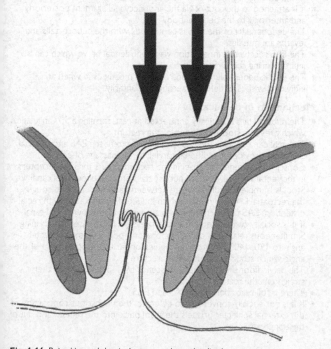

Fig. 1.16 Raised intra-abdominal pressure closes the distal rectum.

Internal anal sphincter

- The IAS is 2–4cm in length and represents a thickening of the inner smooth muscle circular layer of the rectum
- At its thickest point (midcanal) the IAS is 2–3mm and is seen as a hypoechogenic (dark/black) circle on endoanal ultrasound (Fig. 2.35)
- Its lower margin is 1–2cm below the dentate and the groove between it and the lower margin of the external anal sphincter (EAS) is known as the intersphincteric groove
- The IAS is tonically contracted at rest and contributes 80% of resting anal pressure
- The rectoanal inhibitory reflex (sampling reflex) induces relaxation in the IAS on rectal distention. This may allow small quantities of rectal content to enter the upper anal canal and facilitates discrimination between flatus and faeces.

External anal sphincter

- The EAS is a striated muscle tube that envelops the entire IAS and terminates slightly more distal to it at the anal margin
- It is attached to the coccyx via the anococcygeal ligament posteriorly and anteriorly to the perineal body
- The deepest part of the EAS is continuous with the puborectalis and levator ani muscles
- The EAS receives its innervation via the pudendal nerve which can be injured during childbirth
- The EAS is under voluntary control and is mostly used when an individual wishes to defer defaecation voluntarily.

Mechanism of defaecation

- The puborectalis is tonically contracted at rest, forming a 90° angulation which prevents stool exiting out of the rectum
- The anal canal (mainly the IAS, to a lesser extent the EAS and the anal cushions) provide an additional barrier to the passage of stool
- Conscious awareness of stool in the rectum occurs through receptors in the rectal wall, pelvic floor, puborectalis and the upper anal canal
- Stool is 'sampled' to discriminate between flatus and faeces through the rectoanal inhibitory reflex which induces IAS relaxation with rectal distention. EAS contraction prevents opening of the lower anal canal
- If it is socially convenient, intrarectal pressure is increased by straining
- Simultaneous relaxation of the puborectalis opens up the anorectal angle to 110–140°. Squatting or hip flexion facilitates opening up of the angle which straightens out the anorectum
- The pelvic floor simultaneously descends by 1–3 cm which further straightens the rectum
- There is full relaxation of the IAS and EAS
- If it is not socially convenient to defecate, then conscious contraction of the external sphincter propels the stool back into the rectum and out of the upper anal canal.

Colorectal assessment

History and examination

Bowel symptoms have a high prevalence in developed countries (e.g. 20% of adults will experience rectal bleeding in any given year and up to 40% will have experienced rectal bleeding at some time in their life). Furthermore, between 5 and 20% of the population describe symptoms consistent with a diagnosis of irritable bowel syndrome (IBS) (→ Irritable bowel syndrome, Chapter 5, p.244).

Age is a key factor in determining likelihood of serious pathology (e.g. a 75-year-old with a new history of isolated rectal bleeding has 5–10% chance of having colorectal cancer (CRC) while the risk in a 20-year-old is <1 in 1000 (Fig. 2.1). Simple guidelines based on symptoms and age have been developed to guide general practitioners (GPs) making decisions regarding who should be referred urgently for investigation (Box 2.1).

History

Listening to the patient's history remains the key to efficient investigation and diagnosis in patients with bowel symptoms. Although most patients with anorectal symptoms attribute these to 'haemorrhoids', an accurate history will usually enable an astute physician to reach a diagnosis even before an examination is performed.

History taking should be thorough and, once the patient has told their own story, more detailed questioning on the presenting complaint and the history of that complaint is required.

- Take a complete history of the presenting complaint including duration of symptoms, if things are improving and what the patient has done/taken to try and relieve their symptoms
- Ask about systemic symptoms (e.g. fever or weight loss)
- Enquire about a past history of previous surgery, radiotherapy or medical conditions including inflammatory bowel disease (IBD)
- Exclude a family history of colorectal and other cancers
- The drug history should include recent antibiotic usage
- A full review of systems should pay particular attention to a gynaecological history.

Examination

- The head and neck area should be inspected to look for signs of liver or endocrine disease such as thyrotoxicosis, myxoedema, or Cushing's disease. Cervical lymphadenopathy should be excluded
- Patients should be exposed properly to rule out groin or scrotal pathology such as inguinal, inguinoscrotal or femoral hernias, or lymphadenopathy
- The abdomen should be inspected for surgical incisions, abdominal wall hernias, obvious masses, distension, visible peristalsis, dilated veins, caput medusa, etc.
- The basic principles of inspection palpation, percussion, auscultation should be followed
- Visual inspection of the perineum and perianal area will identify haemorrhoids, fissures, fistula, anal tags, ulceration, scars, warts etc. A patulous anus should also be noted

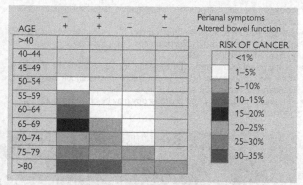

Fig. 2.1 Predictive value of common symptoms in diagnosing colon cancer

The table shows the interaction between age and primary symptoms of colorectal cancer. All patients presented with rectal bleeding and the risk of cancer (as a percentage) is shown for those with additional perianal symptoms or altered bowel function.

Reproduced with permission from Thompson MR, Perera R, Senapati A, Dodds S, Predictive value of common symptom combinations in diagnosing colorectal cancer. *British Journal of Surgery*; 94:1260–1265. Copyright © 2007 British Journal of Surgery Society Ltd. Published by John Wiley & Sons, Ltd. DOI: 10.1002/bjs.5826

Box 2.1 Guidelines for urgent referral of patients with suspected lower GI cancer

Patients >60yrs
- Persistent rectal bleeding ≥6 weeks without change in bowel habit or anal symptom
- Change in bowel habit to loose ± increasingly frequent stool for 6 weeks without rectal bleeding.

Patients >40yrs
- Rectal bleeding and a change in bowel habit towards loose ± increasingly frequent stool for ≥6 weeks.

All patients
- A palpable right lower abdominal mass
- A palpable intraluminal (not pelvic) rectal mass
- Unexplained iron deficiency with a haemoglobin concentration <11g/dl in men or <10g/dl in non-menstruating women.

- Look for evidence of pruritus, inflammation, faecal soiling, or mucus discharge
- Ask the patient to strain and to contract the anus in order to check for prolapsing haemorrhoids, rectal mucosal or full thickness prolapse, and perineal descent (Fig. 2.2)
- Digital rectal examination (DRE) should include assessment of anal tone. Any tenderness, rectal or extrarectal masses should be noted. Evaluate the prostate in males
- A rigid sigmoidoscopy and proctoscopy may be considered for anorectal symptoms.

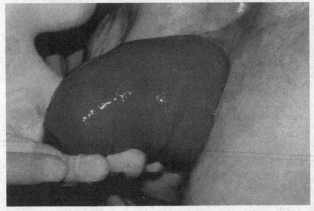

Fig. 2.2 Simple instructions such as asking a patient to strain may reveal a rectal or mucosal prolapse.

Quantitative faecal immunochemical test (qFIT)

Quantitative faecal immunochemical test (qFIT)

qFIT (quantitative faecal immunochemical test) is a sensitive, specific faecal test for human globin. It is used as part of the bowel cancer screening programme and more recently, it has been used to assess/triage patients with new colorectal symptoms (e.g. altered bowel habit, abdominal discomfort, and/or infrequent or isolated episodes of rectal bleeding).

- Lysed red cells release globin. If the blood loss occurs in the stomach or small intestine, the globin is digested and therefore not detected. A positive result implies blood loss from the lower GI tract.
- Theoretically, fresh anorectal bleeding might give a negative result if RBCs are released intact from adenomas. However, a cancer is unlikely to have a negative result.
- It is a quantitative test (range $<10 - >400\mu g$ Hb/g faeces). The threshold for a positive result can be adjusted to alter sensitivity
- When used as part of a bowel screening programme, a value of $80\mu g$ Hb/g faeces is frequently used to denote a 'positive' result
- When used for symptomatic patients, NICE guidelines DG30 (July 2017) recommend $<10\mu g$ Hb/g faeces as the standard for a negative result i.e. higher values are deemed to be 'positive'
- A negative result has a better negative predictive value at excluding significant colorectal pathology (adenomas >1cm/ IBD / cancer) when compared to colonoscopy e.g. symptomatic patients with a qFIT<10 and a normal FBC have a 1 in 1000 chance of having colorectal malignancy. Many such patients can be reassured
- NICE guidelines suggest that 700 of every 1000 colonoscopies currently performed could be avoided with such a strategy
- The actual value of a positive result can predict the likelihood of significant pathology
  - qFIT <10: Minimal risk of significant pathology with a negative predictive value for significant pathology of approximately 94%
  - qFIT 10–400: 20% chance of significant pathology
  - qFIT >400: $>50\%$ chance of significant pathology
- Although qFIT was primarily developed for use in bowel screening and in the triage/assessment of symptomatic patients in primary care, it may also have a role in assessment of patients in secondary care.

Reference

Cubiella J, Salve M, Díaz-Ondina M et al. (2014) Diagnostic accuracy of the faecal immunochemical test for colorectal cancer in symptomatic patients: comparison with NICE and SIGN referral criteria. *Colorect Dis* **16** (8):O273–O282. https://doi.org/10.1111/codi.12569

Radiological investigations: small bowel imaging

The small intestine is challenging to image due to its length and mobility. Multiple different imaging modalities are therefore employed. Findings on imaging are frequently non-specific and need interpretation within the clinical context. The choice of modality for elective investigation will often depend on local expertise and availability. In addition to the following radiological assessments, the small bowel may also be imaged using capsule endoscopy and 'push–pull' enteroscopy.

Plain abdominal radiograph (AXR)

- A simple test which can demonstrate the degree of gaseous distension of the small and large bowel
- Pneumoperitoneum can be identified on a supine abdominal film if Rigler's sign (gas on both sides of the bowel wall) is present or inferred (excess lucency in the upper abdomen) (Fig. 2.3)
- Frequently used as a first-line test in suspected intestinal obstruction
- Limited sensitivity and specificity mainly due to the incomplete depiction of fluid-filled bowel loops
- Still has a role in the monitoring of the degree of bowel distension in cases of obstruction and colitis
- An erect chest radiograph is more sensitive in the detection of free intraperitoneal air.

Barium follow-through

- Variably detailed examination of the small bowel depending on the protocol followed
- Series of plain AXRs obtained at intervals after ingestion of a dilute barium suspension until contrast seen to enter caecum
- Direct fluoroscopic screening is performed to assess terminal ileum
- Relatively insensitive test for mucosal abnormality, compromised by lack of bowel distension and overlapping loops
- Gross structural abnormality and mechanical hold-up usually well displayed
- A modified follow-through exam may be of value in excluding obstruction in patients with conflicting clinical picture
  - Water-soluble contrast (~100ml) taken orally (PO) or via a nasogastric (NG) tube
  - Plain films taken at ingestion and at 1h and 4–6h
  - The contrast is often markedly diluted by small bowel fluid which limits the value of the examination
  - Failure to visualize contrast in the colon at 6h suggests the need for surgical intervention in cases of small bowel obstruction (SBO).

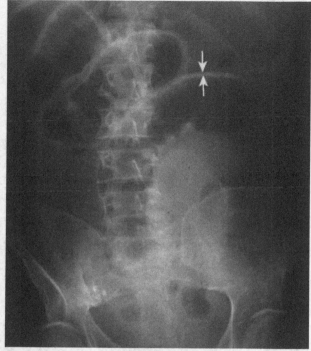

Fig. 2.3 Pneumoperitoneum secondary to perforated distal SBO. Arrows indicate presence of Rigler's sign.

Small bowel enema

This technique was until recently, generally regarded as the gold standard technique for imaging the small bowel. Computed tomography (CT) (Fig 2.4) or magnetic resonance imaging (MRI) enterography are now more frequently performed.

- Nasojejunal tube placed just beyond duodenal–jejunal flexure under fluoroscopic guidance

- Barium injected and then flushed through with a larger volume of negative contrast material such as methylcellulose, polyethylene glycol, water, or air

- Intermittent fluoroscopic screening used to assess distensibility, rate of passage, and mucosal outline

- Can deliver very high spatial resolution of mucosal abnormalities

- Hampered by radiation dose and the lack of direct extramucosal information.

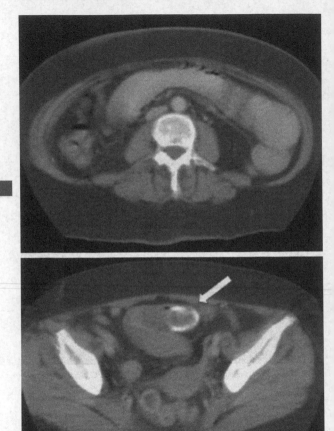

Fig. 2.4 High grade distal small bowel obstruction secondary to a gallstone seen on CT (arrow).

Trans-abdominal ultrasound

Ultrasound (US) is readily available but not commonly used as a first-line imaging technique.

- Advantages include simplicity, availability, low cost, patient acceptability, and safety
- Comparable accuracy in expert hands to CT and MRI in assessing the small bowel (Fig. 2.5)
- Highly operator dependent with reduced reproducibility in comparison with the other techniques
- Complete examination of the small bowel is often difficult or impossible due to the presence of bowel gas and/or the patient's build
- Has potential for monitoring treatment response in established small bowel disease, e.g. Crohn's disease.

Computed tomography

CT provides an overview of the entire small bowel and surrounding structures with high spatial resolution.

- Very useful in the acute setting due to its speed and reproducibility
- Modality of choice in the investigation of:
  - Acute small bowel obstruction (Fig. 2.4)
  - Assessment of intra-abdominal sepsis (Fig. 2.6)
  - Assessment of ischaemic bowel
  - Obscure acute GI blood loss

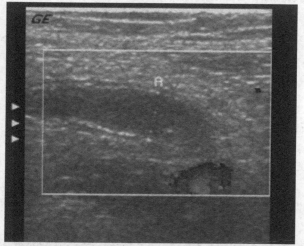

Fig. 2.5 Ultrasound showing tubular fluid-filled structure in RIF in keeping with acute appendicitis.

- Oral contrast is usually given in order to distend the small bowel
  - This is best achieved with a negative (low-density) contrast agent which allows the mucosa to be most easily visualized
  - Water is the simplest agent but is too rapidly absorbed to give satisfactory distal small intestinal distension
  - Agents which are not absorbed by the small intestine such as methylcellulose or polyethylene glycol solution can be administered orally (CT enterography) or via a nasojejunal tube (enteroclysis) to achieve distension
  - Conventional iodinated intravenous (IV) contrast-enhanced CT is then performed
- In suspected small bowel obstruction, no oral contrast is given. The pattern of distension and collapse of bowel can be assessed and, if no focal structural cause is seen, a diagnosis of adhesions can be inferred
- IV contrast is most useful. The patency of the proximal arterial tree can be assessed and areas of relative hypoenhancement identified in cases of ischaemic bowel, but the sensitivity of CT in this setting remains quite low (~60%) (Fig. 2.6).

These techniques can produce highly detailed visualization of the entire small bowel and surrounding structures. The enteroclysis technique results in generally better distension at the expense of time, cost, and patient discomfort of nasojejunal tube insertion. As with all CT there is a significant ionizing radiation dose, of particular relevance in younger patients and those with chronic disease requiring multiple examinations.

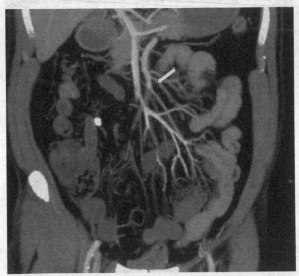

Fig. 2.6 Widespread distal small bowel ischaemia secondary to SMA branch thrombosis as seen on CT (arrow). Note relative hypodensity of distal small bowel with associated absence of mesenteric vessels.

Magnetic resonance imaging

MRI of the small bowel can be performed as an MR enterography or MR enteroclysis procedure.

- Enteroclysis offers consistently better bowel distension
- It provides the opportunity to screen the small intestine as it fills, assessing distensibility and impaired transit
- Spatial resolution is lower than CT but with better contrast resolution
- There is no radiation dose
- Increasingly utilized as primary investigation for Crohn's disease (Fig. 2.7)
- Although MRI scanners are widely available, the procedure is time consuming, both in terms of use of the MRI scanner during the acquisition phase and the length of time required for a radiologist to interpret the images. It tends to be reserved for younger patients and patients with Crohn's disease who are likely to require serial imaging.

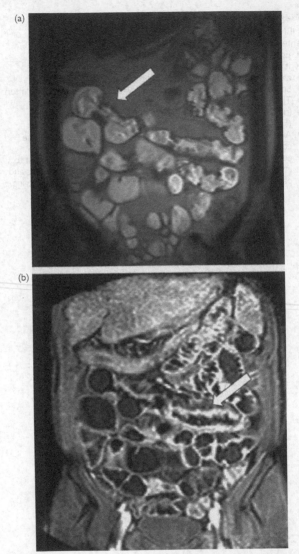

Fig. 2.7 MRI enteroclysis. Multiple Crohn's strictures throughout the small bowel with proximal dilatation on a coronal T2-weighted image (arrows) (a). Coronal contrast-enhanced images show diffuse wall enhancement indicating active disease (arrow) (b).

Radiological investigations: large bowel and rectum

With the advent of endoscopy, the role of radiology in the detection of mucosal pathology in the large bowel was dramatically reduced, with the emphasis turning to staging of malignancy and acute abdominal imaging. Since the introduction of multislice CT, radiology is increasingly employed in both diagnosis and screening of patients with large bowel malignancy. MR has revolutionized staging of rectal cancer and assessment of perianal anatomy. Thus, imaging of the colon and anorectum is now a multimodality approach where the chosen imaging technique is dependent on availability and local expertise.

Plain film

Plain AXR without oral or rectal contrast still has a role in the initial investigation of suspected large bowel obstruction (LBO), trauma, perforation, complications of IBD, or electively with radio-opaque markers in colonic transit studies. It is readily available, quick, and easy to interpret, but may add to overall radiation burden if further ionizing radiation examinations are required.

Barium enema

This has largely been superseded by direct visualization and more recently CT colonoscopy. It was previously widely used in combination with flexible sigmoidoscopy in the investigation of colon cancer (Fig. 2.8).

Fluoroscopy and water-soluble studies

Water-soluble enema

Usually performed in the acute setting on unprepared bowel using slightly hyperosmolar, iodinated contrast. Water-soluble contrast is relatively inert if there is peritoneal spill. Hyperosmolar contrast may have some beneficial effects in functional LBO.

Uses

• Suspected LBO
• Identification of fistula tracks (Fig. 2.9)
• Prior to insertion of self-expanding metal stents (SEMS)
• Elective procedure to confirm integrity of anastomoses or pouch prior to reversal of upstream diverting stoma

Proctography

Semi-solid material is mixed with barium or water-soluble contrast and introduced per rectum (PR); substance is evacuated under fluoroscopy.

Uses

• Functional assessment of incontinence or constipation
• Assessment of the anorectal angle, rectal prolapse, rectocele, or perineal descent during defecation or straining (Fig. 6.2).

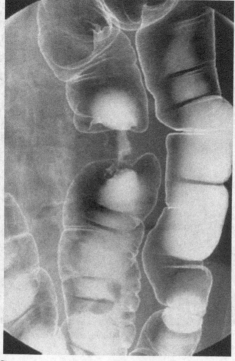

Fig. 2.8 Classic 'apple core' lesion in the distal transverse colon related to an annular carcinoma.

CT scanning

The workhorse of most GI radiology departments is now the multislice CT scanner.

- Scans are acquired using at least 16 rows of detectors collecting data in a continuous helix as the patient moves through the gantry
- Data are processed into isometric voxels creating an image which can be viewed in multiple planes, usually axial, coronal, and sagittal, without loss of image quality
- IV iodinated contrast is usually given unless there are contraindications such as renal impairment or contrast allergy
- Oral iodinated contrast to visualize the bowel is often no longer required due to the multiplanar nature of imaging.

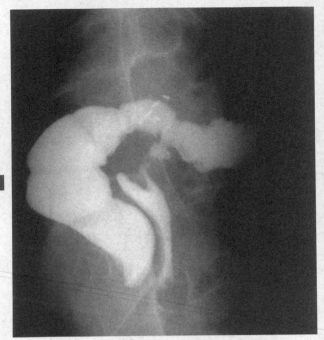

Fig. 2.9 Retrograde water-soluble contrast study showing a colovaginal fistula following a difficult anterior resection.

Uses
- Staging and follow-up of GI tract malignancy
- Investigation of acute lower GI tract blood loss
- SBO or LBO (Fig. 8.5)
- Suspected appendicitis: high sensitivity/specificity at the cost of radiation dose often in young people (Fig. 8.2)
- Diagnosis and management of complicated diverticular disease (Fig. 5.3)
- As part of follow-up protocols although high cumulative dose of radiation.

CT colonoscopy

Increasingly popular and now often the modality of choice in the investigation of large bowel pathology in frail and elderly patients (Fig. 2.10).
- Low risk, requiring minimal patient movement and no sedation or analgesia
- More sensitive than barium enema in the detection of colon cancer and much more sensitive in polyp detection
  - Sensitivity for detection of polyps of <6mm 48%, 6–9mm (70%) and 85% for polyps of ≥10mm

(a)

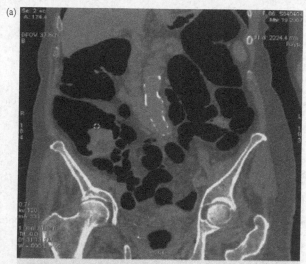

(b)

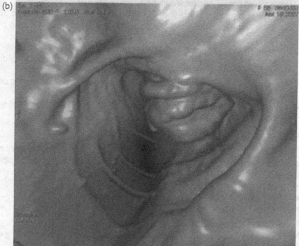

Fig. 2.10 CT colonography. Exophytic polypoidal tumour of caecum with 2D read (a) and the same tumour on 3D read (b).

- Specificity >90% for all groups but best performance shows accuracy comparable with colonoscopy for polyps >6mm
- Therapeutically significant extracolonic lesions detected in 5–10% of older patients
- No additional staging scan is required if pathology demonstrated
- Minimal preparation examinations are highly sensitive in tumour detection in frail population
- Computer-assisted detection may improve diagnostic accuracy
- The technique is not yet routinely available, in part due to demands on CT scanning time and a lack of radiology expertise
- No tissue diagnosis obtained and many patients with pathology will require colonoscopy to confirm the pathology and treat polyps, etc.
- Significant dose of radiation of more concern in younger patients
- Flat polyps usually undetectable
- Angiodysplasia is not seen
- Role in screening for CRC not yet proven.

Technical factors
- Automated CO_2 insufflation via rectal tube
- Low dose scout image ensures adequate large bowel distension prior to formal scan
- Initial supine abdominopelvic scan with portal venous phase timing of iodinated contrast
- Subsequent prone or lateral decubitus scan obtained
- Data processing to produce images in 2D, axial, coronal, sagittal, and 3D planes: a virtual colonoscopy and virtual pathology specimen can also be produced
- Bowel prep determined by radiologist preference and age and mobility of patient. Most commonly a full purgative preparation ± faecal and/or fluid tagging with oral barium or iodinated contrast is performed
- Less invasive bowel prep including 'minimal preparation' with tagging of faeces and fluid without purgative preparation can be considered
- 'Virtual cleansing' post-processing software which removes high density tagged stool.

MRI
MRI now provides a safe and reproducible method of assessing the rectum in both staging of rectal cancer and diagnosis and characterization of peri-anal sepsis. MRI has particular advantages in pelvic imaging.
- Superb contrast resolution
- Smaller field of view allows improved spatial resolution
- Scope for motion artefact is less than in the abdomen.

Rectal cancer staging
MRI has been shown to be an accurate method of pre-operative staging of anorectal cancer. It can be used to:
- Accurately assess T stage of tumour with particular relevance to differentiating T2/early T3 from more advanced T3 tumours (Fig. 2.11). Conventional tumour nodes metastases (TNM) staging is less crucial than assessing tumour distance from plane of surgery. Endoanal US (EAUS) is more accurate in early T staging and also in anal sphincter assessment (Figs 11.21 and 11.22)

- Identify tumour extending to within 1mm of the mesorectal fascia on MR which predicts likelihood of having an involved circumferential resection margin (CRM) at operation
- Identify poor prognostic indicators (extramural spread of >5mm)
- Assess extramural vascular invasion
- Identify suspicious lymph nodes (LNs) within mesorectal fat showing heterogeneity of signal and irregularity of outline suggesting tumour involvement
- Identify the peritoneal reflection and the relationship to the tumour
- Identify disease beyond the surgical field
- Detect bony disease
- Identify very small volume tumour load (as small as 3mm) in nodes using reticuloendothelial agents (ultrasmall particles of iron oxide)
- Assess stage post-radiotherapy. This is more difficult and less accurate in predicting tumour invasion due to the difficulty in differentiating fibrotic tissue and tumour infiltration.

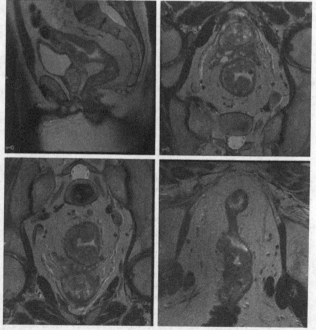

Fig. 2.11 T3 rectal cancer but no threat to mesorectal fascia.

Perianal sepsis
- Due to excellent soft tissue differentiation and fluid-specific sequences the presence of fluid or pus can be identified (Fig. 6.9).
- Relationship of tract to anal canal and sphincter complex visualized
- Presence of deep abscess or supralevator extension demonstrated.

Dynamic MRI
- Uses open-configuration MRI systems
- Provides good visualization of the anorectal angle, opening of the anal canal, and descent of the pelvic floor
- Wide range of morphological variations in healthy individuals and a large interobserver variation limits its usefulness.

Interventional radiology

Interventional radiology involvement in the colon and rectum centres on treatment of malignant LBO with SEMS and investigation and treatment of acute lower GI tract blood loss.

Colonic stenting
- Described in a later chapter (➲ Large bowel obstruction, Chapter 8, p.422).

Selective mesenteric angiography and mesenteric artery embolization
- Usually performed in haemodynamically unstable patient following unsuccessful endoscopic procedure (Fig. 2.12)
- Requires meticulous interrogation of mesenteric arcades with repeated digital subtraction runs with muscle relaxant
- Results significantly better in tertiary centres
- Relatively low risk of ischaemia following embolization
- Repeat angiography and embolization possible if bleeding recurs—access sheath often left in position for 24–48h following initial procedure.

Radionuclide imaging

Images are based on physiology rather than anatomy. A gamma camera is used to acquire images once the agent is given to the patient.

GI bleeding
- Technetium ^{99m}Tc is the radionuclide used in bleeding scans
- ^{99m}Tc can be used to label colloid or RBC. Colloid is rapidly metabolized and best results are with tagged red cells
- If initial scan is negative, a delayed repeat scan at 24h may show site of bleeding although the location of activity on delayed scans does not accurately reflect the site of the bleeding
- Sensitive at a bleeding rate of 0.1–0.2ml/min versus a bleeding rate of 0.5ml/min required for detection at angiography.

Meckel's scan
- ^{99m}Tc pertechnetate is used as it is actively extracted by mucus-secreting cells in gastric mucosa
- Early imaging at 30–60min required to diagnose ectopic gastric mucosa accurately (Fig. 2.13(a)).

Crohn's disease
- Autologous leucocytes are labelled with either indium[111] or ^{99m}Tc-hexamethyl propylene amine oxime (HMPAO)
- ^{99m}Tc-HMPAO offers reduced radiation dosimetry and enhanced image quality
- 3D scanning allows visualization of the entire bowel separate from overlying structures
- Can be used to look for occult disease or assess distribution and activity in known Crohn's disease (Fig. 2.13(b)).

(a)   (b)

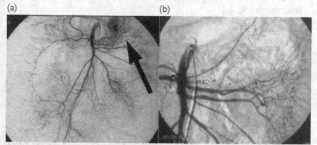

Fig. 2.12 Angiography showing a blush from a jejunal tumour (arrow) (a) and the appearances after embolization with coils (b).

(a)   (b)

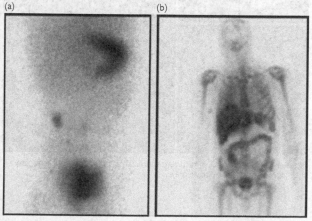

Fig. 2.13 A ^{99m}Tc pertechnetate scan shows a Meckel's diverticulum (a) and a HMPAO-labelled white cell scan in a patient with Crohn's disease showing an active right sided colitis (b).

Positron emission tomography (PET)-CT

- Fluorodeoxyglucose (FDG) analogue taken up by active cellular activity such as tumour
- Used in conjunction with standard non-contrast-enhanced CT scan to correlate anatomical position
- Increased uptake before visible structural abnormalities can be identified radiologically
- Used predominantly as an adjunct to MRI and CT in problem solving in the post-operative pelvis and in the exclusion of occult metastatic disease in patients being considered for radical surgery for local disease recurrence (Fig. 2.14)
- Modality of choice for patients being considered for surgery for locally recurrent CRC
- Detection of non-resectable disease to avert inappropriate surgery
- Improves prognostic stratification in patients with recurrent CRC.

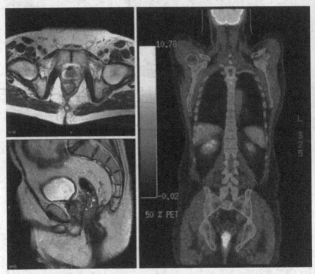

Fig. 2.14 MR and PET-CT of recurrent anorectal cancer prior to salvage surgery showing locally advanced disease only.

Radiological investigations: the liver

Multiple radiological modalities are utilized in liver imaging including, CT, MRI, US, and PET-CT. These are frequently complementary and each has its strengths and weaknesses. Characterization of lesions <7–10mm in size can frequently be difficult by any modality.

CT

Pros and cons
- Quick
- High spatial resolution
- Highly reproducible
- Lacks contrast resolution
- Penalty of exposure to ionizing radiation.

Technical aspects

The use of IV iodinated contrast significantly improves contrast resolution and gives the option of multiple phase dynamic scanning. Readily generated multiplanar images can aid diagnostic certainty and help plan surgical and other interventions. Assessment of segmental anatomy can be easily performed on images acquired in the portal phase of iodinated contrast enhancement (Fig. 2.15).

CT arterial portography

This is an invasive procedure involving multiphase CT acquired before and after direct injection of iodinated contrast into the coeliac artery or its branches. This obtains high quality hepatic arterial phase and portal venous phase scans and provides the highest CT sensitivity for detecting liver metastases. This technique has decreased in use for the assessment of colorectal liver metastases due to its invasive nature and the increasing availability of MRI.

Uses
- Most commonly employed tool to investigate the liver in CRC for both staging and follow-up
- Frequently used in image-guided procedures including biopsy and focal ablative techniques such as radiofrequency ablation (RFA).

Findings

Most CRC metastases are hypovascular and derive their blood supply from the hepatic artery (Fig. 2.16). CT imaging in the portal venous (PV) phase of iodinated contrast enhancement (~60–70s) reveals metastatic deposits to be hypointense relative to surrounding liver with a ring of peripheral enhancement. The PV phase is the most commonly used scanning phase to detect the majority of colorectal liver metastases on CT.

CT imaging of the liver frequently reveals lesions which are either too small to characterize (<1cm) or atypical in appearance. Further investigation with US or MRI is helpful to allow characterization of these lesions.

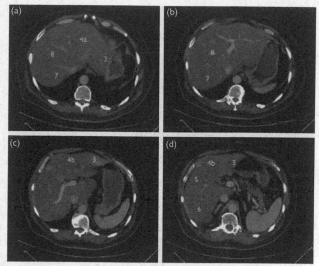

Fig. 2.15 CT liver images demonstrating segmental anatomy. Superior segments identified in relation to the right, middle, and left hepatic veins (a). Division of portal vein into left (b) and right (c) main branches. Inferior segments below portal vein bifurcation (d).

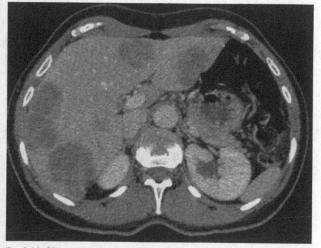

Fig. 2.16 CT scan of liver with bilobar metastatic deposits.

MRI

Pros and cons

- Excellent contrast resolution and good spatial resolution
- Liver-specific contrast agents
- Multiphase dynamic imaging
- No ionizing radiation
- Slow—up to 1h scanning time with some contrast agents
- More prone to artefact
- High cost.

Uses

- Characterize liver abnormalities seen on CT
- Assess the extent of liver disease prior to liver resection or local ablative therapy (Fig. 2.17).

Technical aspects

Dynamic multiphase scanning of the liver is performed with gadolinium (Gd) chelates which act as extracellular contrast agents in an analogous way to the use of iodinated contrast in CT.

- T1 agents increase the signal of normal liver on T1-weighted imaging with metastatic disease appearing of low signal in comparison, e.g. Gd-BOPTA, Gd-EOB-DTPA, Mangafodipir trisodium (Fig. 2.18).
- T2 agents reduce the signal of normal liver on T2-weighted imaging with metastatic deposits appearing of relatively increased signal, e.g. superparamagnetic iron oxide particles (SPIOs).

Improved contrast resolution from administration of 'liver-specific' MR contrast agents has been shown to increase sensitivity of MRI for liver metastases. The two Gd chelates have the advantage that they also provide conventional dynamic contrast scanning which is often helpful in lesion characterization.

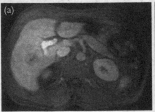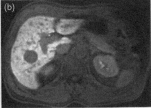

Fig. 2.17 Colorectal liver metastases on MRI. Increased lesion conspicuity with liver-specific contrast (Gd-EOB-DTPA). Low signal metastatic lesion of the right lobe of the liver seen on portal venous phase (a). Multiple additional deposits seen on liver-specific phase (b).

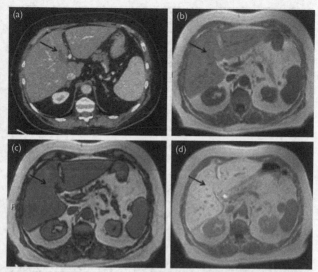

Fig. 2.18 Lesion characterization with MRI. Low-density liver lesion (arrow) on follow-up CT for CRC (a). MRI in-phase T1-weighted image shows lesion (arrow) of slightly increased signal relative to liver (b). Generalized signal loss within liver on opposed phase T1 weighting with marked focal signal loss (arrow) (c). Liver-specific phase (Gd-EOB-DTPA) shows lesion (arrow) isointense to liver (d). MRI characterizes lesion as focal fatty infiltration.

Ultrasound (US)

Transabdominal US is frequently used as a general primary investigatory tool in assessing the liver and biliary tract (Fig. 2.19).

Pros and cons

- Safe, inexpensive, and quick to perform
- Inherent high spatial resolution
- High contrast resolution with the use of US contrast agents and intraoperative scanning
- Complete examination is frequently difficult due to patient build
- Highly operator dependent.

Uses

- Characterization of small low-density lesions identified on CT which can often be confirmed as simple cysts
- Primary investigation of choice for the biliary tract
- Image-guided procedures including biopsies and ablative procedures
- Intraoperative US avoids the problems of access that are experienced with transabdominal US and is highly sensitive. Its principal role is in the assessment of the liver at the time of resection of metastases.

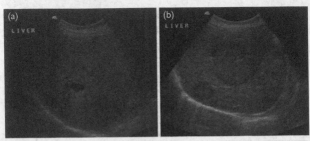

Fig. 2.19 Liver ultrasound. A simple anechoic cyst (a) and colorectal liver metastases with typical hypoechoic appearance (b).

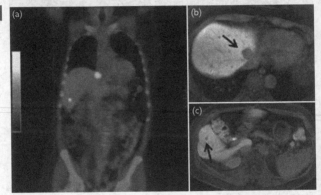

Fig. 2.20 Isolated colorectal liver metastases on PET-CT with MR correlation. Fused coronal PET-CT image showing two FDG-avid lesions within the liver and no distant metastases (a). Liver-specific (Gd-EOB-DTPA) MRI images showing hypoechoic metastases adjacent to the IVC (arrow) (b) and inferiorly within the right lobe (arrow) (c).

PET-CT

PET-CT is a hybrid technology principally used in cancer imaging. The positron-emitting glucose analogue FDG is taken up preferentially by highly metabolically active cells such as cancer cells. Imaging the distribution of this uptake is combined with a conventional CT examination immediately after to aid anatomical localization.

PET-CT's main role in CRC is identification and quantification of metastatic disease (including the liver, Fig. 2.20). This includes investigation of patients with suspected but radiologically occult metastases and assessment of patients considered for resection of recurrent or metastatic disease.

Recent series suggest PET-CT may be the most sensitive test on a per-patient basis for the detection of liver metastases. At present, the resolution of PET-CT is limited to lesions ~7mm or more in size. PET-CT also has a potential role in the assessment of tumour response.

Endoscopic equipment

Structure and function of an endoscope

Flexible endoscopes consist of a control head and flexible shaft. The control head is attached to the light source by an 'umbilical cord' which also conducts the air/water supply and the suction channel (Fig. 2.21). The control head includes:

- Two angling wheels located on the right side which control movement of the tip of the scope in the up/down (~180°) and left/right (~160°) planes. Each angling wheel has a friction braking system which allows the tip of the scope to be temporarily fixed in position
- Two buttons on the anterior aspect, a lower air/water insufflation button, and an upper suction button
- The upper part of the head contains multiple programmable buttons which can be set with variable functions, e.g. freeze frame, image capture, video control, narrow band image control
- An operating channel which is generally 3–4mm in diameter and allows the passage of instruments to the tip of the scope, e.g. biopsy forceps, diathermy snare, injection needle
- The shaft of a standard adult colonoscope is 160–180cm long (flexible sigmoidoscope 60–90cm) and has a diameter of 11–13mm
- Flexibility of the shaft is essential to allow passage of the scope around the angulations within the colon. Stiffness is also important, in order to maintain a straight configuration once the scope has been advanced through a particularly tortuous region of the bowel
- Technologies developed to accommodate these conflicting requirements include:

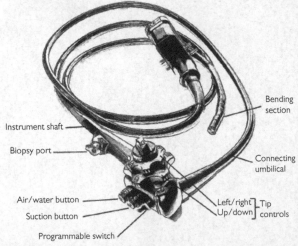

Fig. 2.21 A modern video colonoscope.

- The 'graduated stiffness' colonoscope which has a flexible tip but also increasing stiffness progressing back along the shaft of the instrument
- The 'variable stiffness' colonoscope which allows adjustment of the shaft stiffness using a control ring situated at the base of the head
- The shaft may also contain electromagnetic transmission coils used to display a real-time 3D view of the position/orientation of the colonoscope using a low intensity magnetic field
- The tip of a videoendoscope contains a lens with a field of view of 140–170° which focuses the light reflected from the mucosa onto a charge-coupled device (CCD). This generates electrical impulses transmitted back through wiring to the video processor unit. Many modern CCDs contain 1 million individual pixels, giving high resolution images of the colonic mucosa. In the video processor unit, the information from the CCD is used to create an image which is transmitted to the monitor.

High definition white light flexible endoscopes are now used in most endoscopy units. These systems offer four times the resolution of a standard video system and in combination with electronic magnification in the processor unit allow accurate visualization of minute mucosal structures.

Carbon dioxide insufflator

As carbon dioxide (CO_2) is absorbed into the circulation and excreted by respiration, it is cleared from the colon ~100 × faster than air. When used as the insufflation gas, the bowel is cleared of gas within 20min.
- CO_2 insufflation has been shown to significantly reduce abdominal pain both during and for up to 24h after colonoscopy
- Studies suggest there is no difference in caecal intubation rates
- CO_2 retention does not have any clinically significant adverse effects on patients
- CO_2 insufflation may also reduce the rare complication of gas ignition related to the combination of electrocautery and accumulation of colonic gases.

Diathermy

In endoscopic practice, monopolar diathermy uses electrical current to produce heat and damage tissue, thereby either cutting or coagulating tissue. Although minimal heat is usually generated away from the point of contact of the active electrode, lateral and deep tissue injury may occur due to thermal spread (Fig. 2.22), which may lead to delayed perforation.

The plate should not be placed over metal prostheses which may generate excessive heat.
- Cutting diathermy uses a continuous, relatively low voltage sinusoidal waveform which is less likely to penetrate deeply into the tissue
- Coagulation diathermy uses interrupted pulses of higher voltage in a square waveform which allows a deeper spread of current
- Modern diathermy units use blends of cutting and coagulation current to enhance efficiency while reducing the risk of excess tissue damage

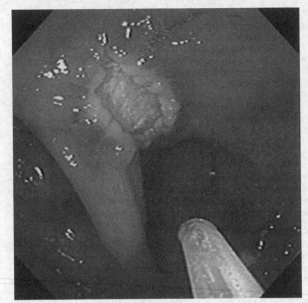

Fig. 2.22 Diathermy burn. A rather deep burn with blanching of the adjacent mucosa following diathermy polypectomy.

- The power settings used are not directly comparable between different diathermy units and so both the power settings and pre-set modes used should be determined from the information provided by the manufacturer.

Argon plasma coagulation

Argon plasma coagulation (APC) is a non-contact thermal method of haemostasis which can also be used to destroy adenomas.

APC sprays a plasma of ionized argon gas, producing an evenly distributed thermal energy field with a limited depth of penetration of energy/heat of ~2–3mm. The argon gas flow rate and thermal wattage delivered can be adjusted to control depth of burn.

Inadvertent direct contact of probe with the mucosa will insufflate argon gas submucosally and into muscle wall. Any subsequent CT scan will show intramural gas and possibly extramural gas, which does not necessarily reflect a 'perforation' of the bowel.

Advantages of APC
- Ease of application and lower cost compared to laser
- Rapid treatment of multiple lesions in the case of arteriovenous malformations or wide areas including the base of resected polyps, tumour bleeding, or bleeding from radiation injury to the rectum
- Safety due to reduced depth of penetration. Care must be taken, however, especially in the right colon.

Advanced endoscopic imaging

Endoscopists now have access to several technical innovations designed to enhance white light endoscopic assessment of the GI tract. Primarily these technologies have been used to differentiate between neoplastic and non-neoplastic lesions of the colon (Table 2.1). These can be broadly grouped as follows:

- *Narrowed-spectrum technologies (virtual chromoendoscopy)*
  - Rely on a narrowed spectral bandwidth (mainly blue light)
  - Narrowed bandwidth achieved through optical or digital filters
  - Available from most endoscope/colonoscope manufacturers
  - High definition endoscopy is required to work properly
- *Autofluorescence imaging (AFI)*
  - Some naturally occurring fluorophores (e.g. collagen and flavins) emit fluorescence after excitation with short-wavelength light
  - The AF signal is altered by changes in mucosal thickness, blood flow, and concentration of endogenous fluorophores
  - A dedicated imaging processor uses these changes to generate an image where thickened tissue (e.g. an adenoma) appears a different colour compared to normal mucosa
  - The resolution of the image is lower than white light endoscopy and prone to degradation with movement of the scope or mucosa
- *Confocal laser endomicroscopy (CLE)*
  - A low powered laser is focused on a single point, up to 250μ below the mucosa. Return light from here is focused on a detector

Table 2.1 Advanced endoscopic imaging

Technique	Company	Notes
Narrow band imaging (NBI)	Olympus	Only blue and green light used. Blue light absorbed by capillaries in mucosa but green light penetrates deeper. NBI produces good contrast between superficial microvasculature and bettter clarity of mucosal surface
Flexible spectral imaging colour enhancement (FICE)/ Fujinon Intelligent Chromoendoscopy)	Fujifilm	Post-processor digital extraction and manipulation of specific wavelengths from digital image.
i-Scan digital contrast (I-SCAN)	Pentax	Post-processor digital extraction and manipulation of specific wavelengths from digital image.
Blue laser imaging (BLI)	Fujifilm	Uses two monochromatic lasers instead of xenon light. More recent advances use an LED light source
Autofluorescence imaging (AFI)	Olympus	
Confocal laser endoscopy (CLE)	Pentax Cellvizio	Requires a contrast agent, administered either IV or topically

- The point of illumination and detection are in the same focal plane giving rise to the term 'confocal'
- An integrated endoscopic version by Pentax is no longer available. A probe-based system which uses the working channel of the endoscope is commercially available from Cellvizio
- Narrow-band imaging (NBI), flexible spectral imaging colour enhancement (FICE), CLE (but not AFI) enable a reliable optical differentiation between neoplastic and non-neoplastic colonic lesions
- Results are not always reproducible outside specialist centres and intensive training/assessment is usually required
- NBI, FICE, i-Scan digital contrast (I-SCAN), and AFI have not been shown to reliably improve adenoma or polyp detection rates
- NBI is not significantly superior to chromoendoscopy which remains the recommended standard of care for colonoscopic surveillance to detect dysplasia in longstanding IBD.

Reference

East JE, Vleugels JL, Roeland P et al. (2016) Advanced endoscopic imaging: European Society of Gastrointestinal Endoscopy (ESGE) technology review: *Endoscopy* **48**;1029–1045

Safe endoscopic practice

Provision of information and obtaining informed consent

To allay anxiety, patients should be provided with adequate written and verbal information prior to the procedure. In obtaining informed consent the patients should be advised of the risks of:

- Discomfort or pain during the procedure
- Bleeding
- Colonic perforation.

The risk of bleeding or colonic perforation with diagnostic colonoscopy is low (<1/500). The risk is higher if any intervention is performed (e.g. polypectomy) (↪ Interventional colonoscopy, discussed later in this chapter, p.84).

Antibiotic prophylaxis

- Current evidence indicates that antibiotic prophylaxis is not required for any diagnostic endoscopy. This also applies to patients having hot biopsy or snare polypectomy performed
- There is no clear evidence to favour the use of antibiotics when performing endoscopic mucosal resection (EMR) (↪ Interventional colonoscopy, discussed later in this chapter, p.84). However, many endoscopists administer prophylaxis for higher risk patients (mitral valve replacement, immunosuppression)
- Prophylaxis is usually given when placing a percutaneous endoscopic gastrostomy (PEG) tube (↪ Interventional colonoscopy, discussed later in this chapter, p.84).

Warfarin, Direct Oral Anti-Coagulant (DOAC), and anti-platelet therapy

Current national and local guidelines should be consulted for advice on management of anti-coagulant and anti-platelet therapy for interventional procedures (Table 2.2).

Sedatives, analgesia, and anti-spasmodics

Conscious sedation is a technique in which drugs are used to produce a state of depression of the central nervous system (CNS) such that treatment can be carried out, but during which verbal contact with the patient is maintained.

Benzodiazepines

- IV midazolam is most commonly used. It is twice as potent as diazepam with a more pronounced amnesic effect
- Maximum recommended dose of midazolam is 5mg but ↓ for elderly patients and patients with significant respiratory or hepatic disease
- Oversedation may be reversed using flumazenil which is a competitive antagonist at the benzodiazepine receptors.

Opiates

- Act in a synergistic fashion with benzodiazepines so doses must be titrated to achieve the desired effect
- Fentanyl is the most commonly used opiate
- Generally, the maximum doses required are 100mcg of fentanyl

Table 2.2 Guidelines on colonoscopy with anti-coagulant and anti-platelet therapy

Drug	Low risk procedure	High risk procedure (polypectomy/EMR)
P2Y12 receptor antagonist anti-platelet agents • Clopidogrel • Prasugrel • Ticagrelor	Continue therapy	**Low risk condition** • Stop 5 days before colonoscopy **High risk condition** • Discuss with cardiology • Consider stopping if possible Continue aspirin if already prescribed
Warfarin	Continue therapy Ensure international normalized ratio (INR) in therapeutic is in therapeutic range	**Low risk condition** • Stop 5 days before colonoscopy • Ensure INR is <1.5 prior to intervention • Restart warfarin evening after procedure and check INR 1 week later **High risk condition** • Stop 5 days before procedure • Start low molecular weight heparin (LMWH) 2 days before procedure • Last dose of LMWH should be >24h before procedure • Restart warfarin evening after procedure and continue LMWH until INR therapeutic
Direct Oral Anti-coagulants (DOAC) • Dabigatran • Rivaroxaban • Apixaban • Edoxaban	Omit morning of procedure	**Rivaroxaban, Apixaban, and Edoxaban** • Last dose >48h before procedure **Dabigatran** • Last dose >48h before procedure. If EGFR is 30–50ml/min, last dose 72h before procedure • If renal function is unstable, consult haematology

Low risk conditions	High risk conditions
Ischaemic Heart Disease (IHD) without coronary stent	Coronary artery stents (when taking anti-platelet agents)
Cerebrovascular disease	Prosthetic metal heart valve in mitral position
Peripheral vascular disease	Prosthetic heart valve and AF
Prosthetic aortic metal or xenograft valve	AF and mitral stenosis
Atrial fibrillation (AF) without valvular disease	<3 months after venous thromboembolism (VTE)
Thrombophilia syndromes (discuss with haematology)	

- The dose for elderly patients and those with respiratory depression should be reduced to 50mcg fentanyl
- Opiate oversedation can be reversed using naloxone, a competitive antagonist at the opiate receptors.

Nitrous oxide
- Nitrous oxide (Entonox: 50% nitrous oxide, 50% oxygen) is increasingly used to provide analgesia during colonoscopy
- A Cochrane review reported that it was as effective as IV analgesia but appeared to be safer as it had a reduced risk of complications

Anti-spasmodic agents
- Bowel spasm can be alleviated for 5–10min using 20–40mg IV hyoscine butylbromide or 0.5–1.0mg IV glucagon.

Propofol infusion
- Can be considered for patients who have had difficulty achieving adequate conscious sedation at previous procedures (e.g. alcoholics, drug addicts) or those who are particularly anxious
- Should always be carried out by an anaesthetist.

Safety and patient monitoring
- All patients undergoing endoscopic procedures should have a pre-procedure check list completed to identify any relevant risk factors
- Resuscitation equipment including sedative reversal agents must be available in the endoscopy room and the recovery area
- One of the two required assistants is dedicated to patient care and has a key role in monitoring the patient's safety, comfort, and well-being
- All sedated patients should have an IV cannula *in situ* throughout the procedure and recovery period
- Oxygen (2litres/min) is administered to all patients prior to receiving conscious sedation
- Continuous pulse oximetry monitoring should be performed throughout the procedure in any patient receiving sedation
- Monitoring in the recovery area should continue for a minimum of 1h following the administration of sedation
- Outpatients should be accompanied home by a responsible adult who should stay with them for a minimum of 12h
- Patients given benzodiazepines should be advised not to drive a car, operate machinery, or sign legal documents in the following 24h.

Reporting the outcome of colonoscopy
An immediate report should be provided to the patient and their GP. Ideally, this should include the following information:
- Indication for the procedure as well as the American Society of Anesthesiologists (ASA) grade
- Type of sedation given and consciousness level
- Quality of bowel preparation
- Extent of visualization i.e. include information on caecal and TI intubation
- Findings and description of any therapeutic procedures
- Duration of procedure including withdrawal time
- Plan for follow-up.

Reference

Veitch AM, Vanbiervliet G, Gerschlick AH, et al. (2016) Endoscopy in patients on anticoagulant therapy, including direct oral anticoagulants: British society of Gastroenterology (BSF) and European Society of Gastrointestinal Endoscopy (ESGE) guidelines. *Gut* **65**:374–389.

Proctoscopy and rigid sigmoidoscopy

These procedures are generally carried out with the patient lying in the left lateral position (Fig. 2.23). Correct positioning is essential to optimize the view obtained.

Prior to insertion of the scope, the perineum is carefully inspected and the perianal area palpated. Anal fissures are normally apparent on inspection alone and, if present, further digital or endoscopic examination should be deferred to avoid unnecessary pain for the patient. A tender fullness in the perianal area on palpation may represent an acute abscess and further assessment may require general or regional anaesthesia. A digital anorectal examination is mandatory prior to any attempt to insert the scope in order to:

- Check that the patient does not have excessive discomfort
- Confirm the presence of an adequate lumen for insertion
- Assess for pathology of the anus or distal rectum.

Proctoscopy

The proctoscope is a relatively short instrument which only allows examination of the distal rectal mucosa and anal canal.

- Insert by gently pushing the well-lubricated instrument in the direction of the patient's umbilicus to the full extent of its length
- The obturator is removed and distal rectal mucosa can be examined
- As the scope is withdrawn, the anorectal junction, anal cushions, and dentate line can all be identified
- Some instruments have a bevelled end which allows the circumference of the anus to be inspected by rotating the scope rather than having to repeatedly reinsert
- Asking the patient to strain may help to demonstrate internal haemorrhoids or rectal mucosal prolapse
- Pathology identifiable at proctoscopy includes:
  - Distal rectal polyps or carcinoma
  - Rectal mucosal prolapse or haemorrhoidal prolapse
  - Internal opening of a fistula in ano or anal fibroepithelial polyp
  - Anal fissure or anal carcinoma.

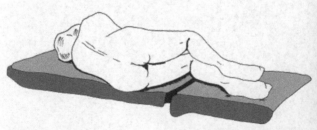

Fig. 2.23 Left lateral position.

Rigid sigmoidoscopy

The value of rigid sigmoidoscopy was reduced with the introduction of flexible endoscopes, but many surgeons still find it useful as an initial screening tool. It has been argued that assessment of the position of lesions such as rectal cancers or polyps is more accurate using a rigid instrument.

Technique
- Prior to the procedure the patient may be prepared with a suppository or a phosphate enema
- The lubricated instrument with the obturator in place is inserted using gentle pressure in the direction of the patient's umbilicus. As the scope enters the rectum a fall in resistance can be felt
- The obturator is removed and the rectum gently insufflated with air
- The scope is further advanced under direct vision. Initially the instrument is angled posteriorly then comes forwards again as it passes round the sacral curve. The top of the rectum is reached at ~15cm from the anal margin. It may be possible to angle the scope anteriorly and to the patient's left to enter the distal sigmoid colon. Often this is not possible and advancement should be terminated if the patient is uncomfortable or excessive pressure is required
- The scope is withdrawn slowly, allowing careful inspection of the entire circumference of the rectal wall. Particular attention should be paid to the areas behind the valves of Houston which are often inadequately visualized
- While obvious pathological appearances should be noted on insertion, the majority of the inspection is performed during retraction of the scope
- Pathology which can be identified includes:
  - Rectal polyps or tumours
  - Areas of inflammation or ulceration
  - Abnormal mucosal vascular pattern including telangiectasia.

Complications
- Complications from rigid sigmoidoscopy are rare
- Perforation rates are <0.01%
- The incidence of significant bleeding is also very low
- It has been suggested that where diffuse pathological processes are biopsied, the samples should be taken from the posterior rectal wall as it is easier to compress this area against the sacrum should significant bleeding occur.

Flexible sigmoidoscopy and colonoscopy

Indications for flexible sigmoidoscopy

- As an adjunct to barium enema, because imaging of the distal part of the large bowel is often obscured due to overlapping loops of colon
- To investigate fresh rectal bleeding in patients <50yrs of age
- To re-assess the distal large bowel after previous intervention.

Indications for colonoscopy

Colonoscopy is currently considered to be the 'gold standard' investigation of the large bowel. It allows careful assessment of the bowel mucosa, provides the opportunity to obtain biopsies for histology, and can be used for therapeutic procedures, e.g. polypectomy. An experienced colonoscopist would expect to reach the caecum in >90% of cases and the terminal ileum in >70% of cases.

There are many indications for colonoscopy (Box 2.2). Careful consideration should be given to the potential risks and benefits of the procedure. Alternatives methods of investigation should be considered in frail patients, those with significant co-morbidity who are unlikely to tolerate/survive a complication, and where the outcome is unlikely to impact on management.

Box 2.2 Indications for colonoscopy

Investigation of symptomatic patient
- Any new history of rectal bleeding in patients >50yrs
- Persistent change in bowel function
- Abnormal CT scan, barium enema, or colon capsule endoscopy
- Iron deficiency (often combined with upper GI endoscopy)
- Evaluation of terminal ileum in Crohn's disease.

Bowel cancer screening, follow-up, and IBD surveillance
- Positive qFIT test as part of a bowel cancer screening programme
- Follow-up after previous colorectal cancer or polyps
- Assessment of extent and severity of disease and screening for dysplasia in IBD.

Therapeutic procedures
- Polypectomy (simple polypectomy, EMR, and endoscopic submucosal dissection (ESD))
- Tattoo lesion/cancer to facilitate localization at surgery or subsequent colonoscopy
- Decompression of sigmoid volvulus and pseudo-obstruction
- Dilatation of colonic and anastomotic strictures
- Insertion of colonic stent
- Treat rectal bleeding (e.g. argon plasma coagulation of radiation injury of rectum).

Bowel preparation

Most patients are required to prepare their bowel prior to attending as an outpatient for the procedure and should be provided with clear, written instructions.

Drug related issues with colonoscopy

- Avoidance of iron preparations for 1 week prior to the scope. Iron produces a black, viscid stool which is difficult to clear and absorbs light, therefore reducing visibility in the colon
- Stopping anti-diarrhoeal agents 1–2 days prior to bowel preparation.
- Plan on stopping or continuing anti-platelet medication and anti-coagulants according to local guidelines which should incorporate the indication/planned procedure (low or high risk), specific drug in question, and the indication for the drug (low or high risk condition) see Table 2.2.
- It is generally safe to continue aspirin, even if a therapeutic procedure is planned

Bowel cleansing preparations

- A high phosphate enema given 20–30min prior to the procedure. This usually gives adequate preparation for flexible sigmoidoscopy
- Oral preparations (e.g. polyethylene glycol, sodium picosulphate) are required to prepare the bowel for colonoscopy and may also be used for flexible sigmoidoscopy (➲ Mechanical bowel preparation, Chapter 10, p.482)
- Patients should take only very low residue foods or fast if possible, for 24h prior to the procedure. They should continue to drink large quantities of clear fluids.
- Oral preparations should not be used in patients suspected of having complete or partial bowel obstruction.

Clinicians learning to perform flexible sigmoidoscopy/colonoscopy should attend an approved course. Many countries now ensure that trainees undergo a rigorous training programme and they must complete a series of assessments before they are allowed to be certified as an independent practitioner. In the UK, the Joint Advisory Group on GI Endoscopy (JAG) supervise the training programme. It is outside the remit of this handbook to give a detailed description of criteria for certification or to provide a detailed description of the practical techniques involved in colonoscopy. However, the following principles should be observed:

- Written informed consent should be obtained
- Prior to starting, the scope should be checked to ensure the light source, control wheels, and insufflation/suction are working
- DRE should always be performed. For colonoscopy via a colostomy, the stoma should be similarly assessed prior to scope insertion
- It is important that the colonoscopist maintains accurate control of the scope during advancement, retraction, and when applying torque. They must master control of the angulation wheels and insufflation/suction buttons with the left hand, leaving the right hand free to manipulate the scope (Fig. 2.24)
- The principles for safe advancement of the scope are to maintain a view of the lumen, to avoid excessive gas insufflation, and to keep the scope as straight as possible

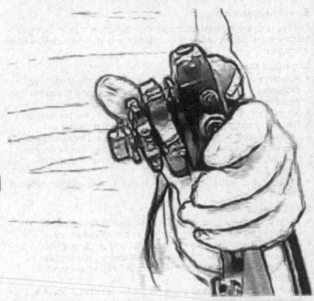

Fig. 2.24 Hand positioning. The correct positioning of the left hand when holding a colonoscope.

- The initial objective is to pass the scope to the caecum/terminal ileum. Large abnormalities should be noted but not dealt with during insertion. Small lesions can prove difficult to re-locate during retraction of the scope and these should be dealt with when identified
- The only reliable way to ensure that the colonoscope has reached the caecum is identification of the ileocaecal valve. Some endoscopists recommend a picture or biopsy of TI biopsy to confirm completion
- The bowel should be carefully examined during retraction of the scope and identified pathology appropriately dealt with
- The scope should be retroflexed in the rectum to assess the anorectal region fully
- An immediate report should be generated (➲ Safe endoscopic practice, discussed earlier in this chapter, p.70).

Tattooing the colonic wall

Between the rectum and ileocaecal valve, the ability to localize the position of the tip of the colonoscope can be highly variable. It is therefore important to mark the location of both cancers and any suspicious polyps that have been removed.

This facilitates subsequent endoscopic review of polypectomy sites and enables surgeons to identify the location of cancers. This is particularly relevant when undertaking laparoscopic surgery as it may not be possible to palpate the bowel before undertaking a resection. All such lesions should therefore be tattooed according to local protocol.

- All suspicious lesions and cancers should be tattooed if they lie outside the rectum or caecum
- Inject at polypectomy site or just distal to lesions or cancers that have not been removed
- For cancers, place at least two tattoos directly opposite each other. If a single tattoo is placed, it might overlie the mesentery and may not be visible at time of surgery
- Preinject the submucosal layer with saline before injecting with a suspension of carbon particles (e.g. SPOT® GI Supply PA USA). This reduces the risk of inadvertent transmural injection, which can be painful. This is also likely to increase difficulty of any subsequent laparoscopic surgery (due to adhesion formation and the presence of black pigment throughout operative field).

Chromoendoscopy

Chromoendoscopy involves topical application of stains, e.g. 0.4% indigo–carmine or 0.1% methylene blue to the mucosal surface to improve tissue characterization (Fig. 2.25). Stains can be injected down the working channel of the scope, but a better effect is achieved with purpose-made catheters which deliver a fine mist to the mucosal surface. Studies are ongoing with regard to use of magnifying endoscopes in conjunction with chromoendoscopy. It is possible to perform detailed surface analysis of small polyps and flat lesions to predict the probable underlying histology ('pit pattern' classification ➔ Colonic polyps, Chapter 7, p.320). Chromoendoscopy may also allow targeted biopsies in IBD surveillance by identifying flat lesions.

A number of new endoscopic systems have been introduced in an attempt to enhance both adenoma/dysplasia detection rates and allow endoscopist to differentiate between adenoma and hyperplastic tissue. However, chromoendoscopy remains the standard of care (➔ Advanced endoscopic imaging, discussed earlier in this chapter, p.67).

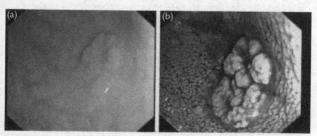

Fig. 2.25 Indigo carmine chromoendoscopy delineating mucosal alteration in the sigmoid: (a) before staining and (b) after staining. Performance of a flexible sigmoidoscopy/colonoscopy.

Reproduced with permission from Trivedi PJ and Braden B, Indications, stains and techniques in chromoendoscopy, QJM: An International Journal of Medicine, 1-6(2): 117-131. Copyright © 2012, Oxford University Press. https://doi.org/10.1093/qjmed/hcs186

Colon capsule endoscopy

- Colon capsule endoscopy (CCE) is a non-invasive diagnostic test that utilizes a disposable capsule to assess the colon. Images are transferred wirelessly to a separate data recorder
- It was first introduced in 2006. An improved, more sensitive version (CCE II) was introduced in 2014
- CCE II has a camera at each end providing a 172° field of view so the total viewing angle is almost 360°. Batteries provide up to 10 hours' recording time
- The frame rate is variable (4–35 frames/sec) and self-adjusts according to position and the speed of travel through the bowel
- More rigorous bowel preparation regimens are usually required. Up to 4 litres of PEG combined with a prokinetic drug (domperidone) and a boost of sodium phosphate is required for good visualization
- CCE II has a sensitivity of 86% for detection of polyps >6mm and 87% for polyps >10mm (with a specificity is 95%)
- CCE II should detect all invasive cancers identified at colonoscopy
- It has a similar sensitivity and specificity to CT colonography although the reading/interpretation time is substantially longer
- The technique may be considered for CRC screening in patients who refuse to undergo colonoscopy, those who have had an incomplete colonoscopy or if colonoscopy is contraindicated
- It is not recommended as a first line investigation for those with a higher risk of colorectal neoplasia, where colonoscopy is investigation of choice
- It may also be used to assess disease activity in inflammatory bowel disease but the lack of ability to take biopsies limits its usefulness
- Overall, the procedure appears to be well tolerated and provides a painless, non-invasive endoscopic colonic examination at the colon.
- Major disadvantages include the need for more rigorous bowel preparation, the cost of the capsule, and time taken to assess images. Patients may also ultimately need to undergo colonoscopy to assess, biopsy, or remove pathology if identified at CCE.

There is an increasing interest in the importance of providing quality colonoscopy and most national gastroenterology societies have developed multiple quality indicators to assist healthcare organizations, endoscopy units, and individual endoscopists to achieve high quality colonoscopy (Table 2.3). Some of the more important indicators are listed.

Colonoscopy completion rate

- Perhaps the most important quality indicator is the most basic i.e. completion or caecal intubation rate
- An incomplete colonoscopy requires an additional intervention/ procedure, increases risk to the patient, and can result in missed cancers, etc.
- Previously, there was wide variability in caecal intubation rates. With appropriate training, ongoing review, and by performing an adequate number of procedures (>100/year), caecal intubation rates of >90% are achievable i.e. there should be no role for the 'occasional colonoscopist'

Table 2.3 UK and American performance indicators and quality assurance standards for colonoscopy

Quality indicator	UK/JAG guidelines*	American guidelines^
Number of procedures/year	100: aspire to 150	
Digital rectal examination	100%	
Unadjusted caecal intubation rate	90%: aspire to 95%	90% for all cases ≥95% when screening
Polyp detection rate	15%: aspire to 20%	25% in patients >50yrs
Polyp retrieval rate	90%	
Withdrawal time	6 mins: aspire to 10 mins	≥6 mins
Biopsies if indication is chronic diarrhoea	100%	100%
Rectal retroversion rate	90%	
Comfort score	<10% moderate to severe discomfort	
Tattoo suspected malignant lesions if outside rectum and caecum	100%	
Perforation rates		<1 in 500 overall <1 in 1000 screening
Postpolypectomy bleeding		<1%

* Source: Data from Rees CJ, Thomas Gibson S, Rutter MD on behalf of the British Society of Gastroenterology, the Joint Advisory Group on GI Endoscopy, the Association of Coloproctology of Great Britain and Ireland, et al., UK key performance indicators and quality assurance standards for colonoscopy. *Gut* 2016;65:1923-1929;

^Source: Data from Rex DK, Schoenfeld PS, Cohen J, et al. Quality indicators for colonoscopy. *Gastrointest Endosc* 2015;81(1):31-53.

- Several improvements and innovations have assisted practitioners in achieving high quality colonoscopy in most patients. These include:
  - Thinner colonoscopes with either graduated stiffness (Pentax®, Fujifilm®) or variable stiffness (Olympus®)
  - Balloon enteroscope-assisted colonoscopy
  - Magnetic endoscopic imaging/fluoroscopy using the ScopeGuide (Olympus®) or Scopepilot (Pentax®)
  - Through-the-scope balloon devices (Vizballoon®)
  - Water-assisted colonoscopy
  - Transparent distal caps
  - Manual compression devices of abdomen, although traditionally, simple manual compression by an assistant has also been used

Adenoma detection rate
- In studies where patients underwent tandem colonoscopies, up to 22% of adenomas were missed
- Rates of interval cancers decline with increasing adenoma detection i.e. risk of interval cancers decreases 3% for every 1% increase in adenoma detection
- Withdrawal time is an important surrogate for quality of colonoscopy and endoscopists with a withdrawal time of ≥6 minutes were 1.8 times more likely to detect one or more polyps.

Reference

JAG trainee certification process Colonoscopy (provisonal and full). Joint Advisory Group on GI Endoscopy. www.thejag.org.uk

Trindale AJ, Lichenstein DR, Aslanian HR et al. (2018) Devices and methods to improve colonoscopy completion (with videos). *Gastroint Endosc* **87**:3; 625–634

Interventional colonoscopy

Snare polypectomy

Endoscopic mucosal resection (EMR)

Interventional colonoscopy

Although simple therapeutic interventions e.g. simple polypectomy can be undertaken by any trained colonoscopist, it may be appropriate to refer patients who require a more complex intervention (e.g. endoscopic removal of large complex polyps) to a specialist endoscopist who has developed a particular skill set. In this circumstance, it is better not to interfere with the polyp at the index procedure as scarring from deep biopsies and unsuccessful attempts at polypectomy may cause mucosa and submucosa to become densely adherent to underlying muscle and increase the risk of perforation at a definitive procedure.

Snare polypectomy

A simple loop snare generally suffices for removal of a pedunculated polyp. Standard snare size is ~30mm diameter although larger/smaller sizes are available. Snare polypectomy is facilitated by obtaining the optimum position for the procedure. Diathermy current can be applied to the snare although it not usually necessary for polyps <7mm (cold snare).
- The scope should be straight, giving optimum control of the tip
- The base of the polyp should lie between 5 and 7 o'clock positions. This can be achieved by rotating the scope ± turning the patient (Fig. 2.26)
- There are occasions when retroflexion of the scope in the rectum or caecum may be useful (Fig. 2.27). Visualization of the polyp may be improved by administering an anti-spasmodic to relax the bowel wall
- Excess fluid/faecal residue should be cleared from the area
- The snare should be fully opened within the lumen of the bowel. It can then be passed over the head of the polyp and around the stalk
- The angle at the base of the loop is positioned against the stalk. A small area of normal-looking mucosa should be left between the base of the polyp and the snare to give an adequate resection margin
- The snare is gently closed around the stalk until it appears snug
- Diathermy is applied until the stalk can be seen whitening. The squeeze can then be increased to encourage the snare to cut through the stalk
- If the polyp cannot be seen after resection, either inject saline or look for the nearest puddle of fluid which usually contains the polyp (Fig. 2.26)
- There may be concern that a thick stalk will ↑ risk of complications
  - Injection of the base with 1:10,000 adrenaline ↓ risk of diathermy injury to bowel wall and bleeding. It is also used to treat active bleeding after polypectomy
  - The base of the stalk can be controlled with a metal clip prior to removal of the polyp to reduce the risk of haemorrhage (Fig. 2.28)
  - The stalk may be snared with a nylon loop either before removing the polyp or following polypectomy.

Endoscopic mucosal resection (EMR)

Sessile polyps up to 2.5cm in diameter may be resected *en bloc*, but larger polyps will require piecemeal resection. The plane of resection is in the mid to deep submucosal layer.
- Where possible the scope should be positioned as described for snare polypectomy of a pedunculated polyp

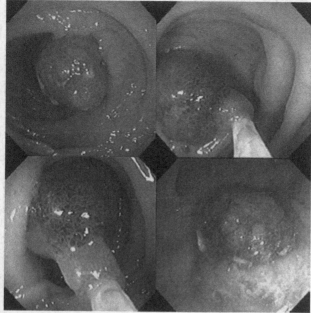

Fig. 2.26 Snare resection of a pedunculated polyp. Note how the colonoscope has been rotated to position the polyp at the 5 o'clock position to facilitate placement of the snare. Following polypectomy, note how the polyp can be found in a nearby pool of fluid which is the most dependent area.

- Submucosal injection of fluid (e.g. 0.9% saline, 1:100,000 adrenaline, colloid) is used to raise the mucosa and create a 'pillow effect' (Figs 2.29 and 2.30). This reduces the risks of bleeding and thermal injury to the bowel wall. Failure of the polyp to lift with submucosal injection must raise suspicion that there is early submucosal tumour infiltration
- A variety of types of snare are available for performing EMR
  - Standard oval snare
  - 'Barbed' snares and 'spiral' snares are designed to improve pick up of the mucosal tissue as they close
  - 'Crescentic' snares are used in piecemeal resection of large polyps. The longer arm of the crescent is placed in the groove created by the preceding resection
- As the snare is closed around the polyp, suction should be applied to decompress the bowel and allow some laxity of the mucosa
- If the patient complains of pain during application of diathermy there may be full-thickness heating of the bowel wall. At this stage there may not yet be a full thickness burn but the procedure should be abandoned before further damage is done

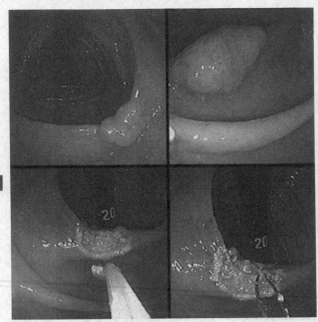

Fig. 2.27 Retroflexion of the colonoscope may facilitate access to polyps lying in awkward positions.

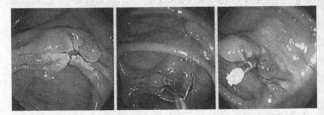

Fig. 2.28 Application of a clip at the site of polypectomy to close the defect.

- Risk of local recurrence following resection has been reported at up to 40%. Treatment of resection margins with APC may reduce this risk
- The site of resection should be tattooed to allow easy identification for future surveillance (◔ Flexible sigmoidoscopy and colonoscopy, discussed earlier in this chapter, p.76)
- The disadvantages of EMR include difficulty in collecting the fragments of tissue, problems in interpretation of histology, and the significant risk of polyp recurrence.

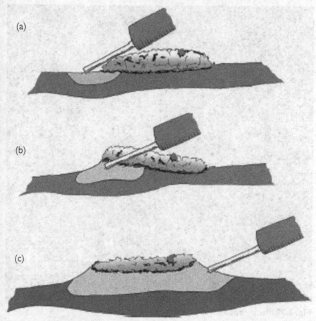

Fig. 2.29 Submucosal proximal injection lifts the flat polyp towards the colonoscope (a). Subsequent lateral (b) and distal (c) injections fully lift the polyp.

Endoscopic submucosal dissection

The technique of ESD is time consuming, but the *en bloc* dissection addresses the disadvantages of piecemeal EMR for larger polyps.

- An endoscopic knife (e.g. insulation-tipped (IT)-knife, hook knife) is used to dissect into the submucosal plane leaving a healthy margin around the lesion
- A transparent cap is placed on the tip of the scope to allow elevation of the polyp and maintain the view of the plane as it is developed
- Effective control of blood vessels is required during dissection using a variety of techniques
- *En bloc* resection rates of up 95–99% are described
- Local recurrence is lower (1–3%) compared to EMR (15–20%)
- The technique is technically challenging and procedure times can range between 60–120 minutes
- Risk of perforation is increased (1–4%) compared to EMR, but can often be managed endoscopically with endoclips
- Risk of bleeding is similar to other techniques and can usually be managed endoscopically
- ESD should only be carried out after appropriate training and accreditation.

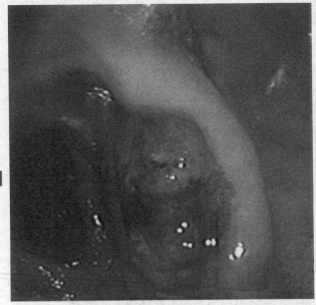

Fig. 2.30 Raising a polyp with saline.

Argon plasma coagulation (APC)
- Mode of action has been discussed (➔ Endoscopic equipment, discussed earlier in this chapter, p.64)
- APC may be used for:
  - Adjunctive therapy to reduce local recurrence after EMR
  - Control of bleeding from neovascularization in radiation proctitis
  - Treatment of arteriovenous malformations in the colon
  - Palliation of colorectal carcinoma.

Laser therapy
The most commonly used laser in colorectal practice is the neodymium: yttrium aluminium garnet (Nd: YAG). Laser therapy may be used to palliate symptoms in patients with advanced rectal carcinoma.
- At lower power settings the laser coagulates the tissues which can be used to control bleeding
- At higher power settings the tissues are vaporized which is more useful for re-canalization of obstructing lesions.

Complications include full-thickness perforation leading to pelvic abscess or fistulae (e.g. enterocutaneous, rectovaginal), bleeding, rectal stenosis, and faecal leakage/incontinence.

Balloon dilatation

Strictures amenable to balloon dilatation may occur as a consequence of IBD, ischaemia, diverticulitis, or non-steroidal anti-inflammatory drug (NSAID) use (Fig. 2.31). They may also occur at the site of an anastomosis (Fig. 2.32). Malignant strictures and those >4–5cm in length generally have a less satisfactory outcome and should not be dilated.

- Most endoscopic dilatation is now done using an 18–20mm balloon which produces a radial dilating force against the stricture
- It is usually possible to place the balloon directly across the stricture
- When traversing a particularly tight or awkwardly positioned stricture it may be necessary to place a guide wire through it first. If required, fluoroscopic imaging can be used to ensure correct positioning of the guide wire
- The balloon dilator system is passed down the working channel of the scope and the deflated balloon is positioned across the stricture
- A hand-held pump with an attached manometer is used to inflate the balloon with water (or dilute contrast medium if fluoroscopy is being used). The pressure measured in the balloon is proportional to the degree of distention and so the dilatation can be performed in controlled incremental stages of 30–60s duration
- Short anastomotic strictures may be dilated to 15–18mm at the first session. Other types of stricture may require a staged treatment over a period of weeks with dilatation to 10–12mm at the first session then repeat sessions to dilate the stricture further up to 18–20mm.

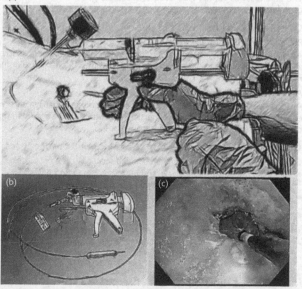

Fig. 2.31 Balloon dilatation. The balloon dilator and syringe are shown in (a) and (b). The balloon being dilated with a stricture is seen in (c).

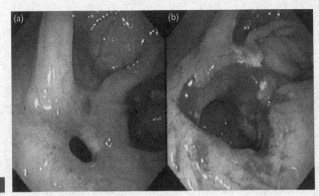

Fig. 2.32 Relatively tight stricture before (a) and after balloon dilatation (b).

Insertion of colonic stents

Colonic stent insertion to palliate malignant obstruction is performed under radiological guidance. Colonoscopy may be used as an adjunct to the procedure. This has the advantage that a radio-opaque marker can be injected into the submucosal layer to mark the distal (and proximal, if possible) extent of the tumour for fluoroscopic imaging during positioning of the stent. The colonoscope can also be used to place the guide wire for the stent deployment system through the malignant stricture.

Use of gastrostomy tubes in the colon
PEG tube fixation of sigmoid volvulus
An alternative to surgical resection is to reduce the volvulus endoscopically, then fix the loop in position by 'tacking' it to the abdominal wall using PEG tubes.

Antegrade colonic lavage
Antegrade saline lavage of the colon has been described to manage chronic constipation secondary to colonic inertia. A PEG tube can be placed in the caecum to create a conduit for the lavage fluid.

Complications of colonoscopy and therapeutic procedures
Complications related to bowel preparation and sedation
- All bowel preparations can have complications related to dehydration, fluid and electrolyte imbalance, vomiting and aspiration
- PEG-based preparation appear to have a lesser impact on fluid and electrolyte imbalance although the larger volume may induce more vomiting
- Cardiovascular complications secondary to sedation and the procedure itself should be uncommon and can be minimized further by appropriate risk assessment of patients before the procedure.

Haemorrhage

- The incidence following snare polypectomy should be <1%
- The reported incidence following EMR ranges from 0.5 to 6.0%
- Primary haemorrhage at the time of polypectomy can usually be treated by application of endoscopic clips (Fig. 2.28)
- Secondary haemorrhage can occur up to 14 days after the procedure
  - It usually settles but patients should be admitted for observation
  - Any coagulopathy should be corrected and transfusion performed as necessary
  - If the bleeding fails to settle, repeat colonoscopy or selective arterial catheterization and embolization may be required.

Perforation

Perforation rates vary depending on the procedure. The pathophysiology may vary

- A linear tear at apex of a loop. This probably occurs due to excessive force when 'pushing through' a difficult loop. The sigmoid colon is the most common area. Incidence is 0.1–0.01% for diagnostic colonoscopy
- Immediate perforation at the time of polypectomy. Electrocautery injury results in full-thickness burn/cut. Incidence is 0.1–0.3% after snare polypectomy and up to 5% with EMR
- Delayed perforation (usually 1–4 days) after polypectomy. Probably occurs as a result of rupture of a full-thickness heat injury to bowel adjacent to a polypectomy site (see 'polypectomy syndrome' below)
- Rupture/tear of colon due to barotrauma. Typically occurs in the caecum. May be submucosal only. Increased risk of perforation if the patient has a stiff colon e.g. collagenous colitis
- Perforation during dilatation of an anastomosis or colonic stricture. Incidence is up to 10%
- If a small perforation is recognized at time of colonoscopy, multiple clips may be applied to seal a small defect. Subsequently, the patient is managed with IV fluids, analgesia, and broad-spectrum antibiotics
- If the polypectomy has involved a relatively large base or the patient's condition is deteriorating, surgical intervention is necessary.

'Polypectomy syndrome'

During polypectomy or EMR/ESD there may be a full-thickness thermal injury to the bowel wall without a perforation. The patient usually develops mild pyrexia and has evidence of localized tenderness/peritonism. There is no radiological evidence of free gas. These patients may be managed conservatively as described above and often settle over a period of a few days. Close observation is, however, required to ensure that the patient does not go on to develop a free perforation requiring surgical intervention.

Reference

Horiuchi A, Tanaka N. (2014) Improving quality measures in colonoscopy and its therapeutic intervention. *World J Gastroenterol*. **20**(36):13027–34. doi:10.3748/wjg.v20.i36.13027

Endoanal and endorectal ultrasound

Endoanal (EAUS) and endorectal ultrasound (ERUS) enable visualization of anorectal structure using a transducer that emits sound at a frequency of 3–10MHz. Changing the frequency also changes the focal length and thus the depth of view. Transducers may produce images with a field of view ranging from 120 to 360°. Direct contact between the transducer and the anal canal is possible when assessing the anal canal. A fluid-filled balloon encompassing the transducer is usually necessary when visualizing the rectum. Although intrinsically a 2D imaging modality, 3D reconstruction is available with newer machines.

EAUS is most widely used to assess anal sphincter morphology in faecal incontinence and in the assessment of anorectal sepsis and fistulae, whereas ERUS is used to assess depth of invasion in rectal cancers.

Faecal incontinence

- EAUS is a simple and safe procedure which is performed without sedation on an outpatient basis
- The IAS and EAS can be clearly delineated (Fig. 2.33)
- The anal canal can be divided into three sections: the proximal canal which contains the puborectalis, the middle section where the IAS is thickest, and the distal canal. Sphincter defects within the distal canal are of particular relevance regarding faecal incontinence (Fig. 2.34)
- Asymptomatic naturally occurring anterior midcanal EAS defects in females can lead to difficulties in interpretation
- EAUS is of limited value in the investigation of neuropathic faecal incontinence
- Although EAUS and ERUS are a subjective assessment, in experienced hands there is good interobserver and intraobserver agreement.

Rectal tumours

- ERUS can have an important role in staging rectal cancer (Figs 2.35–2.37)
- It has an accuracy of 60–95% in evaluating T stage and 60–80% when assessing node involvement
- It is particularly effective when assessing early tumours and can help differentiate between T0 and early T1 lesions
- Although it can usually accurately identify advanced T3 disease, it is not as accurate as MRI when assessing the likelihood of obtaining a positive resection margin
- Errors in interpretation occur, especially between deep T2 and early T3 lesions
- Errors in staging may also occur due to failure to pass the transducer through a stenotic tumour and scarring after previous partial excision or chemoradiotherapy.

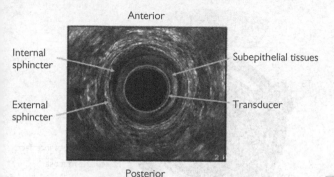

Fig. 2.33 An endoanal ultrasound scan showing an intact sphincter.

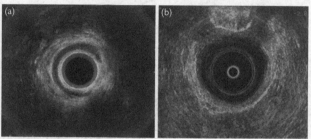

Fig. 2.34 Sphincter defects. Endoanal ultrasound scans of different patients showing a defect in the internal anal sphincter (post-lateral internal sphincterotomy) (a) and a defect in the anterior external anal sphincter (b). The edges of this defect are highlighted by placing a finger in the vagina during scanning.

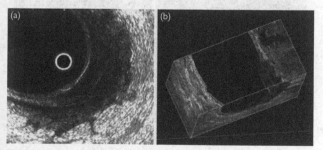

Fig. 2.35 2D (a) and 3D (b) endorectal scans of a T3 cancer of the rectum.

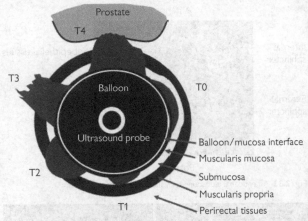

Fig. 2.36 Schematic representation of ERUS and the stages of rectal cancer.

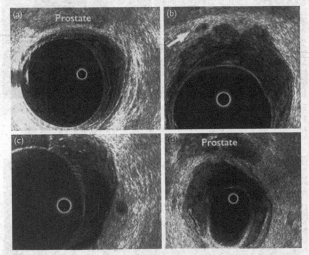

Fig. 2.37 Endorectal ultrasound in patients with rectal cancer. A T2 lesion is seen in (a) with an intact fascia of Denonvilliers. A satellite lesion is marked with an arrow in (b). A T2N1 cancer noted in (c) and a T3/T4 margin threatening cancer with infiltration into Denonvilliers fascia is noted in (d).

Anorectal sepsis

- EAUS may be used as an adjunct to the surgeon during examination under anaesthetic (EUA)
- It may help to identify occult, deep or intersphincteric abscesses (Fig. 2.38)
- Hydrogen peroxide injection into fistula tracts may enhance visualization of smaller fistula tracts and abscess cavities
- EAUS may be used to assess the route and extent that a fistula encompasses the sphincters and can simultaneously assess the sphincter complex prior to sphincterotomy
- EAUS can accurately measure anal wall thickness which can be used to measure disease activity in Crohn's disease.

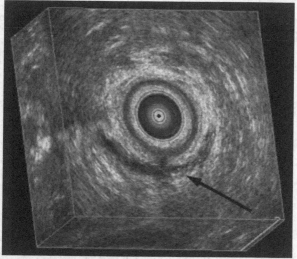

Fig. 2.38 3D US showing a midline posterior fistula with a horseshoe extension (arrow).

Anorectal physiology

The anorectum is responsible for maintaining faecal continence and, when socially appropriate, for defecation. Other factors also play a role in maintaining these functions including stool consistency, mental awareness, and mobility. When assessing individuals with disordered defecation or faecal incontinence, it is essential to take a full history and perform a complete examination.

Thereafter, depending on the complaint, one may perform a number of tests to assess anorectal structure and function. The anorectal physiology laboratory enables an assessment of anorectal pressures, rectal sensation, and compliance, as well as providing an assessment of pudendal nerve function (Fig. 2.39). Complementary investigations include EAUS, defecating proctography, and dynamic MRI.

There is considerable overlap with information that each individual test provides (e.g. anismus or paradoxical contraction of puborectalis may be detected on proctography, manometry, and surface electrode electromyography (EMG) studies). Caution should be exercised when interpreting results of assessments as healthy volunteers can display abnormalities, e.g. anismus, internal intussusception, and sphincter defects.

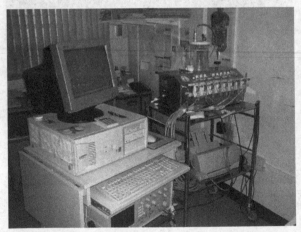

Fig. 2.39 Typical manometry laboratory. Includes a water-perfused manometry system, EMG equipment, and computer for data analysis.

Anorectal manometry
- Performed using a water-perfused or solid-state transducer system
- Pressures are measured simultaneously in the rectum (equates to intraabdominal pressure) and within the anal canal
- Best measured at 1cm intervals from the anal verge (station pull-through technique) and ideally in 4 quadrants
- Pressures at rest, maximum squeeze, and when coughing (Fig. 2.40)

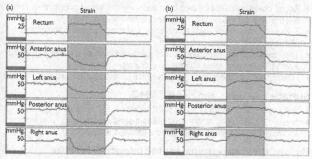

Fig. 2.40 Rectoanal manometry. The top tracing represents rectal pressure. The remaining tracings are from the 4 quadrants within the anal canal. A rise in rectal pressure on strain is followed by a reduction in resting anal pressure i.e. normal (a). With anismus or dyssynergia the resting pressure in the anus rises with strain (b).

- The rectoanal inhibitory reflex is assessed by looking for reduction in resting pressure following rectal distention (Fig. 2.41)
- Values for resting and squeeze vary according to age and equipment, so results should be age- and gender-matched to controls for each lab
- Manometry is used in faecal incontinence, evacuation disorders, and pre-operative sphincter function assessment.

Rectal sensation, compliance, and balloon expulsion tests

- Rectal sensation is assessed by progressively distending a latex balloon which is placed within the rectum
- Balloon volumes are recorded at first perception, first desire to defecate, and when there is an overwhelming desire to defecate
- Impaired rectal sensation may lead to incontinence and preserved rectal sensation improves response to biofeedback therapy

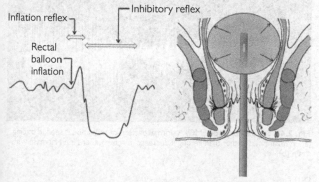

Fig. 2.41 Rectoanal inhibitory reflex. An increase in pressure in the rectum, e.g. inflation of a rectal balloon, leads to a drop in resting anal pressure.

- Rectal compliance is assessed by measuring the rectal pressure–volume relationship using a highly compliant rectal balloon
- Reduced compliance leads to urgency and megarectum is associated with a markedly compliant rectum
- The rectal balloon expulsion test assesses an individual's ability to expel a rectal balloon of fixed volume (e.g. 50ml)
- Failure to expel the balloon may indicate an evacuation disorder.

Surface electrode and needle EMG

- Surface electrode EMG can be used to assess for anismus (Fig. 2.42)
- Needle EMG is now rarely used but is a sensitive measure of enervation and may be used when neurogenic weakness is suspected.

Pudendal nerve terminal motor latency (PNTML)

- PNTML is still performed in some anorectal physiology labs. Prolonged PNTML suggests a neuropathy or injury to the pudendal nerve which innervates the external sphincter
- However, the test has a poor sensitivity and specificity and it is not a good predicator for outcome after surgery.

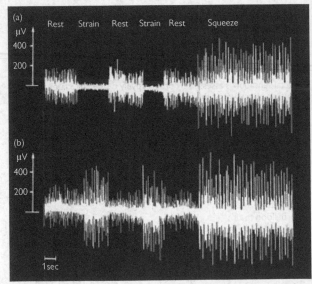

Fig. 2.42 Surface electrode EMG. A normal pattern of relaxation is seen in tracing (a). With anismus, rather than getting a decrease in activity, there is an increase with strain (b).

Outpatient presentations

The outpatient clinic

The clinic is the first point of contact for many patients with a colorectal service and as such their experience of the consultation is important to their ongoing management.

Consultation strategy

- Make at least a differential diagnosis, if not a definitive one. This will help to organize your thoughts when deciding on the appropriate order and modes of investigation
- Advise the patient of the investigative process and how you expect this might achieve a diagnosis. This should include information regarding the sequence of investigations and any related practical issues, what the patient will experience during the process and the risks and benefits related to each investigation
- If a diagnosis has been reached this should be explained to the patient in terms they can understand. A patient who has an understanding of their diagnosis is more likely to comply with treatment
- Treatment options should be discussed including any available alternatives. It may be that you have rejected other treatment modalities for very valid reasons and this also may need explanation
- Information should be given to the primary care physician through the most appropriate method. Usually this will be in the form of a written letter, but often a discussion over the phone about a challenging patient will yield extra information and help to guide the patient's management.

It is important to keep an open mind during the diagnostic process and regularly re-assess the available evidence. Often the initial diagnosis will be incorrect, but what is equally important is to initiate the most appropriate investigation pathway to arrive efficiently at the definitive diagnosis. This is achieved in the majority by listening carefully to the history and taking time to illicit all available signs. There is no substitute for a thorough clinical examination and time spent at this stage will often save valuable time later.

Good communication is one of the cornerstones of medical practice. It is a skill every bit as valuable as the technical aspects of the specialty and, like operative technique, it takes practice to perfect.

Examination

Clinic rooms should be private enough to allow discussion of sensitive subjects without undue embarrassment. Equipment available should include:

- Couch with height and back rest adjustment
- Good light source
- Rigid sigmoidoscope with fibre-optic light source
- Proctoscope with light source adaptor
- Biopsy forceps
- Equipment for banding of haemorrhoids.

Prior to any examination, you should explain what you are about to do to the patient. As a consequence, the patient is more likely to relax and co-operate with the examination.

For anorectal examination the left lateral position is most commonly used in the outpatient clinic, although prone jack-knife can also be utilized if an appropriate examination table is available.

It is recommended that the clinician take the opportunity to sit down when performing an anorectal assessment, having adjusted the examination table to an appropriate height. This will make the patient more relaxed, encourage you to take time with the examination and allows the optimum view as many changes in this region are subtle. Avoid the temptation to rush to spare both your own and the patient's embarrassment.

A chaperone should always be present when performing intimate examinations.

Rectal bleeding

This is a common presentation to the colorectal service and one which worries patients greatly. Patients will associate rectal bleeding either with 'haemorrhoids' or with bowel cancer and will be anxious to seek reassurance that the former is the cause for their symptoms.

The aim of assessment is both to exclude malignancy and to determine the cause of bleeding. Management of acute colonic bleeding is described later (➲ Acute colonic bleeding p.432).

The relevance of patients presenting with GI symptoms and a positive qFIT test is described in an earlier chapter (➲ qFIT for symptomatic patients p.38).

History

A careful history is critical. The patient should be allowed to describe their symptoms in their own words.

Details should include:

- Nature of the blood seen. Is it fresh or dark?
- Is the blood mixed in or streaking the stool (haematochezia) or seen separately (outlet-type bleeding) either on the toilet paper or dripping into the pan?
- The duration, timing and volume of blood
- Is there an associated alteration in bowel habit? Diarrhoea may suggest colitis while either diarrhoea or constipation (and straining) may exacerbate haemorrhoids
- Is there anal pain and what is its association with defecation?
- Is there a swelling, lump or prolapse?
- Is there perianal irritation?
- Are there associated symptoms, e.g. weight loss, anorexia or malaise?

A history of IBD, liver disease and coagulation disorders should be excluded. A drug history should enquire about use of anti-coagulants and NSAIDs and include a brief urological, obstetric and gynaecological history. A personal or family history of CRC or polyps is important.

Examination

The patient should be given time to undress and a cover to maintain their dignity. The first part of the examination should include a search for general signs such as anaemia, jaundice, finger clubbing and lymphadenopathy. The abdomen should be carefully inspected and palpated for the presence of an abdominal mass or organomegaly.

The perineum should be examined in the left lateral position with the buttocks at the edge of the couch (Fig. 2.22). Inspection of the perineum will reveal scars from previous surgery, skin tags, fissures, fistulae, rectal prolapse or haemorrhoids.

The patient should be asked to strain and any evidence of perineal descent noted. During straining, prolapse of haemorrhoids, rectal prolapse, vaginal prolapse or anal polyps may become obvious. A DRE and proctosigmoidoscopy should be performed after careful explanation, looking for haemorrhoids, polyps, strictures, proctitis/colitis and malignancy. Biopsies may be taken when pathology is encountered.

Further investigation

Patient age is one of the most important factors when deciding on further investigation. Differentiation should be made between outlet-type bleeding (blood on the toilet paper, associated with defecation, with no change in bowel habit or alarm symptoms) and more concerning bleeding as the risk of malignancy is quite different (Table 2.1).

Patients under 40 yrs/outlet-type bleeding

If there is a clear history of fresh blood separate from the stool, with associated anal symptoms ± visible pathology at examination, appropriate treatment should be instituted.

In the absence of change in bowel habit, blood/mucus mixed with the stool, abdominal pain, weight loss or anorexia, proctosigmoidoscopy in the clinic may be all that is required. For patients with associated symptoms, flexible sigmoidoscopy is recommended.

Patients over 40yrs/suspicious bleeding

If the patient is >40yrs or where there are associated symptoms of altered bowel habit, further investigation of the colon should be arranged. Those with high risk symptoms should undergo colonoscopy, CT colonography or double contrast barium enema coupled with flexible sigmoidoscopy. The gold standard is colonoscopy. CT colonography has greater sensitivity than barium enema in the detection of small polyps. Choice will depend on local availability and expertise.

Differential diagnosis

- Benign anorectal conditions
  - Anal fissure (➔ Anal fissure p.288)
  - Haemorrhoids (➔ Haemorrhoids p.282)
  - Fistula in ano (➔ Fistula in ano p.296)
  - Rectal prolapse (➔ Rectal prolapse p.270)
- Colorectal malignancy (➔ Colorectal malignancy p.307)
- Proctitis/colitis
  - IBD (➔ Inflammatory bowel disease p.117)
  - Radiation proctitis (➔ Radiation bowel disease p.234)
  - Ischaemic colitis (➔ Mesenteric ischaemia p.230)
  - Infectious colitis (➔ Infectious diarrhoea p.224)
- Diverticular disease (➔ Diverticular disease: background p.214)
- Vascular malformation (➔ Vascular malformations p.242)
- Collagen-vascular disorders (➔ Colitis—other p.236)
- Anorectal ulceration
  - Solitary rectal ulcer syndrome (SRUS) (➔ Solitary rectal ulcer p.280)
  - Trauma (➔ Rectal trauma p.438)
  - Nicorandil (➔ Anal fissure p.288)
  - Anal tumour (➔ Anal cancer p.384)
- Anti-coagulation/coagulation disorders
- Dermatological conditions
- Upper GI source
- Haematuria
- Uterine/vaginal bleeding (➔ Endometrial cancer p.618).

Melaena and occult GI bleeding

Melaena describes black, 'tarry' stool associated with GI bleeding (can be as little as 50ml). The colour change is due to oxidation of iron in Hb as it passes through the GI tract. Melaena is usually due to an upper GI/right colonic source but depends on transit time.

The assessment of melaena will depend on associated haemodynamic compromise which is dependent on the acuteness and volume of the bleed. Initially the history and examination may be a secondary concern to establishing IV access, taking blood for type and cross-matching and commencing resuscitation.

History

- A history of haematemesis indicates an upper GI source
- Associated symptoms of dyspepsia, dysphagia, abdominal pain or change in bowel habit should be explored
- Symptoms of anaemia/blood loss including postural dizziness, syncope, palpitations, shortness of breath
- Constitutional symptoms of anorexia and weight loss
- A past medical history should exclude a history of peptic ulcer, liver disease, coagulopathy/anti-coagulants, NSAIDs, alcohol use/abuse
- Co-existent renal, cardiovascular or respiratory disease may influence management
- Previous GI investigations or surgery may suggest the diagnosis.

Examination

- Abdominal examination for masses organomegaly, previous surgical incisions or aortic aneurysm
- General examination should include signs of liver disease, e.g. palmar erythema, spider naevi, ascites, gynaecomastia, liver flap, etc.
- Examination of the nose and oropharynx should be carried out
- DRE and proctoscopy are essential to exclude an anorectal source.

Investigation

- Bloods include a full blood count (FBC), urea and electrolytes (U&E), coagulation, group and save or a group and crossmatch, iron studies
- Chest x-ray (CXR) and AXR may form part of the initial assessment
- Upper GI endoscopy (UGIE) is the most important initial investigation and may allow therapeutic intervention. Timing should be carefully considered depending on the mode of presentation
- If UGIE is normal, then mesenteric angiography is the most common second-line investigation in acute bleeding (➔ Radiological investigations: large bowel and rectum p.48). Colonoscopy may also be considered depending on availability and experience
- Colonoscopy with ileal intubation is clearly important in the setting of chronic occult bleeding or after acute bleeding has stabilized
- Repeat endoscopy should be considered as pathology is frequently missed on the initial examination particularly if this is in an emergency setting

- Radiolabelled red blood cell (RBC) scan may identify bleeding at a slower rate than angiography (0.1ml/min compared with 0.5ml/min) but localization is less accurate
- Small bowel enteroclysis, wireless capsule enteroscopy, push enteroscopy or double balloon enteroscopy may be required for occult bleeding
- In the acute setting, exploratory laparotomy ± intraoperative endoscopy ± colectomy may still be required.

Differential diagnosis

Upper GI

- Peptic ulcer disease
- Oesophageal/gastric varices
- Oesophagitis/gastritis/duodenitis
- Barrett's oesophagus
- Mallory–Weiss tear
- Portal hypertensive gastropathy
- NSAID-associated ulcers
- Gastric antral vascular ectasia (GAVE)
- Angiodysplasia, e.g. Dieulafoy lesion
- Upper GI neoplasms, e.g. oesophageal, gastric, ampullary, pancreatic.

Small bowel

- Crohn's disease (→ Crohn's disease p.126)
- Radiation enteritis (→ Radiation bowel disease p.234)
- MD (→ Meckel's diverticulum p.416)
- Aortoenteric fistula
- Pancreaticobiliary pathology leading to haemobilia
- Angiodysplasia
- NSAID-associated ulcers
- Small bowel neoplasms, e.g. polyposis, sarcoma, carcinoid, gastrointestinal stromal tumour (GIST), lymphoma, metastasis
- Intussusception.

Large bowel

- Colorectal neoplasms, e.g. polyps, adenocarcinoma (→ Colorectal malignancy p.307)
- Diverticular disease (→ Diverticular disease: background p.214)
- Angiodysplasia (→ Acute colonic bleeding p.432)
- Colitis
  - IBD (→ Inflammatory bowel disease p.117)
  - Ischaemic colitis (→ Mesenteric ischaemia p.230)
  - Infectious (→ Infectious diarrhoea p.224)
- Collagen-vascular disease (→ Colitis—other p.236)
- Iatrogenic, e.g. post-polypectomy, anastomotic line bleeding
- Anorectal conditions (unlikely to cause melaena).

Constipation

Constipation is a less worrying symptom than diarrhoea or increase in bowel frequency and is an increasingly common complaint. It is more common in women than men, particularly in the elderly.

It is important to define what the patient considers normal to be and hence what they mean by constipation:

- Hard stools
- Evacuatory difficulty
- Smaller stools than normal
- Painful evacuation
- Incomplete emptying.

History

- A careful history should detail stool frequency, consistency and duration of symptoms
- Any associated abdominal or anal pain should be noted, along with evidence of rectal bleeding or mucus
- Specific questions may be needed to clarify a history of digitation
- A detailed drug history is important including drug misuse. Specifically use of laxatives, suppositories or enemas should be documented
- A dietary history should be taken
- Numerous extracolonic conditions may contribute to constipation and these should be explored during history taking.

Examination in the clinic should include the abdomen, examination of the perineum, DRE and proctosigmoidoscopy.

Investigation

Blood should be drawn in the clinic to exclude treatable endocrine abnormalities.

- U&E and glucose
- Calcium and phosphate
- Thyroid function tests (TFTs).

In patients <40yrs with no other associated symptoms, further investigation may be unnecessary before commencing a trial of conservative management, e.g. dietary advice, laxatives, reducing constipating medication, treatment of associated medical conditions.

In patients >40yrs and where rectal bleeding is present, colonoscopy, CT colonography or barium enema is required to exclude malignancy.

If luminal pathology is excluded and symptoms are resistant to conservative measures, further investigations, e.g. transit studies, defecating proctography and anorectal manometry should be considered to exclude slow transit constipation and obstructed defecation (⊃ Constipation and slow transit p.250 and ⊃ Obstructed defecation p.274).

Causes of constipation

Dietary

- Poor fibre/fluid intake

Medication

- Anti-depressants
- Anti-cholinergics
- Opiates
- Iron
- Anti-parkinsonian drugs
- Anti-hypertensives (e.g. diuretics, calcium channel blockers)
- Antacids (e.g. aluminium)
- Anti-convulsants
- Bulk laxatives with inadequate hydration.

Colonic

- Colorectal malignancy (➔ Colorectal malignancy p.307)
- Diverticular disease (➔ Diverticular disease: background p.214)
- IBD (➔ Inflammatory bowel disease p.117)
- IBS (➔ Irritable bowel syndrome p.244)
- Hirschsprung's disease (➔ Hirschsprung's disease p.254)
- Megacolon, e.g. Chagas disease
- Collagen-vascular disease (➔ Colitis—other p.236)
- Stricture (➔ Anal stenosis p.292)
- Slow transit constipation (➔ Constipation and slow transit p.250)
- Ogilvie's syndrome (➔ Acute colonic pseudo-obstruction p.426)
- Rectal prolapse/intussusception (➔ Rectal prolapse p.270).

Functional

- Obstructed defecation (➔ Obstructed defecation p.274).

Endocrine, metabolic and connective tissue disorders

- Hypothyroidism
- Hypercalcaemia
- Diabetic autonomic neuropathy
- Hypopituitarism
- Chronic renal failure
- Pregnancy
- Scleroderma
- Amyloidosis.

Neuromuscular disorders

- Cerebrovascular accident
- Parkinson's disease
- Intracranial mass lesion
- Multiple sclerosis
- Cord trauma
- Cauda equina lesion.

Psychological

- Depression
- Anorexia.

Diarrhoea

Diarrhoea describes frequent (>3/day) loose or liquid bowel motions ± an increase in stool weight (>200g/day). Acute diarrhoea is most often due to infectious causes; patients presenting to secondary care usually describe a more chronic history. Chronic diarrhoea (>2–4 weeks) or increased frequency of loose motions is more likely to have a pathological cause than chronic constipation. It is important to define what is normal and what the patient considers to be diarrhoea.

History

- A careful history should be taken, with symptom duration, urgency, frequency and consistency of stool + any associated abdominal pain (intermittent symptoms are suggestive of a functional cause)
- Nocturnal rising or early morning diarrhoea suggests an organic cause
- Bulky stools that are difficult to flush may suggest steatorrhoea and malabsorption
- Direct questioning may be needed to identify incontinence which the patient may confuse with diarrhoea
- Any associated signs of blood or mucus should be detailed and suggest a colonic source
- Changes in appetite and weight should be sought
- The history should include foreign travel, unwell contacts, dietary indiscretion, new drugs and recent antibiotic use or hospitalization
- Details of previous surgery or GI investigations should be clarified
- A family history of GI disorders may be important.

Examination

Examination should exclude signs of sepsis. The abdomen should be examined, assessing for distension, signs of weight loss and any masses. The perineum should be carefully assessed and DRE, proctoscopy and rigid sigmoidoscopy performed.

Investigation

- Bloods including U&E, LFTs, FBC, erythrocyte sedimentation rate (ESR), C-reactive protein (CRP), iron studies, B12, TFTs and anti-tissue transglutaminase (to exclude coeliac disease)
- Stool culture including ova and parasites should be performed to exclude an infective aetiology
- Colonoscopy should be performed with TI biopsies and biopsies to exclude microscopic colitis
- In patients <45yrs with normal initial examinations a trial of treatment for IBS is appropriate
- CT pancreas and faecal elastase if pancreatic insufficiency suspected
- Duodenal biopsy and small bowel enteroclysis to exclude small bowel disease
- In high volume 'secretory-type' diarrhoea inpatient assessment of stool weight and osmolality as well as serum gastrin/VIP, urine hydroxyindoleacetic acid (5-HIAA) and laxative use
- Glucose hydrogen breath test if bacterial overgrowth suspected.

Differential diagnosis

- Infectious (➲ Infectious diarrhoea p.224)
  - Bacterial, e.g. *Campylobacter*, *Escherichia coli*, *Salmonella*, *Shigella*, *Clostridium difficile*
  - Viral, e.g. norovirus, astrovirus, adenovirus, CMV, HSV
  - Parasitic e.g. *Entamoeba histolytica*, *Giardia*, *Schistosomiasis*
- Small bowel
  - IBD (➲ Inflammatory bowel disease p.117)
  - Coeliac disease
  - Radiation bowel disease (➲ Radiation bowel disease p.234)
  - Mesenteric ischaemia (➲ Mesenteric ischaemia p.230)
  - Lymphoma (➲ Colonic lymphoma p.402)
  - Tropical sprue
  - Whipple's disease
  - Intestinal lymphangiectasia
- Malabsorption due to pancreatic insufficiency
  - Chronic pancreatitis
  - Pancreatic cancer
  - Cystic fibrosis
- Colonic neoplasia (➲ Colorectal malignancy p.307)
- Colonic inflammation
  - IBD
  - Collagenous/lymphocytic colitis (➲ Colitis—other p.236)
  - Ischaemic colitis (➲ Mesenteric ischaemia p.230)
  - Diverticular disease (➲ Diverticular disease: background p.214)
  - Radiation proctitis (➲ Radiation bowel disease p.234)
- Functional
  - IBS (➲ Inflammatory bowel disease p.117)
- Post-surgical
  - Ileal resection leading to bile acid malabsorption
  - Gastric or small bowel bypass leading to bacterial overgrowth
  - Post-cholecystectomy
  - Short gut syndrome (➲ Intestinal failure p.264)
  - Colonic resection leading to lack of water reabsorption
  - Fistulae, e.g. ileocolonic
- Endocrine
  - Hyperthyroidism
  - Diabetes e.g. autonomic neuropathy
  - Addison's
  - Neuroendocrine tumour, e.g. VIPoma, gastrinoma, carcinoid (➲ Neuroendocrine tumours p.393)
- Drugs
  - Alcohol
  - Laxative abuse
  - Proton pump inhibitors (PPIs)
- Dietary
  - Lactose intolerance.

Reference

Thomas PD, Forbes A, Green J et al. Guidelines for the investigation of chronic diarrhoea, 2nd edition. *Gut* 2003;**52** (Suppl V):v1–v15.

Anorectal pain

History

- Type, severity duration and periodicity of pain
- Associated bleeding or mucus discharge
- Palpable abnormalities
- Previous anorectal conditions, perianal sepsis, IBS, sexually transmitted diseases, anoreceptive intercourse, diabetes, dermatological conditions and drug history.

Examination

- Inspect the anal verge with gentle traction to separate the buttocks, noting any external fistulous pits or tracts, fissures, herpetic lesions, haemorrhoids or skin tags, perianal haematoma, subtle skin changes or ulceration
- Look for any deformity of the anus. A patulous anus suggests a neuromuscular disorder or receptive intercourse
- Before a DRE is carried out palpate the perianal region for swellings or fluctuance. Tenderness over the ischiorectal fossa may suggest a deep abscess with few other external signs
- Perform a DRE. If this is too painful and an obvious cause is not evident, EUA may be necessary to evaluate the cause further
- Carefully palpate the anal canal (using distal phalanx up to distal interphalangeal (DIP) joint)
  - Palpation may identify swelling and tenderness 2° to an intersphincteric abscess
  - An indurated cord due to a fistulous track can be followed to the internal opening which can be felt like a small grain of rice
  - Assessment can be made of sphincter tone which may be ↑ or ↓. Tenderness on posterior traction may suggest levator ani syndrome
  - Fissures and haemorrhoids may also be diagnosed on gentle palpation
- DRE should include examination of the prostate in men to exclude prostatitis or prostate cancer. In women cervical tenderness should be tested and a vaginal examination performed
- DRE may reveal a rectal tumour or extrarectal mass
- Proctoscopy and rigid sigmoidoscopy should be performed as indicated by findings on inspection and DRE. They are most useful for excluding rectal malignancy or proctitis due to IBD, infection, radiation, etc.
- Asking the patient to bear down on withdrawal of the proctoscope may reveal an occult prolapse
- Further assessment may involve:
  - Pelvic ultrasound to exclude ovarian pathology
  - CT if pelvic malignancy or extrarectal mass is suspected
  - MRI/EAUS for occult sepsis.

Differential diagnosis

- Perianal sepsis (→ Anorectal sepsis p.294)
- Anal fistula (→ Fistula in ano p.296)
- Anal fissure (→ Anal fissure p.288)
- Thrombosed haemorrhoids (→ Haemorrhoids p.282)
- Perianal haematoma (→ Haemorrhoids p.282)
- Rectal prolapse (→ Rectal prolapse p.270)
- Anal/rectal/prostate/gynaecological/presacral tumour (→ Rare anal tumours p.390)
- Pelvic inflammatory process
  - Diverticular abscess (→ Diverticular disease: presentation p.216)
  - Pelvic appendicitis (→ Appendicitis p.412)
  - Endometriosis (→ Endometriosis: introduction p.606)
- Pelvic inflammatory disease (PID)/tubo-ovarian abscess (→ Pelvic inflammatory disease p.610)
- Functional anorectal pain, e.g. levator ani syndrome, proctalgia fugax (→ Chronic anorectal pain p.278)
- Coccygodynia (→ Chronic anorectal pain p.278)
- Degenerative disease of the spine
- Nicorandil-induced perianal ulceration (→ Anal fissure p.288)
- Genital herpes (→ Sexually transmitted infections p.626).

Anorectal mass

The presentation of an anorectal mass requires careful assessment and, although usually due to benign pathology, there are a range of neoplasms which can affect the rectum, anal canal and margin which should be excluded.

History

- Onset, change in size, mode of discovery and pain (painless masses suggest a more suspicious pathology)
- Associated symptoms of bleeding, mucus discharge or pus ± pruritus ani
- Recent change in bowel habit
- Constitutional symptoms including anorexia, weight loss, fever, night sweats
- A full sexual history should be taken
- Previous surgery, particularly anorectal as well as previous GI investigations.

Examination

- Adequate exposure and illumination is vital to perform a thorough examination of the perianal region
- Inspection should determine any skin changes, evidence of discharge, size of the mass and relationship to the anal verge, sphincters and surrounding structures
- Palpation for firmness, fixity, fluctuance, pain and reducibility into the rectum should be followed by DRE, examination of the prostate/vagina and proctosigmoidoscopy as previously described
- An examination of LN groups should be carried out
- Proceed to EUA if examination is not tolerated in the outpatient clinic.

Investigation

- Biopsy of the lesion can be carried out using punch biopsy under LA but may require EUA
- Endorectal US, CT pelvis and MRI may be required for complete assessment depending on likely pathology.

Differential diagnosis

- Haemorrhoids (➲ Haemorrhoids p.282)
- Perianal haematoma (➲ Haemorrhoids p.282)
- Rectal/mucosal prolapse (➲ Rectal prolapse p.270)
- Anal skin tags (➲ Haemorrhoids p.282)
- Perianal abscess (➲ Anorectal sepsis p.294)
- External fistulous opening (➲ Fistula in ano p.296)
- Sentinel tag and anal fissure (➲ Anal fissure p.288)
- Hypertrophied anal papilla

- Condyloma (➔ Sexually transmitted infections p.626)
- Polyps
  - Fibroepithelial
- Adenoma (➔ Colonic polyps p.320)
- Anorectal cancer (➔ Anal cancer p.384)
  - Squamous cell carcinoma (SCC), adenocarcinoma, lymphoma, melanoma, basal cell carcinoma (BCC), verrucous carcinoma, neuroendocrine tumour, GIST, sarcoma
- Retrorectal tumour (➔ Rare anal tumours p.390)
  - Chordoma, bone or soft tissue sarcoma, metastatic carcinoma, teratocarcinoma, neurilemomas
- Congenital abnormalities (➔ Rare anal tumours p.390)
  - Developmental cysts
  - Sacrococcygeal anterior myelomeningocele
- Lipoma
- Sebaceous cyst.

Faecal incontinence

Faecal incontinence (FI) may be defined as the involuntary loss of liquid or stool that is a social or hygiene problem. Anal incontinence is similar but also includes incontinence of flatus.

History

- The type of incontinence should be clearly defined, i.e. flatus, liquid or solid stool, passive and without awareness or urge incontinence
- The timing, nature and degree of patient awareness is also important, e.g. urge incontinence often indicates external sphincter dysfunction whereas passive leakage, especially post-defecation or nocturnal seepage suggests internal sphincter dysfunction
- The frequency of incontinent episodes should be recorded including the effect on lifestyle and whether the patient wears a pad. An incontinence score can then be calculated (Tables 5.1 and 5.2)
- Associated bowel symptoms should be noted including alteration in bowel habit, diarrhoea, abdominal pain, anorectal symptoms
- Assessment should include a full obstetric and surgical history looking for risk factors for incontinence (see below)
- Ask about medications which may affect GI motility including laxative use/abuse
- A dietary history should be taken
- Diabetes and neurological/spinal abnormalities should be excluded.

Examination

- Assess if urge (EAS dysfunction) or passive incontinence (IAS dysfunction) is predominant
- The perineum should be inspected for scars or a patulous anus.
- Assessment should be made of sphincter function with resting (IAS) and squeeze (EAS) pressures documented.
- Ask the patient to bear down to look for rectal/uterine prolapse, intussusception and perineal descent
- Bi-digital examination of the rectum and vagina may be helpful to examine for a rectocele and also the quality of the anal sphincter
- Following DRE, proctosigmoidoscopy should be performed to exclude haemorrhoids, prolapse or other contributory anorectal conditions.

Further investigation

- If the patient's symptoms are troublesome or resistant to conservative measures (e.g. bulking agents, anti-diarrhoeals, pelvic floor physiotherapy and biofeedback) and more invasive interventions are being considered then further investigation may be required
- Anorectal manometry will give information on sphincter pressures, length of the sphincter high pressure zone, perineal descent and rectal compliance/sensitivity
- EAUS can determine muscle thickness as well as any defects
- Pudendal nerve motor latency and defecating proctography may give additional information.

Risk factors

- Female sex
- Obstetric injury
  - Primigravida's (13% have incontinence, odds ratio 9.8)
  - Multigravidas (23% have incontinence, odds ratio 3.4)
  - Forceps delivery (odds ratio 4.8)
  - Vacuum delivery (odds ratio 3.5)
  - Baby's weight >4kg (odds ratio 2.2)
  - Episiotomy
- Increasing age
- Asian race
- Surgical trauma
  - Anal stretch
  - Haemorrhoidectomy
  - Fissure and fistula surgery
- Accidental trauma
- Congenital
- Bowel disorders
  - Colitis, e.g. IBD, diverticulitis, radiation proctitis, etc.
  - IBS (→ Irritable bowel syndrome p.244)
  - Malabsorption
  - Following colonic surgery, e.g. ileorectal anastomosis (IRA), ileal pouch–anal anastomosis (IPAA), segmental resection
  - Rectal prolapse (→ Rectal prolapse p.270)
  - Haemorrhoids (→ Haemorrhoids p.282)
  - Colorectal malignancy (→ Colorectal malignancy p.307)
  - Faecal impaction and constipation
  - Hirschsprung's disease
- Radiation injury
- Neurological disorders
  - Spinal injury
  - Cerebrovascular accident
  - Diabetic neuropathy
  - Spina bifida
  - Cauda equina syndrome
  - Learning difficulties
  - Dementia
  - Parkinson's disease
  - Multiple sclerosis
- Behavioural.

Inflammatory bowel disease

Genetic aspects of IBD

IBD is a multigenic disorder with multiple susceptibility genes, each conferring a small overall susceptibility risk, which interact with environmental stimuli. Compared with other complex diseases, there has been significant recent progress in elucidating the genetic determinants of IBD. It is likely that no single genetic locus confers susceptibility. Multiple separate genetic susceptibility loci have been identified and it is thought that the combined effect of several loci and environmental stimuli are responsible for the development of IBD. Many of these same susceptibility loci have also been implicated in the development of a variety of other autoimmune disorders including ankylosing spondylitis, psoriasis and coeliac disease.

Background evidence

- The importance of genetics in the pathogenesis of IBD was established with data from twin studies and familial association studies
- Familial association studies revealed a much higher incidence of Crohn's disease (CD) and ulcerative colitis (UC) in individuals with a positive family history. This supports the notion that the disease is a polygenic disorder, sharing some, but not all, susceptibility genes
- Twin studies in CD revealed a concordance in 35% of monozygotic twins compared with 7% of dizygotic twins. The concordance is 11% and 3%, respectively, in UC, suggesting that the genetic contribution of CD susceptibility appears to be stronger than that of UC.
- There tends to be familial concordance in CD-related disease location and disease type

Ulcerative colitis

- Abnormalities in the ABCB1, IL10RA, IL10RB, IL23R, IRF5, PTPN2 genes have been implicated in UC
- None of these loci has been consistently shown to be at fault, suggesting that the disorder arises from the combination of multiple genes
- Some of the putative regions encode transporter proteins such as OCTN1 and OCTN2. Other potential regions involve cell scaffolding proteins such as the MAGUK family
- Some human leucocyte antigen (HLA) associations may also be involved. The linkage on chromosome 6 is the most convincing and consistent of the genetic candidates

Crohn's disease

- The disease runs in families and those with a sibling with the disease are 30 times more likely to develop it than the normal population
- Ethnic background is also a risk factor
- Anomalies in the *XBP1* gene on chromosome 22 and related pseudogene on chromosome 5 have been linked to CD. The XP1 protein regulates transcription of genes, important in immune function and the endoplasmic reticulum stress response.
- Mutations in the *ATG16L1*, *IL23R*, *IRGM* and *NOD2* genes, which are involved in immune function, also appear to increase the risk of developing CD.

Recent progress

- It is now believed that >250 genes play a role in IBD, either directly through causation or indirectly via a mediator variable
- Rapid progress has been made as a result of advances in genotyping technology, the HapMap project, international collaboration and genome-wide association studies (GWAS). The latter technique is extremely productive and allows unbiased survey of the entire genome for susceptibility genes.

Key susceptibility genes

IBD1/NOD2 gene

- The nucleotide-binding oligomerization domain-containing IBD1 gene (on chromosome 16) was the first susceptibility gene for CD, identified in 2001
- The IBD1 locus is also called the CARD15 gene or the NOD2 gene
- The NOD2 protein is an intracellular pattern recognition receptor that plays a role in the immune system by recognizing certain bacterial fragments. This response is deficient in mutant form of NOD2, which has led to the hypothesis that reduced ability to clear intracellular pathogens may be central to the development of CD
- Mutations in the IBD1 gene are associated with susceptibility to certain phenotypes of CD location and activity. Specifically, it appears to predispose to ileal disease.

Adaptive immunity (IL23R/1L12B/STAT3/JAK2/TNFSF15/TYK2)

- The IL23R/1L12B/STAT3/JAK2/TNFSF15/TYK2 genes are involved in the adaptive immune response
- The pathway is central to the differentiation of naive T cells, which is associated with both UC and CD
- Ustekinumab, a monoclonal IgG1 antibody with specific activity against IL-12 and IL-23 is used in IBD, thereby targeting the T-helper 1 and T-helper 17 pathways
- Ustekinumab is used as second line therapy in CD

Autophagy pathway (ATG16L1/IRGM/LRRK)

- The ATG16L1, IRGM and LRRK genes regulate the autophagy pathway, which is involved in recycling and removal of intracellular organelles and pathogens/microorganism
- Mutations in these genes lead to problems with the handling of intracellular bacteria and viruses by the innate immune system of the GI tract which has been linked to the development of CD.

IRGM

- IRGM refers to 'immunity-related GTPase family, M', a gene that provides instructions for making a protein that plays an important role in the autophagy
- Autophagy plays a role in the cellular response to intracellular bacteria and viruses
- Changes in the IRGM protein may disrupt the autophagy process, preventing the immune system from destroying harmful bacteria effectively and leading to chronic inflammation within the intestinal wall.

Major histocompatibility complex (MHC)
- It has long been appreciated that specific MHC loci confer increased risk of developing IBD
- Several human leukocyte antigens (HLAs), are especially important
  - HLA-DR2 is associated with UC
  - HLA-A2, HLA-DR1 and DQw5 are associated with an increased risk of extra-intestinal manifestations of CD
  - The importance of other HLA loci appears to differ within ethnic groups and some may show opposite effects in CD and UC.

References

Turpin W, Goethel A, Bedrani L, Croitoru Mdcm K. Determinants of IBD Heritability: Genes, Bugs and More. *Inflamm Bowel Dis* 2018;**24**(6):1133–1148.

The role of infectious agents and environmental factors

The role of infectious agents and environmental factors

IBD is the result of complex interactions between the environment and the host immune system, in a genetically susceptible individual. It is understood to have a large environmental component, as evidenced by the higher number of cases in Western industrialized nations. Numerous key environmental factors have been identified.

It is increasingly recognised that IBD may develop because of an aberrant response to the resident microbiome of the gut. We are only beginning to understand how bacteria, viruses and environmental factors modulate our innate and adaptive immune responses, which in turn are governed by our inherited genome.

Bacteria

The bacterial host luminal flora in the GI tract is central to the pathogenesis of IBD. Supportive evidence comes from the following observations:

- A reduction in the biodiversity of the colonic flora in IBD subjects compared with healthy subjects has been noted, with a reduction in anaerobic bacteria in IBD patients
- Colitis in animal models can be prevented by raising the animal in a sterile environment and can be treated with various antibiotic regimens
- Antibodies to specific microbial antigens can be detected in the serum of those with CD who tend to develop aggressive penetrating disease
- The onset of IBD has been associated with bouts of viral and bacterial gastroenteritis
- The risk of developing IBD appears greatest in the first year after gastroenteritis but may persist for up to 15 years
- Antibiotics can be effective in the treatment of perianal CD
- Enteroinvasive *E. coli* have been shown to colonize the ileal mucosa of those with CD as opposed to healthy subjects
- Treatment with antibiotics has been documented to precipitate flares in IBD and a meta-analysis suggested that antibiotic exposure was associated with an increased risk of developing CD
- Some studies have suggested that *Mycobacterium avium* subsp. *paratuberculosis* plays a role in CD, in part because it causes a very similar disease (Johne's disease) in cattle.

Smoking

- Smoking is the strongest environmental risk factor thus far identified in the development of IBD, although the mechanism remains unclear
- Smoking appears detrimental to CD but protective for UC
- The onset of UC has been linked to the cessation of smoking
- Smokers with UC tend to have a more benign course with fewer flares, less hospitalization, less need for corticosteroids and reduced colectomy rates
- Smokers with CD have more aggressive disease, with penetrating complications, faster and more aggressive post-surgical relapse and higher rates of failure of medical therapy.

Helminths and the hygiene hypothesis

- This hypothesis proposes that the rise in IBD in 'Westernized' countries is due to a healthier lifestyle with a reduction in microbial exposure to the GI tract
- The reduced exposure causes failure of the priming of the mucosal immune system, resulting in loss of tolerance to normal flora
- Widespread use of antibiotics, vaccines, refrigeration of food, water sanitation and reduced parasitic infection have all been implicated in support of this hypothesis
- It has been suggested that certain forms of IBD can be effectively treated by therapeutic use of helminths
- Helminths decrease immune responsiveness and treat colitis in some animal models
- Initial open-label studies in humans have suggested that ingestion of the ova of *Trichuris suis* improved symptoms in patients with CD. Further research is required.

Dietary factors

- High dietary fibre is associated with ↓ risk of CD
- High total fat, animal fat and polyunsaturated fats associated with ↑ incidence of UC and CD

Appendicectomy

Appendicectomy in childhood for appendicitis or mesenteric adenitis has been shown to be associated with a reduction in the risk of subsequent development of both of the main forms of IBD.

Others

- Numerous other factors have been implicated, including, drugs (NSAIDs, antibiotics), sleep deprivation, and emotional stress
- Physical activity may have a protective effect by ↓ risk of CD
- The introduction of hormonal contraception in the USA in the 1960s was linked with a dramatic increase in the incidence rate of CD. However, a causal linkage was never conclusively demonstrated.

References

Zhang YZ, Li YY. Inflammatory bowel disease: pathogenesis. *World J Gastroenterol*. 2014;20(1):91–99.

Epidemiology and pathogenesis

The incidence of UC in North America and Europe is ~10 new cases/year/100,000 population. The mean reported prevalence rate of IBD is ~150/100,000 although prevalence rates as high as 1 in 125 have been reported from recent datasets in Lothian. Onset has been described at all ages; however, the peak incidence is in patients aged 15–25yrs, impacting negatively on growth, schooling, employment potential and overall quality of life.

Prevalence estimates for CD in Northern Europe have ranged from 27 to 48/100,000 with an incidence of 2–8/yr/100,000 population. Scotland has one of the highest world-wide incidences of CD. The condition tends to present initially in the teens and twenties, with another peak incidence in the fifties to seventies, although the disease can occur at any age. Smokers are three times more likely to develop CD.

- IBD affects males and females equally
- IBD appears to have a higher prevalence in those with a more affluent background
- UC and CD are more common in Northern Europe compared with southern regions
- There has been a 4-fold increase in the incidence of CD in the Western world over the last few decades whilst the incidence of UC has remained stable
- Incidence and prevalence of IBD is lower in South America, Asia and Africa compared with Western societies. It is now increasing in incidence, probably secondary to urbanization and improved diagnostic methods
- IBD is more common in people of Jewish descent in all geographical locations
- The incidence in Jewish, Chinese and Asian people resident in the UK and USA is higher than those living in Israel, Hong Kong and India/Pakistan, respectively, suggesting that environmental factors play an important role.

Aetiology

- Both UC and CD are related chronic IBDs which occur in a genetically susceptible host after appropriate environmental stimulation
- Some genetic loci confer risk for both disorders, yet others seem specific to CD or UC. There have been several recent advances in the field of genetics (→ Genetic aspects of IBD p.118)
- Numerous environmental determinants have been identified which are likely to affect susceptibility, phenotype and disease course (→ The role of infectious agents and environmental factors p.122).

Pathogenesis

- Both UC and CD are characterized by a loss of mucosal tolerance so that instead of downregulating the luminal response to antigens, antigen-presenting cells and macrophages secrete a profile of cytokines that leads to a prolonged and excessive mucosal inflammatory response
- This is amplified by recruitment of leucocytes
- In CD, the major response is a T helper 1 (Th 1)-induced cell-mediated response
- In UC, a non-Th1 cytokine response produces a mainly humoral reaction with local release of cytokines, growth factors and reactive oxygen metabolites (Table 4.1).

Table 4.1 Immune and inflammatory response in inflammatory bowel disease

	Ulcerative colitis	Crohn's disease
Humoral immunity		
Association with autoimmune disease	Strong	Weak
Autoantibody production	Common	Rare
Cell-mediated immunity		
Mucosal infiltrate	Non-granulomatous, neutrophils prominent	Granulomatous, T lymphocytes prominent
T-cell reactivity	Normal	Increased
Cytokine profile		
Th response	Non-Th1 (IL-10, IL-4, IL-5, IL-13)	Th1 (IL-2, IFN-γ, IL-12, IL-18, TNF-β)

Reference

Armitage EL, Aldhous MC anderson N, Drummond HE, Riemersma RA, Ghosh S, Satsangi J. Incidence of juvenile-onset Crohn's disease in Scotland: association with northern lattitude and affluence. *Gastroenterology* 2004;**127**:1051–1057.

Jones G, Lyons M, Plevris N et al. IBD prevalence in Lothian, Scotland, derived by capture-recapture methodology Gut 2019;**68**:1953–60

Crohn's disease

Introduction

CD is an inflammatory condition which can occur anywhere in the GI tract, from the mouth to the anus. Crohn et al. described a series of patients in 1932 with 'a disease of the terminal ileum, affecting mainly young adults, characterized by a sub-acute or chronic necrotizing and cicatrizing inflammation'. In 1960, Lockhart-Mummery and Morson were the first to report a case of CD affecting the large intestine.

The pathognomonic feature of the condition is transmural inflammation. Classically there is segmental involvement or 'skip lesions' with normal bowel in between (Table 4.2). It also gives rise to extraintestinal manifestations (EIMs) in ~40% of patients and may affect the liver, eyes, skin and joints (◑ Extraintestinal manifestations p.198). Complications include perforation, stenosis, fistula formation, bleeding and malignant change.

It is important to differentiate between CD and UC. Surgical options appropriate for UC may be contraindicated in CD. No feature is absolutely specific for either condition. The diagnosis is made on history, clinical examination, investigation with endoscopy and radiology, gross operative appearances and histology.

In ~10–15% of cases of colitis, it is not possible to differentiate confidently between CD and UC. Such cases are labelled indeterminate colitis (◑ Indeterminate colitis p.196).

Clinical manifestations relating to disease location

Specific symptoms relate to the site of involvement, but in general patients have abdominal pain and may have diarrhoea and weight loss.

Mouth

- Oral ulceration is present in 6–9% of patients
- Thought to be specific to the disease process and not a sign of general debility
- There may be cobblestoning of the buccal mucosa and aphthous ulceration.

Oesophagus

- Rare, presenting with painful, progressive dysphagia.

Gastroduodenal

- A rare manifestation affecting 1–4% of patients
- Duodenal involvement is more common than gastric disease
- In most cases, ileocolic disease is also present
- May be difficult to distinguish from peptic ulcer disease and erosions caused by NSAIDs.

Gastric disease

- Presents with epigastric pain unrelieved by antacids or PPIs
- Obstructive symptoms are common with weight loss and malnutrition
- Fistulating disease from stomach is very rare
- Surgery for gastric outlet obstruction is the most common indication for surgery and occurs in ~30%
- Gastrojejunostomy for outlet obstruction is usually successful, but reoperation (mostly for other areas of the GI tract) is common.

Table 4.2 Comparison of various factors in Crohn's disease and ulcerative colitis

	Crohn's disease	Ulcerative colitis
Terminal ileum involvement	Commonly	Seldom
Colon involvement	Usually	Always
Rectal involvement	Rectal sparing common	Always
Perianal involvement	Anal disease in up to 40%	Seldom
Disease distribution	Segmental distribution	Confluent disease from the anus
Depth of inflammation	May be transmural, deep into tissues	Mucosa and submucosal involvement only
Ulceration	Fissuring ulceration, associated with cobblestone mucosa	Epithelial ulceration and regeneration
Endoscopy findings	Aphthous ulcers, discreet longitudinal ulcers, deep geographic and serpiginous (snake-like) ulcers, skip areas, strictures, fissures and fistulae	Confluent granular mucosa, developing in continuous ulceration with no skip areas. Rectum is worst affected (unless local steroid/ 5ASA suppositories and enemas have been used to treat)
External appearance of bowel	Fat wrapping of affected bowel	Usually normal
Fibrosis and strictures	Fibrosis and stricture are common	Fibrosis rare. Strictures very rarely
Mucosal histology/ biopsy	Non-caseating granulomas (40%) with multinucleate giant cells, micro abscesses and deep fissured ulcers. Chronic inflammatory infiltrate with lymphoid hyperplasia	Polymorphonuclear infiltration with crypt abscess formation and depletion of goblet cell mucous. Proliferative granulation with pseudopolyp formation
Cytokine response	Th1 (IL-2, IFN-γ, IL-12, IL-18, TNF-β). Vaguely associated with Th2	Non-Th1 (IL-10, IL-4, IL-5, IL-13)
Bile duct involvement	No increase in rate of sclerosing cholangitis	Higher rate
Smoking	Higher risk for smokers	Lower risk for smokers

Duodenal CD
- Involves the 2nd part more that the bulb
- Fistulating disease is common and such patients may get bacterial overgrowth and malabsorption
- Treatment is with steroids, immunosuppressive drugs and PPIs
- Up to 30% will require surgery for pain, bleeding or fistulation
- Surgery for duodenal CD carries a high morbidity.

Small bowel disease
- Small intestine alone is involved in ~30% of patients with CD
- In the majority, the disease is located in the TI
- Presents with weight loss, colicky abdominal pain and altered bowel habit. In active disease there may be anorexia, malaise and diarrhoea
- Associated signs include anaemia and finger clubbing
- Symptoms of subacute obstruction with abdominal pain and bloating after food may indicate stricturing disease (Fig. 4.1)
- ↑ incidence of peptic ulcer disease, gallstones and renal stones in patients with ileal disease
- ↑ incidence of liver disease
- ~65% will ultimately require surgery. The most common indication is obstruction
- Following resection, 25–59% will require a second operation within 10yrs.

Those with isolated jejunal disease tend to have diffuse macroscopic involvement which can be a difficult management problem (Fig. 4.2). The presentation can be one of obstruction, malabsorption or steatorrhoea. Patients may also have anaemia, anorexia, malnutrition, weight loss, diarrhoea and abdominal pain.

Ileocolonic disease
- The ileocaecal region is the most common site of inflammation (~40%)
- Symptoms include diarrhoea, spasmodic abdominal pain and low-grade fever
- Examination may reveal tenderness in the RIF with a mass
- >90% of patients with ileocaecal disease ultimately require resection for internal fistulation, abscess or obstruction. Localized abscesses may obstruct the ureter or fistulate into bladder, sigmoid colon, mesentery or skin
- Those with stenotic disease will present with symptoms of obstruction.

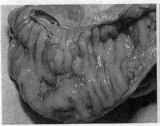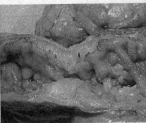

Fig. 4.1 Crohn's disease. Ulceration and stricture formation of the small intestine.

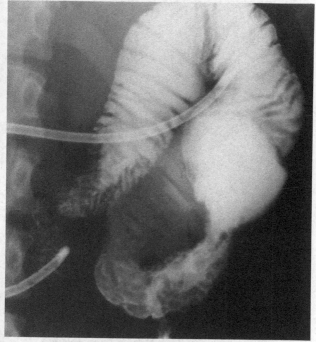

Fig. 4.2 Severe cobblestoning of the jejunal mucosa secondary to Crohn's disease.

Colonic disease

- Most patients will have diarrhoea, abdominal pain and weight loss. The diarrhoea may or may not be bloody
- The disease may be segmental or pan-colonic affecting ~25% of patients (Figs 4.3 and 4.4).
- Perianal disease is more common if the rectum is involved
- ~10% of women with Crohn's colitis will develop a rectovaginal fistula
- Obstruction may occur in fibrostenotic disease and fistulae to and from the colon frequently occur
- ~50% of patients with Crohn's colitis will require surgery, the most common indications being perianal disease and LBO
- Recurrence after colectomy is lower with end ileostomy compared with ileorectal anastomosis
- Mean age of onset is ~30yrs although it is also seen in children
- Elderly patients may develop a segmental colitis which can be difficult to differentiate from complicated diverticular disease.

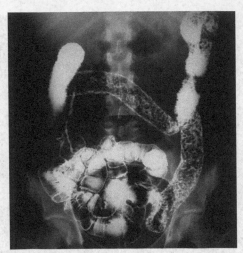

Fig. 4.3 Pan-colonic Crohn's disease. Cobblestoning of the colonic mucosa with loss of haustration.

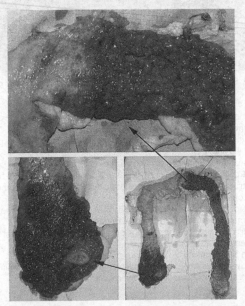

Fig. 4.4 Segmental Crohn's colitis.

Anorectal disease
- Presents with perianal discomfort, itch and irritation
- Abscess formation with fistulae, deep anal fissures and anal/distal rectal stenosis can all occur
- Large 'elephant ear' skin tags with a purple/blue discoloration are not uncommon
- Perianal symptoms may precede the development of intestinal disease by many years
- Isolated perianal or anorectal disease occurs in only 3%.

Systemic symptoms
- CD may give rise to a variety of systemic symptoms
- In children, growth failure is common and may be the main presenting feature
- In adults, weight loss is not uncommon. This may be related to a reduction in food intake due to pain. Patients with active disease are also likely to be hypercatabolic.
- Those with extensive small bowel disease or those who have undergone extensive small bowel resections may have a degree of malabsorption
- Fever is not uncommon in the presence of active disease although a fever >38.5°C should raise suspicion of an abscess or collection.

Other disease sites
In addition to GI and systemic symptoms, CD can affect a number of other systems. Non-deforming reactive polyarticular arthritis is the most common alternative presenting complaint. Others include oral ulceration (with granulomas), cutaneous manifestations including erythema nodosum or pyoderma gangrenosum, cholestatic liver disease, acute pancreatitis or even choledocholithiasis.

EIMs are described in full later (➔ Extraintestinal manifestations p.198).

Pattern of disease

CD usually follows the same pattern of disease which may be categorized by its behaviour into the following groups
- Stricturing disease which may lead to obstruction
- Penetrating disease which presents with fistulae and abscesses
- Inflammatory disease which typically causes thickening and inflammation but not necessarily strictures (Fig. 4.5).

Although patients may have more than one pattern of disease, a single pattern tends to predominate and aggressive disease tends to remain aggressive whereas indolent disease progresses slowly (Table 4.3).

It is important to remember that CD is characterized by exacerbations and remissions and between 10 and 40% of patients with active disease will undergo a spontaneous remission within 6 months. In up to a fifth of patients with indolent disease, remission may be long lasting (>20yrs). In patients with aggressive disease, 30% will relapse within 1yr and 40% will relapse within 2yrs.

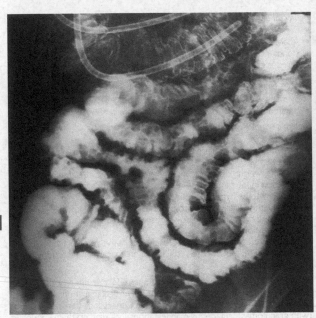

Fig. 4.5 Jejunal Crohn's disease with widespread thickening of circular folds, cobblestone ulceration and pseudoseparation of loops due to mural thickening.

Table 4.3 Comparison of aggressive and indolent disease pattern in Crohn's disease

Characteristic	Aggressive disease	Indolent disease
Disease type	Inflammatory	Fibrostenotic
	Perforating	
Symptom duration before surgery	Short	Long
Surgical indications	Inflammatory mass	Obstruction
	Fistula	Stricture
	Perforation	Refractory to medical therapy
Recurrence rate after surgery	High	Low
Duration of remission	Short	Long
Need for second surgery	High	Low

Post-operative recurrence

- The clinical pattern of post-operative recurrence is similar to the pre-operative disease state, i.e. the natural history is rarely altered by surgery
- Reoperation rate is ~50% for all disease sites and higher still for fistulous and perianal disease
- ~20% develop symptoms and 75% will have endoscopic anastomotic recurrence within 1yr of surgery. The respective figures for 3yrs are 35 and 85%
- Risk factors for early recurrent disease include
  - Extensive resections
  - Multiple anastomoses
  - Inflammatory or aggressive disease
  - Short disease duration before surgery
  - Smoking
- Microscopic disease at the resection margins or age at first resection are not risk factors for disease recurrence.

Quality of life

Issues regarding quality of life and psychology frequently have a significant impact on patients suffering from CD although psychological factors are not felt to play a direct role in the aetiology. Living with a chronic illness can result in lower self-esteem and limit the ability to form healthy relationships and socialize normally. This in turn can lead to depression.

Up to half of children with CD show signs of significant depression and anxiety and psychiatric symptoms may correlate with severity of disease.

Adults with CD lose more time off work although this does not seem to affect the proportion employed or career achievement. The rate of long-term unemployment is higher among sufferers. Stressful events tend to correlate with worsening disease activity and periods of major stress may be associated with a doubling in the risk of suffering from an exacerbation. Complications of CD and reduced sexual intimacy correlate with poorer psychological well-being and greater stress.

Measuring disease activity

Indices for disease activity in CD are numerous and frequently complicated. Inflammatory activity and symptomatology frequently do not correlate and some symptoms, e.g. diarrhoea, may be secondary to previous surgery rather than active disease.

Disease activity indices

The Crohn's Disease Activity Index (CDAI) was developed by Best et al. in 1976. Eight variables are collected over a 7-day period, giving a total CDAI from a negative value to >600. The following variables are recorded:
- Stool frequency, abdominal pain and general well-being
- The presence or absence of arthritis, iritis, skin complications, anal fissure, fistula, fever and an abdominal mass
- Use of anti-diarrhoeals, deviation from standard weight and reduction in haematocrit

One of the major flaws is the subjective nature of scoring for some variables which can heavily influence the final score. The index is heavily biased by stool frequency, which can remain elevated after resection even with quiescent disease. Therefore, a number of alternative indices have been proposed, although none has attained universal acceptance.

In 1980, Harvey and Bradshaw published their index based on 5 of the original 8 parameters (Table 4.4). The Harvey-Bradshaw Index (HBI) correlated well with the original CDAI and has seen widespread use in clinical trials, but also suffers from the weighting given to the number of bowel motions per day.

Faecal calprotectin
- This is a biomarker protein derived from neutrophil granulocytes and is measureable in faeces
- It has a sensitivity of 100% and a negative predictive value of 100%
- It is a good marker of response to treatment
- It has been compared with clinical scoring and correlates well with the CDAI as a marker of mucosal inflammation.

Radiological diagnosis

Plain x-rays
- Play a role in the diagnosis of complications, e.g. obstruction, perforation and toxic megacolon, but do not contribute to diagnosis of CD.

Small bowel investigations
- The barium meal or follow-through is the traditional examination. Small bowel enema may provide better imaging (Fig. 4.6).
- MRI enteroclysis has recently been adopted in many centres as the investigation of choice when assessing small bowel disease. The absence of radiation and the additional information about extraluminal disease make MRI attractive (Fig. 2.6)
- Good quality double contrast barium enema can provide information in chronic disease but is contraindicated in the acute setting
- CT is useful when assessing extraluminal disease. Abscesses, lymphadenopathy and strictures can be well delineated
- Fistulogram may be used to assess the extent and direction of fistulae by direct instillation of water-soluble contrast (Fig. 4.10)
- MRI pelvis is the investigation of choice for assessment of anorectal disease.

Table 4.4 Harvey and Bradshaw Modified Activity Index

General well-being	0–4 (0 very well, 4 terrible)
Abdominal pain	0–3 (0 none, 3 severe)
No. of loose stools per 24h	No. of loose stools on previous day
Abdominal mass	0–3 (none, dubious, definite, tender)
Complications	0–8 (1 each for arthralgia, uveitis, erythema nodosum, aphthous ulcers, pyoderma gangrenosum, anal fissure, new fistula, abscess)

Reproduced with permission from Harvey RF, Bradshaw JM. A simple index of Crohn's disease activity. *The Lancet*;1; 514. Copyright © 1980 Published by Elsevier Ltd. DOI:https://doi.org/10.1016/S0140-6736(80)92767-1

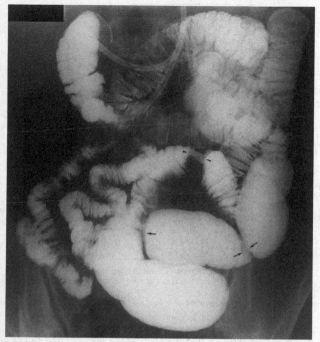

Fig. 4.6 Small bowel enema in Crohn's disease showing at least three strictures and dilated segments.

General radiological features

- Oedema of the deep layers of the bowel leads to a thickened 'hose pipe' appearance (Fig. 4.3)
- Strictures may produce a long narrow segment, the 'string sign of Kantor' appearance
- There is separation of loops of thickened small bowel (Figs 2.6 and 4.5)
- As ulceration progresses, cobblestoning may be visible. If there are deep penetrating ulcers these produce a spike or 'rose thorn' appearance. Deep ulcers may undermine the mucosa, to produce a collar stud appearance (Fig. 4.7)
- Fibrosis produces contraction. As the disease tends to be asymmetric involving the mesenteric border, this can lead to pseudosacculation
- Enteric fistulae may be identified with contrast radiology as either a single or complex track.

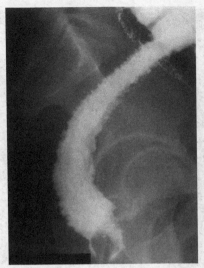

Fig. 4.7 Crohn's disease of the rectum. Severe, diffuse, rose thorn ulceration, marked loss of distensibility and an increase in the pre-sacral space due to oedema.

Endoscopic appearances

- Classically the disease is discontinuous, with skip lesions and rectal sparing in up to 50% of those with colonic involvement
- The mucosal surface is granular or nodular in appearance with friability and contact bleeding
- There may be erosions and aphthous ulceration (Fig. 4.8)
- In severe colonic disease there are deep linear ulcers and a lack of colonic distensibility
- Colonoscopy is contraindicated in the severe acute attack because of the increased risk of perforation.

Laboratory findings

The following abnormalities may be seen:
- ↑ ESR and CRP
- ↓ serum iron
- Microcytic hypochromic anaemia.

In an acute attack, there is a leucocytosis, with raised monocyte and eosinophil counts. There is also a thrombocytosis. Biochemical derangement is rare, but hypoalbuminaemia, hypokalaemia and hypomagnesaemia can been seen. In an attack of fulminant colitis, liver function tests may be deranged with elevated aspartate transaminase (AST) and alkaline phosphatase.

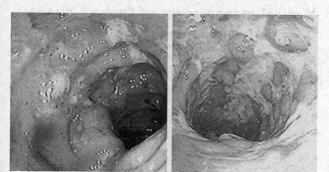

Fig. 4.8 Typical endoscopic appearances of a Crohn's colitis.

References

Crohn BB, Ginzburg L, Oppenheimer GD. Regional ileitis. *JAMA* 1932;**99**:1323–1329.

Lockhart-Mummery HE, Morson BC. Crohn's disease (regional enteritis) of the large intestine and its distinction from ulcerative colitis. *Gut* 1960;**1**:87–105.

Best W, Becktel JM, Singleton JW et al. Development of a Crohn's disease activity index. *Gastroenterology* 1976;**70**:439–444.

Harvey RF, Bradshaw JM. A simple index of Crohn's disease activity. *Lancet* 1980;**1**; 514.

Medical management of Crohn's disease

CD is a significant diagnosis with long-term implications for health, work and relationships. Patients should be principally managed by an interested gastroenterologist with close contacts with a colorectal surgeon. At different times in the natural history of the condition, medical or surgical therapy will be at the forefront of management. MDT review plays an important role when assessing patients with complex problems, fistulating or stricturing disease and multiple radiological investigations.

Low versus moderate/high risk patients

- Clinical decision making may be helped by stratifying patients into low risk or moderate/high risk categories. The following relate to patients in the low risk category
  - No or minimal symptoms
  - Normal or minimal elevation in CRP and faecal calprotectin
  - Limited disease distribution with no or superficial ulceration only
  - No perianal disease
  - No previous intestinal resection
  - No penetrating or stricturing disease
  - No extra-intestinal manifestations of the disease
  - Age > 30 years
  - Non-smoker
- All other patients should be viewed as moderate/higher risk. It also includes patients who are refractory to corticosteroids or who have relapsed after an initial remission with corticosteroids

Review

- Asymptomatic patients should be reviewed 6–12 monthly
- Patients should be encouraged to make contact for early review if symptoms recur
- Assessment of symptoms and physical examination should be coupled with laboratory assessment of indices of disease activity (FBC, U&Es, albumin, CRP and liver function tests (LFTs), faecal calprotectin)
- Specific complications may require prompt review by a surgeon
- Early colonoscopy/imaging may need to be considered if there is concern regarding a relapse.

Non-specific interventions

Replacement therapy

- Patients with chronic diarrhoea are often sodium and water depleted. Total body potassium is also often depleted. Patients with high ileostomy output or chronic diarrhoea may require sodium, chloride and potassium supplementation
- Glucose–electrolyte solutions are helpful in maintaining fluid balance in those with short gut
- Magnesium supplementation may be necessary. Oral magnesium salts may induce diarrhoea so IV supplementation may be needed.

Correction of anaemia
- Chronic blood loss is common, particularly in Crohn's colitis
- Anaemia may be multifactorial, so assessment should include estimations of serum iron, folate and vitamin B12
- Vitamin B12 is absorbed in the distal ileum. Those who have active terminal ileal disease or who have had a distal small bowel resection will require supplementation.

Metabolic complications
- Vitamin D is absorbed in the proximal small bowel. Extensive resection or active disease may impair absorption leading to osteomalacia
- Corticosteroid therapy may suppress calcium absorption
- Resection of >100cm of distal ileum impairs bile salt absorption and may cause steatorrhoea. Supplementation with bile acids is unsatisfactory as the bile acids themselves can cause diarrhoea.

Symptomatic measures
- Anti-diarrhoeal and anti-cholinergic treatments are widely used
- Cholestyramine or other drugs to sequester bile can help in patients who have CD-related diarrhoea
- Patients should be actively supported in efforts to stop smoking
- It may be advisable to avoid NSAIDs.

Nutrition
- Malnutrition is common in CD. This may be due to decreased oral intake, malabsorption from active small bowel disease, nutrient loss through diarrhoea, restrictive diets and anorexia
- In adults, energy deficit presents as weight loss. In children it presents as growth retardation
- Diets should be rich in protein with plenty of energy content to maintain or restore weight. A multivitamin supplement is helpful
- Lactose intolerance is common with small bowel disease. True malabsorption should be documented before removing dairy products
- A low residue diet may be helpful to those with stricturing disease
- Advice should be sought from a dietician with an interest in the management of CD.

Nutritional therapy
Enteral nutrition
- In patients with severe diffuse small bowel disease or multiple resections, it may not be possible to maintain nutritional requirements by diet alone
- Enteral feeding may be used as the entire nutritional intake or as supplementation
- Patients may use fine-bore NG feeding overnight
- Enteral feeds are commonly low in fat and contain the required nutrients in an easily absorbed form
- Feed may induce diarrhoea which can usually be controlled using appropriate anti-diarrhoeal agents
- Exclusive enteral nutrition (EEN) is as effective as corticosteroids in induction of remission and is the favoured induction therapy in children with Crohn's disease.

Parenteral nutrition
- This has a role to play in the support of those with severe diffuse small bowel disease leading to intestinal failure and those with enterocutaneous fistulae
- Patients with severe disease may experience a decrease in symptoms during a course of total parenteral nutrition (TPN) and bowel rest. However, there will be mucosal atrophy with prolonged bowel rest
- Patients with established small bowel failure can be maintained on home TPN. Success requires a motivated patient with excellent education, supported by an experienced and motivated team of nurse specialists, surgeons, gastroenterologists and biochemists (❥ Intestinal failure p.264).

Probiotics & antibiotics
- There has been a great deal of interest in probiotic preparations. Probiotics such as *Lactobacillus* and *Bifidobacterium* appear to exert direct effects on intestinal mucosal function. However, no good data has been produced to suggest that probiotics can induce or maintain remission in CD
- Antibiotics appear to have a modest benefit by inducing remission and improving symptoms in patients with active luminal and perianal CD. The mechanism of action of antibiotics is not clear.
- Antibiotics also have a role in the management of penetrating complications of CD disease such as abscess formation.

Drug therapy
- The aim of drug therapy is to induce and maintain remission, in order to improve the quality of life of patients and, if possible, avoid hospitalization and surgery for complications
- A **step-up approach** (i.e. starting with less powerful drugs that have fewer side-effects and working up to more powerful drugs if required) is usually adopted for low-risk patients. Initial therapy might include a six week course of EEN or a short course of systemic corticosteroids.
  - In event of a clinical remission with corticosteroid therapy, maintenance therapy with a thiopurine should be considered
- **A top-down approach** is increasingly used as initial therapy for moderate/high risk CD patients i.e. start with more powerful biologic or immunomodulator therapy. The aim is to quickly control disease activity with a view to altering the natural history of the disease
- Consider biologic monotherapy in moderate/severely active uncomplicated CD (no fistulation). Options include
  - Ustekinumab
  - Vedolizumab
  - Anti-TNF (infliximab (IFX) or adalimumab) +/- thiopurine
- Combination therapy (anti-TNF & thiopurine) is often considered in moderate/severely active fistulating CD. Combination therapy may also reduce immunogenicity against the biologic, thereby reducing risk of developing anti-drug-antibodies (ADAs) (see below)

- Indications for second line therapy include
  - Relapse after initial response (check peak and trough anti-TNF drug levels and ADAs). Dose escalation or adding in a thiopurine may overcome low level ADAs
  - Non-responders
  - Side-effects from first line therapy
- Second line therapy will usually be a different class of biologic e.g. . ustekinumab or vedolizumab if an anti-TNF drug was initially used. A thiopurine or other immunosuppressive may be added if biologic monotherapy was initially used for induction of remission
- Previously, both biologics and thiopurines were continued in combination as maintenance therapy in the long-term. However, increasing anxiety about risk of lymphoma with long-term use of thiopurine drugs has resulted in a shift to try and discontinue after 1-2 years.
- See ➲ Drug therapy in IBD p.180 for a more detailed description of the drugs used in the management of CD.

Mesalazine

- Mesalazine and 5-amino-salicylic acid (5-ASA) drugs have little if any effect on the disease course of CD
- They are, however, frequently used, especially in the light of evidence that regular use may reduce the incidence of CRC in those with Crohn's colitis. However, there is no good evidence that 5-ASA drugs reduce relapse rates when used as maintenance therapy in low-risk patients with colitis
- They can be used in enema or suppository form for distal Crohn's proctocolitis.

Corticosteroids

- Systemic steroids are effective in inducing remission in CD but do nothing to alter the natural history of the disease process and have a host of significant side effects
- Budesonide is an effective alternative. It has a high first-pass metabolism in the liver, thereby reducing its systemic steroid profile
- Budesonide is effective for ileitis and right-sided colonic CD (9mg/day)
- Topical steroids are useful for distal Crohn's proctocolitis.

Thiopurines

- Azathioprine and 6-mercaptopurine (6-MP) are immunosuppressant drugs that are effective in 2/3 of patients with CD
- They have a disease-altering and steroid-sparing effect
- Drug intolerance is not uncommon and more serious although rarer side effects also occur (➲ Drug therapy in IBD p.180)
- Regular and careful monitoring is required
- 3-5-fold increased risk of lymphoma with prolonged use

Methotrexate
- Randomized controlled trials (RCTs) support its use as an effective steroid- sparing immunosuppressant in the management of CD
- It is given as a 25mg intramuscular (IM) injection on a weekly basis. Oral folic acid is given on alternate days to reduce systemic side effects
- Close monitoring is required and the most serious side effects include myelosuppression, hepatotoxicity and pneumonitis
- There is a theoretical advantage to methotrexate compared to a thiopurine in patients with CD-related arthropathy.

Infliximab (IFX)
- The first licensed biological for the treatment of CD. Licensed for refractory, steroid-dependent and fistulating perianal disease
- Given as an IV infusion. It can induce immunogenicity which may manifest as an anaphylactic reaction, delayed type hypersensitivity reaction and loss of response to the drug, which is frequently due to the development of antibodies.
- Low-level anti-TNF antibodies may be overcome by dose escalation or adding in an immunomodulator such as a thiopurine. As a consequence, rather than considering monotherapy with IFX, many gastroenterologists now consider starting with dual therapy of IFX and a thiopurine to reduce risk of developing anti-IFX antibodies
- Other well described side effects include sepsis, reactivation of tuberculosis (TB) and onset of demyelinating disorders.
- Use is associated with an increased risk of lymphoma

Adalimumab
- This is a fully human anti-tumour necrosis factor (TNF) antibody
- It is administered by a subcutaneous (SC) injection every 2 weeks
- It is less immunogenic and SC administration allows patient self-administration outside the hospital setting
- Data suggest it is as effective as infliximab.

Vedolizumab
- This is a humanized monoclonal antibody which is active against $\alpha 4\beta 7$ integrin
- Used in moderate/severely active CD, where patients have failed treatment with immunomodulators and/or an anti-TNF
- 50% – 60% clinical response rate and clinical remission in 25-35%
- 35% – 55% will lose response during maintenance therapy

Ustekinumab
- A monoclonal IgG1 antibody with activity against IL-12 and IL-23.
- Used in moderate/severely active CD, where patients have failed treatment with immunomodulators and or an anti-TNF
- Generally well tolerated
- Initial response rates ~85%; induction of remission in ~1/3 and loss of response during maintenance therapy in ~1/3
- May be used as monotherapy in patients who are biologic naïve and in combination with an immunomodulator in patients who have relapsed/failed previous biologic therapy

Site specific therapy

Terminal ileum/right colon disease

- Budesonide is widely recommended as first line therapy in low risk ileocolonic disease. Maximum duration should be 8-12 weeks, then stop. If not possible to taper/stop, consider a thiopurine or biologic.
- Prednisolone is also effective but associated with side-effects
- Although 5-ASA drugs are used, there is some evidence that they are not as good as budesonide at inducing remission
- Randomised clinical trial data suggests that a limited resection of TI/caecum is equivalent to medical therapy for CD limited to this area.

Pancolitis/left colon disease

- Low risk patients should be treated with a tapering course of prednisolone
- 5-ASAs and sulphasalazine have also been used and although better than placebo, they are not as effective as steroids in inducing remission

References

Gomollón F, Dignass A, Anneseon V et al on behalf of ECCO. 3rd European Evidence-based Consensus on the Diagnosis and Management of Crohn's Disease 2016: Part 1: Diagnosis and Medical Management, J Crohn's & Colitis 2016; **11**: 3–25

Martins R, Carmona C, George B, Epstein J. Management of Crohn's disease: summary of updated NICE guidance BMJ 2019; 367 :l5940

Crohn's complications

Acute complications

Acute complications requiring surgery occur in 710–20% of patients with CD.

Perforation
- Usually occurs in patients with known long-standing CD
- Presents with peritonism ± signs of sepsis and hypovolaemia
- Perforation due to transmural ulceration most commonly occurs in a strictured TI. Jejunum and sigmoid are less common sites (Fig. 4.9)
- An abscess complicating a Crohn's mass may also give rise to a free perforation producing a similar picture
- Patients should be resuscitated with IV fluids and antibiotics administered. If possible, they should be seen by a stoma therapist and marked for an ileostomy before proceeding to laparotomy.

Operative management
- The safest policy is to resect the obstructed/perforated segment
- It can be difficult to decide on whether to perform a primary anastomosis: if colon is involved, a stoma is advisable
- If there is a small bowel perforation but with significant contamination and/or significant co-morbidity (malnutrition, steroids, multiorgan failure), formation of a stoma and mucous fistula is appropriate
- In a young person with an early presentation, minimal contamination and no sepsis, an anastomosis may be acceptable.

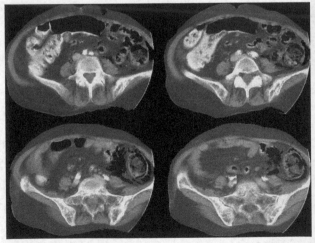

Fig. 4.9 Retroperitoneal perforation of sigmoid colon secondary to Crohn's disease.

Exsanguinating haemorrhage
- Profound persistent or recurrent blood loss from ileal disease is rare
- Presentation is with significant hypovolaemia and rectal bleeding
- More common causes of acute GI blood loss, particularly an upper GI source in those taking steroids, must be excluded
- Bleeding is usually from a small ulcer on the mesenteric border of the small bowel
- Rarely bleeding arises from linear ulceration in the colon
- Management of acute GI haemorrhage is discussed later (➔ Acute colonic bleeding p.432).

Ruptured abscess
- Presents with sudden onset abdominal pain, signs of sepsis and peritonitis
- The diagnosis of CD is usually well established and the patient may have experienced an increase in symptoms prior to presentation
- Pneumoperitoneum is not always present and a mass may be present on CT
- Most abscesses originate within complex terminal ileal disease, although the descending and sigmoid colon may also be involved
- The abscess may be part of an inflammatory mass, often with an enteroenteric fistula and transmural inflammation
- If the patient requires laparotomy then resection of the source segment is required. Drainage and washout alone are not appropriate
- Primary anastomosis is not recommended and a stoma and mucus fistula should be created.

Intestinal fistula
The development of an enterocutaneous fistula is not an indication for emergency surgery, unless it is to manage and drain intra-abdominal sepsis. Fistulae in CD tend to be either spontaneous or post-operative.

Spontaneous fistulae
- Usually originate in a segment of active disease adherent to the abdominal wall, often under scars from previous surgery (Fig. 4.10)
- May be associated with an abscess
- Tend to be due to small bowel rather than colonic disease and are often associated with a degree of distal obstruction (Fig. 4.11)
- Should be aggressively managed by an experienced gastroenterologist, who will consider immunomodulation with azathioprine and an anti-TNF drug
- The ACCENT-II trial showed that 36% of patients had complete response to IFX at 12 months compared with placebo
- If medical management is unsuccessful then elective surgery and resection is indicated.

Post-operative fistulae
- Rarely due to residual disease and should be managed as any other post-operative small bowel fistula including
  - Resuscitation and control of fistula output with skin protection
  - Drainage of intra-abdominal sepsis either radiologically or at laparotomy with a defunctioning stoma if possible
  - Nutritional support
  - Definition of the anatomy, i.e. fistulous track, the origin of the fistula and any mass
  - Planned definitive treatment, if necessary, should be when the patient is optimized and as an elective procedure.

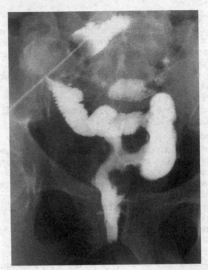

Fig. 4.10 Crohn's fistula from ileum to strictured and ulcerated rectum.

Acute intestinal obstruction

Acute obstruction from active CD is uncommon and other pathologies such as adhesions, volvulus around a band or an internal hernia should be considered. If obstructive symptoms fail to settle promptly, laparotomy may be required to avoid loss of healthy small bowel due to ischaemia/infarction.

Chronic subacute obstructive symptoms with intermittent distension, colicky abdominal pain, intermittent vomiting and weight loss are more common. This may be against a background of known CD or may be the primary presentation. Such patients need careful assessment and should be jointly managed with a gastroenterologist. Many will settle with medical management, but patients who fail to settle or with a history of repeated episodes should be considered for surgery.

Severe acute colitis and toxic megacolon

Discussed in detail in section on ⮕ Severe acute colitis and toxic megacolon p.186.

Growth retardation

Pre-pubertal CD is associated with a high morbidity and longer-term mortality. Many of the typical features seen in adults may not be obvious and diagnosis can be difficult. Weight loss and malnutrition commonly occur without specific abdominal symptoms.

- Growth failure is specific to childhood CD and is present in 35–40%
  - In up to 50% growth failure is permanent
  - Degree of growth failure is related to disease severity and activity

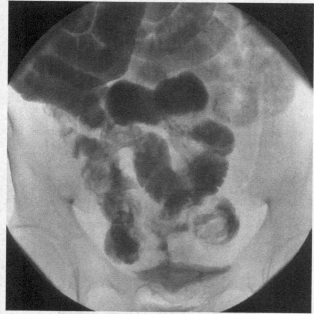

Fig. 4.11 Ileal Crohn's disease with bladder filling with contrast via an enterovesical fistula.

- Thought to be due to lack of dietary energy which may be related to chronic obstructive symptoms with pain and anorexia
- Additional factors include protein loss from chronic active colitis and malabsorption of fats, carbohydrates, vitamins and minerals
- Steroids have a catabolic effect and may exacerbate growth failure
- Careful monitoring of nutritional state is important. The aim of disease management in children is to reduce steroid use to a minimum while keeping the disease fully under control and ensuring optimal nutrition.
- Growth rates can be improved by enteral feeding via a fine-bore NG tube with an elemental diet in suitable patients
- Immunomodulation has an important role in keeping disease activity under control
- Early diagnosis of nutritional failure is vital to prevent growth retardation
  - Children should have height and weight charted at every clinic visit, to identify those who are falling off their growth curve early
  - This allows aggressive management of active disease and nutritional supplementation.

Crohn's disease and the urinary tract

- The urinary tract may be involved at any level as a result of fistulation. Fistulae to bladder (Fig. 4.11), renal pelvis, ureters and urethra have all been described. A rectourethral fistula may produce the classical 'watering can' perineum
- Ureteric obstruction can also occur (Fig. 4.12)
  - Extensive Crohn's may induce retroperitoneal fibrosis, particularly at the pelvic brim, producing hydroureter and hydronephrosis. The same may be seen after extensive pelvic surgery
  - Symptoms may be minimal although patients frequently suffer from concomitant urinary sepsis
  - Treatment involves resection of any Crohn's mass which should lead to resolution of the obstruction. The presence of hydroureter on pre-operative imaging should alert the surgeon to the need for meticulous dissection. Ureteric stents should be considered.
- Renal and bladder calculi are seen in >5% of individuals with IBD
  - Contributing factors include ↓ urine volume, ↑ crystalloid concentration, pH changes, recurrent/chronic urinary tract sepsis and ↑ absorption of oxalate in ileal disease withs 2° hyperoxaluria
  - Sufficient oral intake of water should be encouraged to keep urine adequately dilute without compromising stoma output
  - It may be necessary to alkalinize the urine and reduce the oral intake of oxalates.

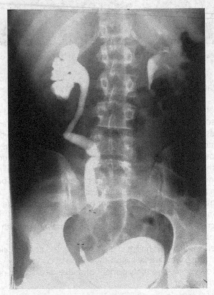

Fig. 4.12 Intravenous pyelogram in a patient with known Crohn's disease who developed a pelvic inflammatory mass associated with right ureteric obstruction.

References

Present DH, Rutgeerts P, Targan S et al. Infliximab for the treatment of fistulas in patients with Crohn's disease. N Engl J Med 1999;**340**:1398–405.

Sands BE anderson FH, Bernstein CN et al. Infliximab maintenance therapy for fistulizing Crohn's disease. N Engl J Med 2004;**350**:876–885.

Sands BE, Blank MA, Patel K, Van Deventer SJ. Long-term treatment of rectovaginal fistulas in Crohn's disease: response to infliximab in the ACCENT II Study. Clin Gastroenterol Hepatol 2004;**2**:912–920.

Principles of surgical management of Crohn's disease

CD is a pan-enteric disease which cannot be cured by surgery. However, 85% of patients will require surgery at some point and of these, 50% will require a further operation within 10 years of the index procedure. An MDT approach is vital to management of these often complex patients. The team should include a surgeon, gastroenterologist, radiologist, pathologist, stoma therapist, microbiologist and nutritional support.

Indications for surgery

Elective surgery is indicated for
- Symptomatic lesions causing pain, weight loss, anorexia and malaise
- Malignancy
- Failure of medical management.

Indications for emergency surgery have previously been discussed ($\ominus$ Crohn's complications p.144) and include
- Perforation
- Obstruction
- Exsanguinating haemorrhage
- Abscess
- Fistula
- Fulminant/toxic colitis.

In patients with complex disease, the longer surgery is delayed, the greater the risk of a more extensive resection with a higher risk of post-operative complications. It is therefore important to consider early surgical intervention once a complication has developed.

The following points should be considered in all patients.
- Surgery is for symptoms, not for radiological abnormalities. If the patient is asymptomatic despite dramatic radiological appearances surgery should be avoided
- The primary aim is to avoid extensive resection
- Destructive procedures around the anal canal should be avoided as this may lead to incontinence
- A stoma may always be necessary and the patient should be prepared appropriately
- Careful pre-operative planning with reference to radiology is important.

Extent of resection

- With small bowel disease the aim is to resect as little as possible
- There is no difference in recurrence rates if there is microscopic disease at the resection margin or not
- Strictureplasty is used for fibrotic strictures to preserve length
- Colonic disease may be best managed by a subtotal colectomy. although segmental resection is possible.

Pre-operative preparation

- If possible, nutrition should be optimized. Albumin may be abnormal in the presence of sepsis, but obvious malnutrition is unacceptable
- Pre-operative prophylactic antibiotics may need to be continued for 48–72h post-operatively in the presence of sepsis
- Deep venous thrombosis (DVT) prophylaxis should be used
- All patients should be seen and counselled by stoma therapist, with sites marked for both ileostomy and colostomy.

Intraoperative considerations

- The patient should be positioned on the table in Lloyd–Davies position. Access to the perineum may be necessary in any Crohn's procedure
- A midline incision is used. This avoids scarring across potential stoma sites and is easier to reopen and close in any subsequent procedure.
- Absorbable suture material is used to avoid potential foci of sepsis
- The small bowel should be freed from duodenojejunal (DJ) flexure to the TI to ensure no strictures have been missed
- The mesentery is often thickened with enlarged rubbery nodes. It should be divided between Kocher toothed clamps and suture ligated. This avoids vessels retracting into a mesentery, producing a mesenteric haematoma.

Elective surgery for small bowel disease

The most common indication for small bowel surgery is obstruction, but enteroenteric or enterocutaneous fistulae also occur.

Resection

- This should be a minimalist resection of the segment causing the complication. Wide resection is inappropriate. Surgery cannot cure the disease and wide resection can lead to short bowel complications in later life
- The presence of granulomas or inflammatory cells at the resection margin has no influence on the risk of recurrence. Even in the presence of complex enteroenteric fistulae large *en bloc* resection should be avoided if at all possible, to avoid sacrificing length of uninvolved bowel
- The best point for resection can be judged by palpating the junction between the mesentery and the small bowel. An indistinct thickened junction suggests fat encroachment and active disease, whereas a clearly defined junction suggests no active disease (Figs 4.13 and 4.14).

Strictureplasty

- Heineke–Mikulicz strictureplasty is the most common type of strictureplasty performed, typically for short (<10cm) strictures. Multiple strictureplasties may be required (Figs 4.15 and 4.17)
- Longer (10–20cm) strictures can be treated with a Finney strictureplasty. However, this type of strictureplasty carries a small risk of bacterial overgrowth and is generally reserved for patients who have undergone multiple previous resections (Figs 4.16 and 4.17)
- A variety of other strictureplasty operations have been described in including the Michelassi side-to-side isoperistaltic strictureplasty and the D'Hoore modification of this operation for use over the ileocaecal valve.

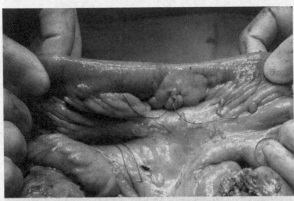

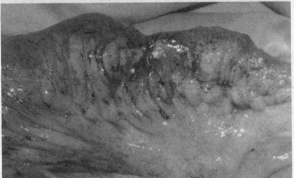

Fig. 4.13 Early and more advanced fat encroachment of the small intestine in Crohn's disease of the small intestine.

By-pass procedures

These are of historical interest only and have no place in modern management of CD. The technique has been abandoned because of metabolic sequelae from the blind loop, the high incidence of recurrent disease and the risk of malignancy developing in the blind loop.

Post-operative complications

- Wound sepsis
- Intra-abdominal sepsis
- Urinary tract infection (UTI)/chest sepsis
- Anastomotic breakdown
- Fistulation.

Pre-operative use of steroids and the intraoperative presence of an abscess are important factors in determining post-operative sepsis. All patients must be encouraged to stop smoking. It is worth noting that 70% will have evidence of recurrence at the anastomosis at 1yr if they are investigated with endoscopy.

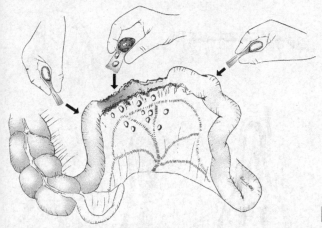

Fig. 4.14 Palpation of the junction between the mesentery and the bowel to look for fat encroachment. An indistinct thickened junction suggests fat encroachment and active disease, whereas a clearly defined junction suggests no active disease which is suitable as a point for resection.

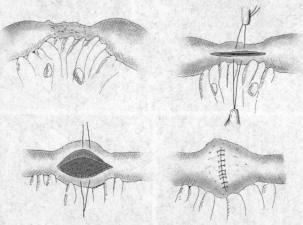

Fig. 4.15 Heineke–Mikulicz strictureplasty. Short strictures (<10cm) are opened longitudinally and closed transversely.

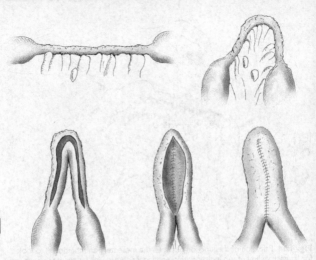

Fig. 4.16 Finney strictureplasty for longer (10–20cm) strictures.

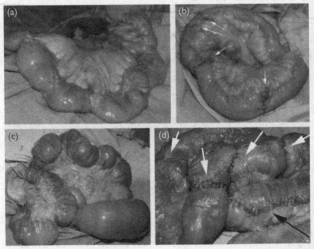

Fig. 4.17 Multiple strictures before (a and c) and following resection (b and d). The white arrows indicate Heineke–Mikulicz strictureplasties and the black arrow a Finney strictureplasty.

Anorectal Crohn's disease

Anorectal Crohn's disease

Isolated perianal disease is the presenting symptom in 10% of patients with CD. Overall, it is seen in up to 30% of patients and is more common in those with concomitant rectal or colonic disease.

The primary manifestations are anal fissures, oedematous (elephant ear) skin tags and cavitating ulceration (Fig. 4.18). This in turn leads to abscesses, strictures and fistulae (anorectal, ano and rectovaginal).

Anorectal disease is one of the more challenging aspects in the treatment of CD. Surgery has an important but limited role in management. Many lesions heal spontaneously. Aggressive intervention in the asymptomatic patient is unwarranted and can lead to more morbidity than CD itself.

Given that perianal CD may appear in isolation or precede intestinal disease by many years, it is important to consider other conditions that may cause similar appearances. The differential diagnosis includes:
- Complex perianal fistula (Fig. 4.19).
- Hidradenitis suppurativa (Fig. 4.20)
  - Involvement at other sites including the groin or axillae is common
  - Careful examination of the anal canal may be helpful
  - In hidradenitis the endoanal skin is preserved
- Anal carcinoma or Paget's disease of the anus
  - Any suspicious areas should be biopsied
- Sexually transmitted diseases, including human immunodeficiency virus (HIV)-related sepsis (Fig. 4.19)

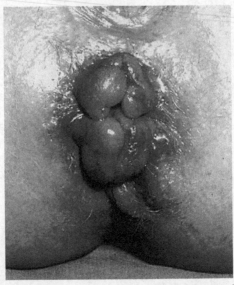

Fig. 4.18 Elephant ear skin tags in Crohn's disease. Commonly mistaken for haemorrhoids.

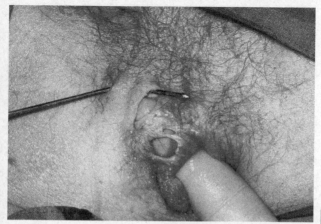

Fig. 4.19 Extensive perianal fistulation secondary to HIV-related sepsis.

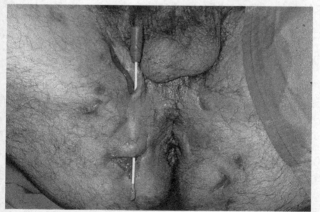

Fig. 4.20 Extensive perianal hidradenitis suppurativa mimicking Crohn's disease.

- Haematological condition, e.g. leukaemia, myeloma and changes seen following cytotoxic therapy
- TB and actinomycosis
- Nicorandil
  - Can cause deep cavitating anal and colonic ulcers (Fig. 4.21)
  - Ulcers usually heal after cessation of therapy
  - Dose reduction does not usually help.

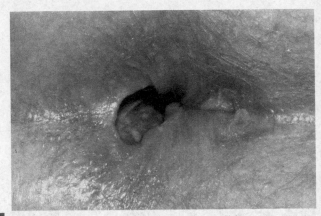

Fig. 4.21 Deep cavitation ulceration secondary to nicorandil therapy.

Natural history

Many patients with significant anal disease are asymptomatic. Many perianal lesions will heal with time or with the effective management of disease elsewhere. Anorectal disease falls into two broad groups:
- Those with a benign course, i.e. skin tags, low fistulae and fissures, which rarely require surgical intervention
- Progressive disease irrespective of medical therapy and disease activity elsewhere, such as deep cavitating ulcers, strictures, high complex fistulae and rectovaginal fistulae.

Management

- Direct examination of the perianal region and DRE is essential to obtain a proper assessment
- Endorectal ultrasound (ERUS), CT and MRI (Fig. 6.9) of the anorectal region may be considered if sepsis or fistulae are suspected
- A full assessment of the proximal GI tract should also be considered before embarking on medical or surgical treatment.

Medical therapy

- Oral metronidazole ± ciproxin can significantly improve perianal disease. Care must be taken to monitor patients on long-term metronidazole because of the possibility of peripheral neuropathy. A reduced dose of 400mg twice a day (bd) may reduce the risk
- Immunosuppression with azathioprine, 6-MP or infliximab may also be beneficial
  - Up to 70% of fistulae and 80% of ulcers and fissures will heal with immunomodulation
  - Continued therapy is necessary and reactivation/reopening of fistulae may occur, especially after cessation of infliximab therapy.

Local surgical procedures

- Any anorectal surgery requires careful patient selection and thorough pre-operative counselling

- Patients should be warned that wounds may not heal and that there could be a significant impact on their continence
- Some patients may need to be counselled regarding a stoma for faecal diversion, to reduce the risk of sepsis. Diversion is not advisable in those with an anal or rectal stricture, as this will deteriorate while diverted.

Treatment of proximal disease

The precise role that active proximal disease plays in fuelling perianal disease is unclear. Most perianal lesions will settle spontaneously. It has been reported that the outcome of perianal disease is determined in large part by the extent and severity of proximal disease. Subsequent studies have reported a similar association, particularly for colonic disease. It is therefore reasonable to consider aggressive treatment of symptomatic proximal disease before embarking on surgical management of symptomatic anorectal disease.

Specific conditions

Skin tags

- These are usually only prominent if there is active intestinal disease
- Typically, they have a bluish discoloration and are frequently misdiagnosed as haemorrhoids
- Present in up to 70% of patients with CD and usually painless, but can cause problems with hygiene
- 25% will resolve completely without treatment. Intestinal disease elsewhere should be aggressively managed. The remainder are usually asymptomatic
- Surgery should be avoided. Wounds may not heal; they may generate sepsis or post-operative scarring may lead to anal stenosis.

Haemorrhoids

- These are uncommon in CD, but may occasionally cause significant symptoms
- Conservative management is the best approach. Topical measures and an attempt at normalization of bowel habit should be the first treatment. If unsuccessful, rubber band ligation may be indicated
- Haemorrhoidectomy should be approached with great caution. Both patient and surgeon should be cognizant of the significant complication rates including the risk of unhealed wounds.

Metastatic Crohn's disease affecting the perineum

The perineum may be affected by so-called 'metastatic' CD. This can give rise to extensive oedema and swelling and ulceration of the perineum, scrotum and vulva (Fig. 4.22). It is important to ensure that there is no direct communication with anorectal fistulae. An MRI scan of pelvis can be helpful in this regard.

Anal fissures

- These are common, often multiple, deep, off midline and often associated with oedematous skin tags
- A high percentage will heal spontaneously, with <20% persisting. However, they may heal by fibrosis, causing stenosis and induration
- If the fissure is painful it must not be assumed that pain is simply due to the fissure. The patient must be carefully examined, under general anaesthetic (GA), to exclude sepsis or a cavitating ulcer

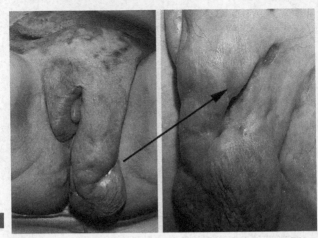

Fig. 4.22 Marked swelling and skin ulceration secondary to Crohn's disease. EUA and MRI scans showed no abscess or connection with internal fistulae.

- If EUA does not reveal sepsis or an ulcer, then chemical sphincterotomy may be helpful. Oral metronidazole may also be helpful
- Destructive procedures such as surgical sphincterotomy have been reported to be successful but should be approached with great caution as they may lead to incontinence.

Ulcers
- These lesions have a poor prognosis
- They tend to be deep and destructive, eroding through the anal canal and into the sphincter complex
- They cause sepsis, complex fistulae, induration and strictures. They are usually painful
- Ulceration can be present in up to 40% of those with anal disease and most have associated proctitis and large bowel involvement
- Many ultimately require proctectomy or proctocolectomy although simple faecal diversion with a loop colostomy may produce symptomatic improvement.

Perianal sepsis
- ~50% of all patients with perianal CD will develop at least one perianal abscess
- Sepsis is almost always associated with an underlying ulcer or fistula
- Prompt early drainage with antibiotic cover is mandatory to prevent further tissue destruction
- On occasion, a mushroom-tipped catheter can be left in place to facilitate extended drainage (Fig. 4.23)
- If a fistula is identified it is better to drain with a Seton as fistulotomy carries additional risks of incontinence in patients with CD

- Long-term metronidazole may have a role but may not be tolerated due to nausea, a metallic taste, neurotoxicity and paraesthesia
- In some patients with persistent or recurring sepsis, faecal diversion may be appropriate.

Low anorectal fistula

- Some surgeons treat uncomplicated low fistulae in a conventional manner by laying open, provided that there is no evidence of rectal disease
- It should be remembered that some of these fistulae will heal spontaneously. Even limited surgery can have significant morbidity, with poor wound healing rates and possible compromise to continence
- It is the author's preference to be conservative, aiming to drain sepsis combined with the liberal use of long-term loose Setons.

High anorectal fistula

- When the fistula is high or more complex, pre-operative imaging with MR should be considered
- A variety of procedures have been described for the management of high anorectal fistulae. These include sphincterotomy, advancement flaps and use of staged cutting or loose Seton drains
- Single or multiple long-term loose Seton drains frequently offer the best compromise by providing symptomatic improvement and maintaining continence (Fig. 4.23)
- Outcome for any local procedure is poor if there is active intestinal disease, with colonic disease carrying a worse prognosis
- Endorectal advancement flaps should be reserved for symptomatic patients with no active rectal disease. Healing rates of up to 87% have been reported when there is no active small bowel disease compared with 25% in the presence of active small bowel disease
- Faecal diversion may be appropriate and patients should be counselled that proctectomy may ultimately be necessary.

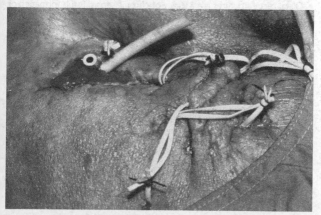

Fig. 4.23 Insertion of a mushroom catheter and multiple Seton drains in extensive perianal fistulae secondary to Crohn's disease.

Rectovaginal fistula

This is an uncommon but potentially devastating complication affecting ~10% of women with anorectal CD. Patients present with passage of flatus or stool from the vagina. Patients require careful assessment of rectovaginal disease, continence and sphincter integrity, as well as assessment of the activity of distant intestinal disease.

Low rectovaginal fistulae
• Begin in infected anal glands. The internal opening is therefore at the dentate line
• May be superficial, trans-sphincteric or supra-sphincteric
• Low rectovaginal fistulae may also originate in a Bartholin's gland abscess
• Can be persistent and difficult to manage, even after faecal diversion.

Mid-vaginal fistulae
• Usually 2° to deep cavitating ulcers or fissuring from severe rectal disease
• Prognosis is generally poor.

High vaginal fistulae
• Usually 2° to rupture of an abscess in the pouch of Douglas which develops as a consequence of active disease in the terminal ileum or sigmoid colon.

Closure rates of up to 45% have been reported with infliximab. Others have found the presence of a rectovaginal fistula as a poor predictor for response to immunomodulator therapy.

Local repair can be attempted in well selected patients. The use of advancement flaps, based in the rectum or the vagina, is well described. Faecal diversion may be necessary to optimize outcome. Despite optimum local therapy, many patients eventually require proctectomy.

Stricturing disease
• Distal rectal strictures are a legacy of chronic sepsis, fistula formation or deep cavitating ulceration
• Present with urgency, incontinence, tenesmus and frequency of defecation
• May be associated with vulval lesions, proctitis, rectovaginal fistula or complex anorectal fistula
• Short annular strictures can be found in the anal canal. These may resolve with repeated dilatation and aggressive management of rectal disease
• Longer more proximal rectal strictures are usually secondary to deep progressive disease and, despite aggressive medical management, frequently require either faecal diversion or proctectomy.

References

Hannaway CD, Hull TL. Current considerations in the management of rectovaginal fistula from Crohn's disease. *Colorectal Dis* 2008;**10**:747–755.

Joo JS, Weiss EG, Nogueras JJ et al. Endorectal advancement flap in perianal Crohn's disease. *Am Surg* 1998;**64**:147–150.

McKee RF, Keenan RA. Perianal Crohn's disease. Is it all bad news? *Dis Colon Rectum* 1996;**39**:136–142.

Ulcerative colitis

UC is one of the two common forms of IBD. It is characterized by a chronic relapsing and remitting inflammation of colonic mucosa, of unknown aetiology. The disease always affects the rectum and extends proximally for a variable distance. It affects the entire colon (pan-colitis) in 20% of patients.

Clinical presentation

The clinical presentation of UC depends on the extent of the disease process. Patients typically present with diarrhoea mixed with blood and mucus, faecal urgency, tenesmus and varying degrees of abdominal pain, from mild discomfort to severe cramps. It is also important to enquire regarding FI which may not be volunteered by the patient and is a sign of significant urgency/inflammation.

UC may be accompanied by systemic upset with fever, tachycardia, weight loss and anorexia. The disease may be associated with a number of EIMs (➲ Extraintestinal manifestations p.198) although the condition cannot be diagnosed with confidence until the onset of intestinal manifestations.

Diagnosis

- A careful history including drug history (e.g. use of antibiotics and NSAIDs), history of foreign travel and ingestion of raw meat or fish
- Bacterial infection must be actively excluded. Stool for culture and sensitivity to exclude *C difficile*, *Salmonella*, *Shigella*, *Campylobacter* and *Yersinia* in all new colitic patients and if there is a flare
- Stool should also be sent for faecal calprotectin
- In moderate and severe colitis, a plain AXR should be performed to exclude dilatation (see below)
- Routine blood tests including FBC, U&Es, LFTs and CRP should be performed. There may be a rise in platelet count and CRP. In severe cases there may be hypoalbuminaemia
- The diagnosis is made on the macro- and microscopic appearances of the colonic mucosa
- Flexible sigmoidoscopy is usually sufficient for diagnosis
- Endoscopy typically shows a loss of vascular pattern, contact haemorrhage, ulceration and luminal mucus and pus
- Histological features include crypt architectural distortion, chronic inflammatory cell infiltrate, cryptitis and goblet cell depletion.

Differential diagnosis

A combination of history and endoscopic examination, histology, blood tests and stool samples is normally sufficient to confirm the diagnosis. Amoebiasis and bacillary dysentery should be considered if there is a history of foreign travel. If there is concern in this regard, a freshly voided stool sample should be sent directly and without delay for microscopic examination. Gonococcal infection and lymphogranuloma venereum proctitis may also closely resemble UC proctitis. CMV infection in patients with AIDS (acquired immunodeficiency syndrome) or other immunodeficiency may give rise to endoscopic appearances that are easily confused with UC. Histology reveals giant cells with intranuclear inclusion bodies.

The differential diagnosis includes
- Crohn's disease (◐ Crohn's disease and Table 4.2 p.126)
- Infectious colitis including pseudomembranous colitis and sexually transmitted disease (◐ Infectious diarrhoea p.224)
- Ischaemic colitis (◐ Mesenteric ischaemia p.230)
- Radiation colitis (◐ Radiation bowel disease p.234).

Complications
- EIMs (◐ Extraintestinal manifestations p.198)
- Colorectal carcinoma (◐ Colorectal cancer p.308)
- Acute severe ulcerative colitis (◐ Severe acute colitis and toxic megacolon p.186).

Assessment of disease severity

It is important to be able to assess disease severity accurately in order to initiate appropriate management which may include the need for hospital admission. Although first published in 1955, modified versions of the Truelove and Witts index continue to be used today (Table 4.5).
- Patients may be stratified into low or high risk for long-term sequelae if they only have the following low risk characteristics
  - Mild or moderate disease (see above)
  - No systemic symptoms
  - Mild/moderate endoscopic disease activity (no deep ulcerations)
  - Normal or mild elevation in EST, CRP or faecal calprotectin
  - No extraintestinal manifestations
  - Diagnosis age > 40 years
  - Normal albumin
- Patients may also progress to the high-risk category if they do not respond to medication, have recurrent flares or develop complications including CMV and *C difficile* infection.

Approximately 15% of patents will develop a severe attack of UC requiring hospital admission and intensive inpatient treatment. Up to 30% of this cohort will require emergency colectomy. Laboratory markers indicating a severe attack include a leucocytosis, hypoalbuminaemia and raised CRP and ESR.

Second-line medical therapies for severe acute UC (ciclosporin and infliximab) have been employed with limited short- and long-term success, in those failing to respond to corticosteroids (◐ Drug therapy in IBD p.180).

Risk scores exist to stratify those patients with a severe acute attack. Mean stool frequency, CRP, albumin and the presence or absence of colonic dilatation on plain AXR are of major prognostic significance in this cohort (◐ Severe acute colitis and toxic megacolon p.186).

Disease assessment prior to treatment
- Many of the investigations performed to obtain a diagnosis may need to be repeated to assess disease extent and disease activity in the event of a relapse (e.g. blood tests and stool for culture and faecal calprotectin. See above)
- Assessment of disease severity and extent are the major factors in determining appropriate therapy for each individual patient.

Table 4.5 A modified version of the Truelove and Witts' index of disease activity in ulcerative colitis

Clinical features	Severity
≤ 4 bowel motions per day	MILD
No systemic upset	
Normal CRP	
Mild crampy abdominal pain with diarrhoea or constipation. Bowel motions make contain blood	
4-6 bowel motions/day	MODERATE
No or minimal systemic toxicity, weight loss or nutritional deficiencies	
Bowel motions usually bloody	
Mild anaemia	
CRP < 30	
Six or more bloody motions daily plus at least one of the following	SEVERE
• Pulse >90bpm	
• Fever >37.5°C	
• Hb <10.5 g/dl	
• ESR >30mm/h or CRP > 30	
• Severe cramps, systemic toxicity, weight loss and or nutritional deficiencies	
10 stools/day	FULMINANT
Continuous bleeding, need for transfusion	
Toxicity	
Abdominal distention or tenderness	
Colonic dilatation on x-ray	

Source: Data from Truelove SC, Witts LJ. Cortisone in ulcerative colitis. Final report on a therapeutic trial. *Br Med J* 1955;ii:1041–1048. Original criteria in *italics*

- There is a positive correlation between severity and extent of disease. Disease extent is also closely related to the risk of complications including cancer
- In general, 'distal disease' refers to proctitis or proctosigmoiditis, with more extensive disease including 'left-sided colitis', 'extensive colitis' (to the hepatic flexure) and 'pan-colitis' (affecting the whole colon)
- Distal disease may extend to involve the proximal colon in ~30% of patients.
- Rigid sigmoidoscopy will confirm disease limited to the rectum
- A full colonoscopy with bowel preparation may be considered in mild/ moderate relapsed disease if it is > 6 months since last assessment. It provides histological confirmation and allows for an accurate assessment of the extent of the disease
- A careful flexible sigmoidoscopy (no preparation) may also be considered in moderate/severely active disease in order to assess disease activity and possibly extent. Ideally, insufflation should be with CO_2 and no attempt should be made to progress beyond the sigmoid colon if there are deep ulcerations
- A CT may also give a reasonable estimation of the extent of disease in the acute setting

References

Truelove SC, Witts LJ. Cortisone in ulcerative colitis. Final report on a therapeutic trial. *Br Med J* 1955;**ii**:1041–1048.

Travis SPL, Farrant JM, Ricketts C et al. Predicting outcome in severe ulcerative colitis. *Gut* 1996;**38**:905–910.

Ho GT, Mowat C, Goddard CJ et al. Predicting the outcome of severe ulcerative colitis: development of a novel risk score to aid early selection of patients for second-line medical therapy or surgery. *Aliment Pharmacol Ther* 2004;**19**:1079–1087.

Management of ulcerative colitis

The goal of therapy is to induce and maintain remission (both clinical and endoscopic), improve quality of life and avoid emergency hospital admission. Although clinical remission is very important for patients, it is increasingly understood that it is also important to aim for complete mucosal healing.

Ideally remission should be achieved with the least toxic medical therapies available. Drugs used to induce and maintain remission overlap, but treatment regimens differ. The mode of action and side effects of drugs used in IBD are discussed in more detail elsewhere (→ Drug therapy in IBD p.180). Care should be discussed at an MDT.

Proctitis, proctosigmoiditis and left-sided colitis
- ~30% of UC patients present with proctitis
- First-line treatment in mild to moderately active proctitis is topical mesalazine suppositories (1 gram daily). If no improvement after 2 weeks, the dose is increased to 1 gram bd for 4 weeks and then reduced again to 1 gram daily
- Patients with mild to moderate disease limited to the rectosigmoid should be treated with mesalazine enemas (1 gram daily). This can also be increased if no response after 2 weeks
- Topical rectal corticosteroids, 5-ASA orally and or oral corticosteroid (budesonide MMX) may be added after 2-4 weeks in low risk patients who do not respond to the above
- Topical rectal mesalazine is preferred for maintenance therapy
- Low-risk patients with mild to moderately active disease extending into left colon should be treated with a combination of a 5-ASA drug, combined with topical rectal mesalazine
- Oral 5-ASAs (e.g. mesalazine, olsalazine or balsalazide) require 4–6 weeks to work. Higher dose therapy is most effective (e.g. mesalamine ≥ 2.4 grams/day in single dose)
- If oral 5-ASA therapy combined with local 5-ASA therapy is ineffective, an oral glucocorticoid can be added e.g. budesonide MMX (9 mg daily for 8 weeks)
- As an alternative, prednisone (40–60mg/day for a week and then tapered by ~5mg/week until it can be stopped) may also be considered but associated with higher risk or adverse effects
- Corticosteroid therapy should take effect within 10–14 days
- Biologic agents may need to be considered with corticosteroid-refractory disease (no improvement with 2 weeks corticosteroids)
- Once remission is induced, plan for maintenance 5-ASA therapy

Pancolitis
- Patients with mild to moderately extensive or pancolitis should be treated with an oral 5-ASA, e.g. mesalazine (≥ 2.4 grams/day) combined with topical rectal mesalazine
- If oral 5-ASA therapy is ineffective, a glucocorticoid can be added e.g. budesonide MMX (9 mg daily for 8 weeks) or oral prednisone (40–60mg/day)
- Once remission is induced, 5-ASA maintenance therapy is used

- Steroid refractory patients with moderately active colitis may be considered for the following
  - Anti-TNF therapy (infliximab, adalimumab, golimumab)
  - Anti-integrin therapy (vedolizumab)
  - Anti-interleukin 12/23 therapy (ustekinumab)
  - JAK kinase inhibition (tofactinib)

Severe/fulminant colitis (⊕ Severe acute colitis and toxic megacolon p.186)
- Patients with severe disease should be hospitalized and started on IV steroids (e.g. hydrocortisone 100mg IV 4 times a day)
- Mesalazine or hydrocortisone enemas daily or bd can be given, although many avoid oral 5-ASA drugs initially until the colitis has started to respond to steroids
- A gastroenterologist and surgeon should be jointly involved in the care of patients with severe colitis
- Antibiotics should only be considered if patient clinically septic or felt at risk of spontaneous colonic perforation
- Patients with toxic megacolon (patients with toxic colitis and transverse colon dilatation >5.5cm) who do not respond to IV hydrocortisone therapy within 72h should be considered for colectomy
- After 3-5 days, non-responders with less severe disease may be considered for salvage therapy with IV ciclosporin or infliximab
- If no improvement following 4-7 days of salvage therapy, colectomy should be considered
- Long-term maintenance therapy should be given to responders. Therapy depends on agent used to induce remission. Drugs used include
  - Anti-TNF with azathioprine/6-MP
  - Anti-TNF monotherapy
  - Azathioprine/6MP monotherapy
- Responders to ciclosporin should be switched to oral ciclosporin for 3–4 months while azathioprine/6-MP therapy is established
- A cholesterol level should be checked in patients taking ciclosporin as low cholesterol may predispose to seizures. In addition, prophylaxis against *Pneumocystis carinii* pneumonia is advised.

Steroid-dependent active ulcerative colitis
- Steroid dependency is defined as the inability to wean systemic steroids below 10 mg prednisolone within 3 months without recurrent active disease or symptomatic relapse of IBD within 3 months of stopping steroids
- Patients should be treated with azathioprine/6-MP, an anti-TNF, vedolizumab or methotrexate.
- Infliximab may be best combined with azathioprine/6-MP
- Second line therapy includes an alternative anti-TNF, vedolizumab or surgery

Additional drug related issues
- Small doses of loperamide may be considered in mild to moderate disease with no systemic toxicity
- Cholestyramine may also be beneficial in mild diarrhoea
- Avoid opiates (risk of megacolon) and NSAIDs
- Heparin has anti-inflammatory effects and reduces the risk of DVT. Its role in acute colitis is unclear

Patient monitoring
- Many patients with IBD are anaemic. If identified, anaemia should be investigated to exclude causes other than iron deficiency
- Patients on 5-ASAs can develop impaired renal function and the eGFR should be monitored
- Patients taking azathioprine and 6-MP require monitoring of the FBC and LFTs
- Faecal calprotectin is useful to monitor disease activity in IBD
- Screening for CRC based on extent/duration of their disease

Surgery
Unlike CD, UC is cured by removal of colon and rectum. Surgery is indicated in the following circumstances
- Exsanguinating haemorrhage or frank perforation
- Carcinoma or dysplasia
- Toxic megacolon or severe colitis not responding to medical therapy
- Disabling symptoms unresponsive to medical therapy
- Side effects limiting medical therapy

Alternative treatments
- Dietary fibre may be helpful
- Lactose intolerance may exacerbate symptoms in some patients
- Some patients with cramping/diarrhoea may benefit from avoiding fruit, caffeine, carbonated drinks, and sorbitol-containing foods
- Some parasites inhibit the intestinal immune response, which facilitates colonization of the gut. It has been postulated that this response might be used to treat IBD. Helminthic therapy using the whipworm *Trichuris suis* has been shown to improve symptoms in UC
- Faecal bacteriotherapy (infusion of human probiotics through faecal enemas) may induce sustained remission in some patients

References
Rubin DT, Ananthakrishnan AN, Siegel CA, Sauer BG, Long MD. ACG Clinical Guideline: Ulcerative Colitis in Adults. *Am J Gastroenterol.* 2019;**114**(3):384.
Lamb CA, Kennedy NA, Raine T, et al. British Society of Gastroenterology consensus guidelines on the management of inflammatory bowel disease in adults. *Gut* 2019;**68**:s1–s106

Surgery for ulcerative colitis

Excision of the colon and rectum cures the intestinal manifestations of UC. Indications for surgery may be divided into elective and emergency (Box 4.1). Approximately 1/3 of patients with UC will come to surgery.

Elective surgery

- In adults, ongoing symptoms despite medical therapy is the most common indication for surgery
- Side effects of therapy or inability to reduce drugs, e.g. steroid therapy, is also an important indication
- Risk of colon cancer with pancolitis is 5% at 10yrs and 20% at 20yrs and the risk of cancer is increased in the presence of dysplasia
- Ileal pouch anal anastomosis (IPAA) or proctocolectomy and end ileostomy are the two most commonly performed operations
- Colectomy and ileorectal anastomosis may rarely be considered in order to avoid a stoma in patients with cirrhosis or ascites or to avoid a reduction in fecundity in women of child-bearing age
- Continent ileostomies (e.g. Kock pouch) have a high failure rate and are not usually considered in primary surgical management.

Emergency surgery

- Patients with toxic colitis are best managed under the combined care of a colorectal surgeon and gastroenterologist (⊃ Severe acute colitis and toxic megacolon p.186)
- Plain AXR, CXR and CT can be helpful in excluding perforation, toxic dilatation or delineating the extent of disease
- Emergency surgery should be considered in acute or fulminant disease if no clinical improvement after 5 days of maximal medical therapy
- A deteriorating clinical picture, localized tenderness or toxic dilatation may precipitate earlier surgery
- Toxic megacolon is characterized by the presence of transverse colon dilatation of >5.5cm in a patient with toxic colitis
- Toxic dilatation has an increased risk of perforation which has a mortality of 30% vs 1% for surgery in non-perforated acute colitis

---

Box 4.1 Indications for surgery in ulcerative colitis

Emergency indications

Acute/fulminant disease not responsive to maximal medical therapy
Colon perforation
Uncontrolled haemorrhage

Elective indications

Ongoing symptomatic disease refractory to medical therapy
Unacceptable side effects or complications with medical therapy
Colonic dysplasia or cancer
Extraintestinal manifestations of the disease
Growth retardation in children

- Colectomy and end ileostomy is the emergency operation of choice
- The rectum is left untouched to facilitate subsequent surgery and to reduce the high morbidity of proctectomy in an emergency setting.

Areas for consideration

Quality of life

- A number of studies have shown that IPAA confers a greater improvement in quality of life compared with proctocolectomy and end ileostomy or Kock pouch. Other than a minor deterioration in continence, this improvement is sustained over time
- Dietary influences on quality of life are significant for patients with an IPAA or end ileostomy.

Fertility and pregnancy

- Women with active colitis have only a minor reduction in fertility which is related to disease activity
- IPAA is associated with a 50% reduction in fecundity, whereas women with UC who do not undergo surgery have similar fertility compared with age-matched controls in the general population
- Up to 1/3 of females who get pregnant after IPAA do so only after *in vitro* fertilization (IVF)
- Consideration should be given to delaying surgery in women of child-bearing age when it is safe to do so
- Pregnancy does not usually present a problem for patients who have undergone IPAA or proctocolectomy and end ileostomy
- One third of patients with an ileal pouch will experience a transient disturbance in bowel function towards the end of the pregnancy
- Vaginal delivery following IPAA appears to be safe but may be associated with a higher incidence of anterior sphincter defects and reduced anal pressures, although this does not necessarily translate into impaired pouch function or incontinence
- For a more detailed discussion of these issues see ➲ Reproduction and IBD p.208.

Age

- Traditionally IPAA was not felt to be appropriate for older patients and most were offered a conventional proctocolectomy and end ileostomy
- Poor continence and nocturnal seepage is more common after IPAA in patients aged >65yrs, but this appears to have a lesser impact on quality of life compared with younger patients
- Increasingly, age alone is no longer considered a valid reason to limit the surgical options for older patients and many in their sixties and occasionally in their seventies cope well with IPAA.

One-stage restorative proctocolectomy

Traditionally, ileal pouches have been defunctioned in order to minimize the clinical impact of an anastomotic leak. A number of surgeons now consider performing the one-stage procedure in selected patients. The following points should be considered.

- Pre-operative steroids are associated with an increased risk of leak after non-diverted IPAA
- The leak rate is as high as 12% with a uniform policy of non-diversion IPAA and as low as 4% with selective non-diversion in low-risk patients (e.g. well nourished and not on steroids/immunosuppressives)
- Single-stage IPAA without diversion is associated with fewer episodes of SBO and reduced need for re-laparotomy
- Overall hospital stay is shorter after a one-stage IPAA although inpatient stay for the primary operation may be longer.

Ileal pouch complications

Ileal pouch complications

IPAA is a safe operation with a low mortality rate (0.5%). It offers improved quality of life compared with end ileostomy; however, it is associated with a morbidity rate of 30%, many of whom will require re-operative surgery. Pelvic sepsis is one of the most serious early complications, occurring in 5–15% of patients. Risk factors include use of immunosuppressive drugs including long-term steroids and poor nutrition. The use of a diverting stoma may be protective.

Pouch failure

- Incidence of pouch failure (the need to remove or defunction the pouch with a permanent stoma) increases with time and rises from 5% at 5yrs to 10% at 10yrs and 15% at 20yrs
- ~25% of failures occur in the first year
- Causes of pouch failure include pelvic sepsis, usually following on from post-operative sepsis (50%), poor pouch function (30%) and pouchitis (10%)
- Long-term steroid use and malnutrition are associated with an increased risk of pelvic sepsis.

Pouch function

- Long-term (25yrs) function after IPAA is stable
- Most patients will have a stool frequency of 4–8 movements/24h, with 50% needing to evacuate at night
- Urgency and daytime faecal leakage occur in <5% of patients and is generally stable over time
- Leakage at night may increase from 4% at 10yrs to 9% at 25yrs
- Anti-diarrhoeals are required by 30% at 10yrs and 45% at 25yrs.

There are a number of causes of poor pouch function and pouch failure (Box 4.2). Patients frequently present with a similar symptom complex. A careful clinical assessment including a review of the primary diagnosis, endoscopic and occasionally radiological evaluation of the pouch may be necessary in order to come to an accurate diagnosis. (Table 4.6)

Pelvic sepsis

Early post-operative sepsis

- Occurs in 5–10% and is responsible for a 5-fold increase in the pouch failure.

Late problems

- Rectovaginal fistula (incidence 5–10% at 10yrs) is usually related to a leak from the anastomosis and can present at any time after surgery. Low fistulae may be treated with perineal/transanal flaps, but high fistulae may require pouch advancement
- Rarely, pelvic sepsis may present years after surgery and treatment by drainage may be effective.

Box 4.2 Complications of IPAA surgery

Early complications (occur in 15–20% of patients)
Small bowel obstruction
Anastomotic or pouch leak
Pelvic sepsis

Late complications
Small bowel obstruction
Anastomotic stricture (may start early on after operation)
Pouch–cutaneous or pouch–vaginal fistula (may follow on from early pelvic sepsis)
Pouch dysfunction (pouchitis, Crohn's disease, irritable pouch syndrome)
Erectile/bladder dysfunction
Reduced fecundity
Pouch failure (need to excise or permanently defunction a pouch with a stoma)

Table 4.6 Features of pouchitis, irritable pouch syndrome and cuffitis

Group	Pouchitis	Irritable pouch syndrome	Cuffitis
Symptoms	Frequency, urgency, cramps, systemic upset, flu-like symptoms	Frequency, urgency and cramps	Frequency, urgency, cramps and bleeding
Endoscopy	Oedema, contact bleeding, ulceration	Normal	Typical UC-like inflammation of the cuff below the anastomosis
Histology	Acute and chronic inflammation with ulceration and villous atrophy	Normal	Ulceration, erythema
Treatment	Metronidazole ± ciprofloxacin for 2 weeks	Manage as for IBS	Topical 5-ASA, hydrocortisone or budesonide

Pouchitis

Pouchitis is a non-specific inflammation of the pouch. It is the most common late complication of IPAA, affecting 20–60% within 5yrs of surgery. 60% develop recurrent attacks and 10% suffer refractory or chronic pouchitis. Risk factors include a history of UC, backwash ileitis, sclerosing cholangitis (doubles the risk), non-smokers and use of NSAIDs.

Presentation
- Symptoms include frequent loose stool, urgency, occasional rectal bleeding, abdominal cramps, malaise, anorexia and low grade fever
- Endoscopic findings consist of oedema, contact bleeding, a granular mucosa and ulceration not related to staple lines and anastomosis

- The diagnosis requires the clinical picture and typical endoscopic and histological findings, as up to 90% of pouch biopsies taken 6 months after surgery will shown some degree of inflammation (Table 4.8)
- Severity may be assessed using the Pouchitis Disease Activity Index (PDAI). A score of 7 is diagnostic
- Pouchitis may be classified into (1) acute antibiotic-responsive, (2) relapsing antibiotic-dependent and (3) chronic antibiotic-refractory.

Aetiology
- The precise aetiology is unclear, although it appears to be related to bacterial overgrowth within the pouch
- Sulphate-reducing anaerobic bacteria are produced exclusively in the pouches of patients with preceding UC. These bacteria produce hydrogen sulfide gas which appears to be toxic to the pouch mucosa
- The proinflammatory cytokine IL-8 is an important mediator of inflammation and expression correlates with the grade of pouchitis.

Management
- Treatment is with antibiotics (metronidazole ± ciproxin)
- Probiotics (e.g. VSL 3® (Ferring Pharmaceuticals Ltd)) inhibit the growth of enteropathic bacteria and can maintain remission in up to 85% of patients
- Other therapies include topical 5-ASAs, topical steroids, budesonide.

Cuffitis
- Similar symptoms to pouchitis. Rectal bleeding is more common
- Endoscopic changes of mucosal inflammation and ulceration limited to the rectal mucosa (below the anastomosis). The pouch is uninvolved
- Treated with topical steroids or mesalazine.

Irritable pouch syndrome
- Presents with increased stool frequency, stool urgency and pain
- The PDAI is <7 so they do not satisfy the criteria for pouchitis
- Such patients are felt to have a form of IBS
- Treatment as for IBS with anti-spasmodics, dietary manipulation, etc.

Crohn's disease
- The overall likelihood of pouch loss for all patients undergoing IPAA is 10–12%. Risk increases to 33% for patients with CD
- In the absence of ileal or perianal disease, pouch failure rate for Crohn's patients is similar to the overall pouch failure rate of 10–12%.

Mechanical causes of poor pouch function
Outflow obstruction
Stricture of the ileoanal anastomosis or a long retained rectal stump may cause mechanical obstruction. Symptoms include difficulty with defecation and frequent small volume stools. Diagnosis is confirmed at EUA and on contrast radiology. Anastomotic strictures may be dilated.

Weak sphincter

A weak anal sphincter may lead to FI. This may have been present at the time of surgery or may be secondary to birth-related injury. Management is difficult and conservative measures such as biofeedback and anti-diarrhoeal drugs form the mainstay of care.

Small volume pouch

A standard J-pouch will be 7400ml. Smaller volume pouches will result in frequent defecation. Diagnosis is made on contrast radiology.

Risk of cancer and need for follow-up after IPAA

A small number of patients may develop dysplasia following IPAA although the risk of developing frank adenocarcinoma is very small. A recent systematic review reported the incidence of pouch-related adenocarcinoma was 0.35%, 20 years after IPAA. A recent large meta-analysis reported that the only definite risk factors were a history of dysplasia or CRC in the preceding colectomy specimen. It is clear that such patients should undergo regular (annual) pouch surveillance.
* Some studies however also have reported ↑ risk of pouch related cancer if there was Co-existing primary sclerosing cholangitis
* Villous atrophy and type C ileal pouch mucosa
* Family history of CRC
* Long retained rectal cuff

Although there is little hard evidence to support regular surveillance in patients who did not have preceding dysplasia or CRC, most guidelines now also include these factors as an indication for regular (annual) surveillance. It may be that 3-5 yearly surveillance is appropriate in asymptomatic patients with an ileal pouch and none of these risk factors.

Ileal pouch carcinoma has also been described after IPAA for familial adenomatous polyposis (FAP). The risk of developing polyps in the pouch at 5, 10 and 15yrs is 7, 35 and 75%, respectively. Between 10 and 30% of patients also develop polyps in the anorectal mucosa below the anastomosis, whether or not they have had a mucosectomy. A mucosal proctectomy halves the risk and should be considered at the time of surgery. Follow-up for FAP should include:
* Annual endoscopic screening of the pouch and anastomosis
* Biopsy of all abnormal areas
* Fulguration of small polyps
* Transanal resection of large polyps.

References

Selvaggi F, Pellino G, Canonico S, et al. Systematic review of cuff and pouch cancer in patients with ileal pelvic pouch for ulcerative colitis. *Inflamm Bowel Dis* 2014;**20**:1296–308s.

Cairns SR, Scholefield JH, Steele RJ et al. Guidelines for colorectal cancer screening and surveillance in moderate and high risk groups (update from 2002). *Gut* 2010;**59**:666-690.

Drug therapy in IBD

Corticosteroids

- Effective for induction of remission in active IBD
- They do not alter the natural history of the disease and have significant side effects
- The aim of systemic steroid treatment is to achieve remission quickly and then maintain the patient on an alternative form of therapy
- For distal colitis, topical steroids can be combined with topical 5-ASAs, as their mechanism of action is different.

Mechanism of action

- Steroids passively diffuse into the cell cytoplasm where they bind with cytoplasmic receptors and move into the nucleus. This produces transcription and translation effects on signal proteins
- This in turn affects the production of interleukins and arachidonic acid metabolites including prostaglandins E2 and F2α
- Capillary integrity is enhanced, leading to reduced fluid efflux and reduced oedema
- They inhibit margination, leading to increased levels of circulating neutrophils and diminished recruitment in the inflammatory response.

Side effects

- Inhibition of adrenal function
- ↑ protein catabolism and ↓ protein synthesis, leading to poor wound healing and growth retardation in children
- ↑ gluconeogenesis with inhibition of glucose transport into cells leading to diabetes
- Induction of hypercholesterolaemia and hypertriglyceridaemia
- Redistribution of body fat leading to moon face and a buffalo hump
- Ocular complications—subcapsular cataract formation and glaucoma
- Osteoporosis occurs in up to 50%. Pathogenesis is multifactorial, related to dose and duration of use.

Route of administration

- IV in an acute attack, e.g. 100mg hydrocortisone qid for 5 days
- Orally in the form of prednisolone for maintenance
- Topical enemas or foams for distal proctocolitis. There may be significant systemic absorption.

Aminosalicylates

- 5-ASA works as a topical anti-inflammatory and has been shown to be twice as effective as placebo for inducing remission in UC. The number needed to treat is ~10 to achieve complete remission compared with 2 for corticosteroids
- Mesalazine products are the mainstay of treatment for maintenance of remission in UC
- There is evolving epidemiological evidence that regular dosing with mesalazine products provide protection against the development of colorectal carcinoma. This may be related to control of inflammation rather than a specific chemo-preventative property of 5-ASA drugs

Mechanism of action

- Sulphasalazine consists of a sulphapyridine linked to 5-ASA via an azo bond which is cleaved in the colon to sulphapyridine and 5-ASA
- The sulphapyridine is absorbed in the colon and acetylated in the liver. 5-ASA, the active moiety, is acetylated by colonic luminal bacteria
- Newer 5-ASA compounds use alternatives to the sulphasalazine moiety which causes most of the side effects
- The precise mechanism of action of 5-ASAs remains unclear
- It is thought there is modulation of arachidonic acid metabolism
- 5-ASA has an inhibitory effect on cyclo-oxygenase (COX) and lipoxygenase pathways and inhibits platelet activation factor.

Side effects

- Tolerability of sulphasalazine therapy is related to a patient's genetically determined acetylation status (slow vs fast)
- 10–45% report nausea, dyspepsia headache and fatigue
- Can lead to male infertility, with 80% of men developing sperm motility changes and changed morphology
- Mesalazine has a good safety record. Renal dysfunction is well described but reversible
- Skin eruptions range from a maculopapular rash to toxic epidermal necrolysis and Stevens–Johnson syndrome
- Haematological toxicity includes agranulocytosis, leucopenia, thrombocytopenia and impaired folate absorption leading to anaemia
- Can cause an exacerbation of colitis symptoms and, if so, should be stopped immediately.

Route of administration

- Most clinicians withhold 5-ASAs in the first few days of managing severe acute colitis
- In mild or moderately active colitis, a combination of prednisolone 40mg daily and mesalazine 800mg three times a day (tid) orally is a common regimen
- 5-ASAs are most commonly used in oral maintenance therapy
- There is no evidence that one 5-ASA product is more effective than another. An available once-daily preparation increases compliance and reduces daily pill burden with no apparent loss of efficacy
- Topical 5-ASA preparations are available for the treatment and maintenance of mild to moderate distal proctocolitis
  - Proctitis can be well controlled using suppositories
  - Liquid/foam enemas can be used to treat sigmoid disease.

Thiopurines

Azathioprine and 6-MP are effective steroid-sparing immunosuppressants which can be used to maintain remission in UC and CD. They are the most common immunomodulators used to treat IBD. Approximately 66% of patients will respond to treatment.

Mechanism of action

- Azathioprine and 6-MP are imidazole purine analogues that have multiple effects on the cascades controlling inflammation
- After oral administration, azathioprine is converted to 6-MP in RBCs

- Mercaptopurine is converted to the active metabolite thioinosinic acid which inhibits purine nucleotide synthesis, causing inhibition of cell proliferation
- It also affects cytotoxic T cells and natural killer cell activity
- Thioinosinic acid is deactivated by methylation by thiopurine methyltransferase (TPMT). This enzyme is lacking in 1 in 300 individuals, leading to increased susceptibility to adverse effects.

Adverse effects
- ~1/3 of patients are intolerant, with GI upset and nausea the most common side effects. 6-MP may be better tolerated than azathioprine
- Fever, rash, hair loss, hepatitis and peripheral neuropathy have also been reported
- Pancreatitis occurs in 3–15% of patients. This appears to be an allergic-type reaction and if it occurs with azathioprine, it will also occur with 6-MP. It usually resolves after discontinuing the drug
- Bone marrow suppression is an expected, dose-related effect. It may be delayed in onset. Blood counts should be monitored regularly
- The drugs do not start to exhibit an effect for at least 6 weeks after administration and a final assessment of the efficacy should not be made before 12 weeks
- The immunosuppressive action also persists for some weeks after cessation of therapy, which may be of relevance when considering cessation of therapy before surgery
- Cessation of the drug is not usually associated with an immediate rebound increase in disease activity.

Route of administration
- These are oral medications based on a dose–weight regimen
- Their main use is in maintenance treatment allowing reduction in the use of corticosteroids
- Should be prescribed in the setting of a specialist gastroenterology clinic with regular blood monitoring required
- Thiopurine S-methyltransferase (TPMT) activity is usually measured before starting a thiopurine as 10% of patients have moderately reduced TPMT activity which requires a dose reduction. An additional 1% display almost no TPMT activity and should not be given a thiopurine.
- 6 thioguanine nucleotide (6-TGN) levels can be checked to ensure compliance and to tailor dosing in the maintenance phase..

Methotrexate
Used to treat both steroid-dependent and steroid-resistant CD.

Mechanism of action
- Folic acid inhibitor with anti-inflammatory and immune-modulating effects
- Metabolites of methotrexate inhibit DNA synthesis
- It may also inhibit leukotriene B4 and IL-1 production.

Adverse effects
- Common side effects include nausea, abdominal pain, diarrhoea and stomatitis. Fatigue, headache and dizziness have also been reported.

- Bone marrow suppression is less common than with azathioprine or 6-MP, particularly at low dose. Blood counts still need careful monitoring
- Hypersensitivity pneumonitis has also been reported. This is a rare but serious complication which can occur even on a low dose.
- There is a risk of hepatotoxicity and liver enzymes should be monitored routinely
- Women should be advised to use contraception and avoid pregnancy.

Route of administration
- Can be administered orally or by IM or SC injection
- Bioavailability is good orally in low dose
- Higher doses may be better absorbed and better tolerated when administered parenterally.

Ciclosporin

This drug has a role in the management of acute fulminant colitis.

Adverse effects
- Common side effects include hypertension, hypertrichosis, gingival hyperplasia, paraesthesia, headaches and electrolyte abnormalities
- Renal insufficiency is also common and dose reduction or cessation of treatment is mandatory if there are signs of nephrotoxicity.

Relative contraindications
- Hypertension
- Significant renal impairment
- History of seizures
- Low magnesium or albumin

Route of administration
- Mostly used as an IV infusion in severe acute IBD non-responsive to corticosteroids
- Careful monitoring of serum drug concentration is required, as well as monitoring electrolyte levels and renal function.

Infliximab

- The first licensed biological agent for the management of CD, later proven to be effective in UC
- Mainly used in the management of refractory and fistulating CD

Mechanism of action
- It is a chimeric (part murine, part human) Ig1 monoclonal antibody directed against TNF-α
- Binds to circulating TNF and to cells expressing TNF on their cell membrane, causing lysis or apoptosis.

Adverse effects
- Generally, well tolerated, common side effects include headache, nausea, fatigue and upper respiratory tract infection
- Other side effects include sepsis, reactivation of TB and onset of demyelinating disorders.
- Probably does increase the risk of lymphoma and other malignancies

- Acute and delayed infusion reactions risk Contraindications
  - Active infection or evidence of latent TB
  - Malignancy
  - Demyelinating disorders (e.g. MS, optic neuritis)
  - Heart failure

Route of administration
- Given by IV infusion (5 mg/kg) at 0, 2 and 6 weeks and then 8-weekly thereafter.

Adalimumab
- An anti-TNF-alpha antibody

Mechanism of action
- This is a human IgG1 kappa monoclonal antibody which is specifically neutralizes TNG-alpha

Route of administration
- Initial 160 mg SC, then 80mg in 2 weeks and then maintenance of 40mg every 2 weeks thereafter

Adverse effects
- Generally, well tolerated. Common side effects include headaches, skin rashes, infections, upper respiratory tract infections. Hypersensitivity reactions are rare. Autoimmune disorders, demyelination, malignancy and increased risk of lymphoma

Vedolizumab
This gut selective biologic is often used in older patients and those with a history of malignancy and infectious complications. It is thought to have a lesser systemic impact on immune function compared to other biologics.

Used in moderate/severely active CD and UC, where patients have failed treatment with immunomodulators and/or an anti-TNF. Also used as monotherapy in patients who are biologic naïve and in combination with an immunomodulator in patients who have relapsed/failed previous biologic therapy
- 50% - 60% clinical response rate and clinical remission in 25-35%
- 35% – 55% will lose response during maintenance therapy

Mechanism of action
- This is a humanized monoclonal antibody which is active against $\alpha 4\beta 7$ integrin
- It is primarily active in the GI tract and blocks movement of inflammatory cells into the gut in both CD and UC

Route of administration
- Induction therapy given (300 mg) by IV infusion on week 0, 2 and 6 and then maintenance every 8 weeks

Adverse effects
- Generally, well tolerated, common side effects include nasopharyngitis, headaches, arthralgia, GI upset, fever, lethargy and skin reactions

Ustekinumab

Used in moderate/severely active CD, where patients have failed treatment with immunomodulators and or an anti-TNF. It has recently been licensed for use in UC. Increasingly used as monotherapy in patients who are biologic naïve and in combination with an immunomodulator in patients who have relapsed/failed previous biologic therapy.

Mechanism of action
- A monoclonal IgG1 antibody with activity against IL-12 and IL-23.
- Targets the T-helper 1 and T-helper 17 pathways

Route of administration
- Induction therapy given by IV infusion and then maintenance dosing SC 8 weekly.

Adverse effects
- Generally, well tolerated. Common side effects include arthralgia, infection and nasopharyngitis, headache, lethargy

Anti-drug antibodies (ADA)

- ADAs are increasingly recognized as one of the most important reasons for loss of efficacy and allergic reactions to anti-TNF drugs
- Neutralizing antibodies most commonly develop against infliximab (directed against the mouse portion of the chimera) and a lesser extent adalimumab, golimumab and biosimilars
- ADAs typically develop within 2-6 months of initial exposure
- Patients who develop ADAs are less likely to respond and have lower serum levels of the relevant biologic
- Reduced efficacy due to low level ADAs may be overcome by either dose escalation or adding in an immunomodulator e.g. thiopurine
- 50 -60% of patients receiving infliximab will develop an ADA

Other biologics

- Golimumab is a human IgG kappa monoclonal against TNF-alpha.

Biosimilars

- Biosimilars are copies of the original biologic therapies. Most show similar activity but usually have a price advantage
- Although similar, there may be some differences in efficacy, side-effects and immunogenicity
- Currently, biosimilar drugs are on the market for both infliximab and adalimumab and it is likely that others will follow.

Reference

Cohen BL, Sachar DB. Update on anti-tumor necrosis factor agents and other new drugs for inflammatory bowel disease *BMJ* 2017; **357**:j2505

Severe acute colitis and toxic megacolon

Toxic colitis and toxic megacolon represent one end of a broad spectrum of disease activity in IBD. The conditions are closely related and should be viewed as different stages in the same disease process. Optimal management is through the joint care of a gastroenterologist and colorectal surgeon. In less urgent cases, care pathways may be discussed at an IBD-MDT which would also include a GI radiologist, stoma therapist, pathologist and nutrition team.

Incidence

- Incidence of acute severe colitis and toxic megacolon is falling
- This is partly due to a change in disease distribution as 50% of all new patients now present with only distal colitis
- 6–10% of patients with IBD develop an episode of toxic colitis and ~30% of cases occur as part of the initial presentation
- CD accounts for ~50% of cases
- In UC acute attacks are more likely to occur after a longer duration of disease and at an older age than with CD
- Lifetime risk of toxic megacolon is ~1% for patients with IBD
- The risk of developing toxic dilatation is highest early in the disease: 30% of cases occur within 3 months of diagnosis of IBD; 60% of cases occur within the first 3yrs.

Factors associated with the development of toxic colitis

- Sudden cessation or rapid taper of corticosteroids or 5-ASA drugs. This is not the case for azathioprine and 6-MP
- Use of certain drugs and medications
  - Barium sulphate
  - Narcotic analgesics (e.g. codeine)
  - Anti-diarrhoeal drugs (e.g. loperamide)
  - Anti-cholinergic drugs (e.g. buscopan)
- Electrolyte imbalance (especially hypokalaemia)
- Cessation of smoking may be a trigger of disease activity in UC
- In patients with IBD, infection with the following organisms
  - *Salmonella*, *Shigella*, *Campylobacter* and pathogenic *E. coli*
  - Amoebiasis
  - *C. difficile*-induced pseudomembranous colitis
- These pathogens may also precipitate a fulminant colitis *de novo* (Table 4.7)
- CMV colitis. In one series of 46 patients undergoing colonic resection for UC, CMV was found in 5/6 patients with toxic dilatation but only 2/40 patients without dilatation (Cooper 1977). CMV may also precipitate toxic megacolon in patients with AIDS.

Pathology

- The usual clinical pathological features that distinguish UC and CD become less distinct in toxic colitis and toxic megacolon
- Rectal sparing is not a consistent finding in CD-related toxic colitis
- In cases of UC, inflammation extends into the submucosa
- In toxic colitis/dilatation, transmural inflammation with necrosis can make differentiation between UC and CD impossible. A diagnosis of indeterminate colitis is much more common after emergency surgery
- Toxic colitis is associated with extensive ulceration which exposes large areas of the submucosa and muscularis propria (Fig. 4.24)
- Granulation tissue and oedema may extend through to the subserosa
- With progressive inflammation the muscle loses contractility and the colon dilates and becomes thinned, leading to toxic dilatation
- Colonic dilatation correlates closely with the depth of ulceration
- Myocyte death is a prominent feature in cases of toxic megacolon. Despite this, the submucosal and myenteric plexus are well preserved until late in the disease, suggesting a neuropathic process is unlikely to be an important factor in development of dilatation
- NO may play a role in the development of toxic megacolon.

Presentation

Although there are a number of definitions of a toxic colitis, a modified version of Truelove and Witt's grading of colitis continues to serve the basis for most clinical diagnoses. This relies on the presence of at least 6 bloody stools per 24h in a patient with established colitis in association with at least one sign of systemic toxicity (Table 4.5).

Toxic megacolon is characterized by the presence of total or segmental colonic dilatation (>5.5cm), occurring in association with a toxic colitis. The transverse colon is frequently the area of the colon where the colonic distension is most apparent.

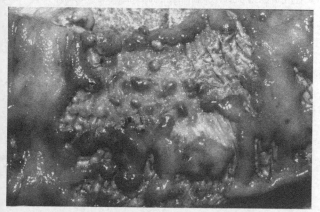

Fig. 4.24 Fulminant colitis showing confluent ulceration and visible mucosal islands.

Clinical features

- Patients are frequently systemically unwell. Tachycardia, hypotension and confusion may be present
- Abdominal examination may show generalized colonic tenderness
- Localized tenderness/rebound suggests impending/actual perforation
- Abdominal distension is a cause for concern as both small bowel and colonic dilatation are poor prognostic features
- Clinical findings may be modulated by the treatment and disease
  - High dose steroids may mask symptoms and signs of perforation
  - Bloody diarrhoea may not be present after rectal 5-ASA compounds
  - Diarrhoea may be suppressed with narcotic analgesia
  - Those developing toxic megacolon may experience a reduction in stool frequency despite having a very severe colitis.

Initial assessment

- Bloods for FBC, ESR, U&Es, LFTs, blood gases and coagulation screen. Results may show ↓Hb, ↓albumin, ↑CRP, ↑ESR and electrolyte imbalance. Metabolic alkalosis suggests profound fluid and potassium depletion and is a poor prognostic indicator.
- Stools for culture & sensitivity and *C. difficile* infection (CDI)/toxin
  - CDI may be a cause of acute severe exacerbations in UC
  - CDI increases the likelihood of a patient requiring a colectomy
- Colonoscopy is usually not indicated. A limited flexible sigmoidoscopy in unprepared colon may be helpful when the diagnosis is uncertain.

Radiology

- Plain AXR can be helpful in both diagnosis and providing a serial assessment of transverse colon diameter to exclude toxic megacolon
- Free air may be seen under the diaphragm or in the retroperitoneum
- An absence of colonic air may limit the usefulness of plain radiology
- CT can be helpful in confirming a clinical diagnosis of colitis and delineating the extent of disease
- CT will also exclude localized perforation or abscess formation.

Features of acute colitis on plain AXR

- Mucosal oedema/thickening → loss of the normal haustral pattern
- Ulceration → irregular mucosal pattern and thumbprinting (Fig. 4.25)
- Confluent ulceration → visible oedematous mucosal islands
- Multiple loops of distended small intestine is a worrying feature and may be an indication for surgical intervention.

Differential diagnosis

Superadded infection in known IBD patients should be excluded. A more extensive differential diagnosis is considered for a first presentation. (Table 4.7)

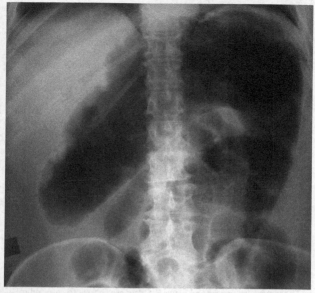

Fig. 4.25 Plain abdominal x-ray showing toxic megacolon with thumbprinting, mucosal islands and small bowel dilatation.

Table 4.7 Differential diagnosis in toxic colitis

Group	Specific condition
Inflammatory	Ulcerative colitis
	Crohn's disease
	Indeterminate colitis
Infectious	C. *difficile* pseudomembranous colitis
	Salmonella-typhoid
	Shigella, Campylobacter, Yersinia enterocolitca
	Entamoeba histolytica
Viral	Cytomegalovirus colitis (especially in immunosuppressed patients)
Other	Kaposi's sarcoma
	Drug induced (penicillin, quinolones, methotrexate)
	Glutaraldehyde

Management

- IV fluid resuscitation and correction of electrolyte abnormalities
- Transfusion as necessary
- Anti-cholinergics, anti-diarrhoeals, NSAIDs and narcotic analgesics are avoided
- Corticosteroids (e.g. IV hydrocortisone 4mg/kg) form the mainstay of therapy
- After 5 days of treatment 60% will be symptom free, 15% will be significantly improved and 25% will have failed to respond
- In patients who do respond, IV corticosteroids can be tapered and the patient switched to oral steroids (prednisolone 40mg orally daily)
- Only 1/3 of patients with severe colitis avoid colectomy in the long term
- An anti-TNF biologic may be considered as first line treatment if corticosteroids are contraindicated/not well tolerated

Other therapies

- LMWH to reduce the risk of venous thromboembolism
- Bowel rest does not appear to offer any proven advantage
- Antibiotics may be considered but there is no supportive evidence
- Nutritional supplementation should be considered but there is little evidence to support the use of either parenteral or enteral nutrition
- Most clinicians avoid using 5-ASA drugs in acute situation but consider introduction once the patient shows signs of improvement.

Escalation of medical therapy

- Those who fail to respond within 3-5 days are unlikely to respond to corticosteroids and should be considered for an anti-TNF, ciclosporin or undergo colectomy

Infliximab (IFX)

- Anti-TNF therapy, which is active in both UC and CD, has increasingly become the preferred second line drug to use in IV steroid-resistant UC (IVSR-UC)
- IFX is given at initial dose of 5mg/kg (➔ Drug therapy in IBD p.180). Patients usually respond within 3-5 days.
- A second infusion (10mg/kg) may be considered within 5 days if there is an inadequate response to initial infusion, although consideration should also be given to surgical intervention
- A recent Swedish–Danish study reported that single dose IFX as rescue therapy in IVSR-UC halved the colectomy rate from 67 to 29% at 3 months
- In an observational study of 211 patients with acute severe UC who were treated with IFX, surgery was avoided in 64% at 1 years and 53% at 5 years
- IFX should be used in those who are predicted to have a poor outcome at day 3 of conventional IV corticosteroid therapy (Table 4.8)
- Those with less active disease on day 5 may benefit most from IFX (perhaps because those with more active disease at this point will inevitably progress to colectomy)
- At 6 months, response rates fall to 30% (cf. 60% initial remission rate). Of these late responders, at least 40% still require steroids

- Concern regarding potential for neoplastic change, risk of infection (pneumonia, TB, histoplasmosis) and neuropathy means that its role should be carefully considered
- IFX continues to work for weeks after a dose which may ↑ septic complications if recipients need to undergo emergency surgery
- Ciclosporin has a very short half-life. In the event of a patient not responding, surgery can be performed with less concern regarding its immunosuppressive actions.

Ciclosporin

- Ciclosporin (CsA) is a helpful rescue therapy for IV steroid-resistant UC (IVSR-UC) where it may act as a bridge to thiopurine therapy
- Average response rate of 80% (➲ Drug therapy in IBD p.180)
- Side effects have limited its acceptability. A dose reduction from 4 to 2mg/kg/24h reduces early toxicity
- IV treatment is followed by oral therapy (5-8mg/kg/24h)
- Mean time to respond is 7 days and response is maintained for up to 6 months in 50% of patients
- Azathioprine and 6-MP improve response rates to78% although dual therapy should be maintained for at least 8 weeks until the thiopurine is fully effective
- Early colectomy rate is ~10%, although up to 60% of initial responders ultimately require colectomy
- Side effects include paraesthesia (51%), hypertension (43%) and hypomagnesaemia (42%). Major toxicity also occurs including renal insufficiency (23%), infections (20%), grand mal seizures (3%), death (2%) and anaphylaxis (1%). Opportunistic infections (e.g. *Aspergillus* sp. and *P. carinii*) may occur during crossover therapy when patients are being treated with both CsA and a thiopurine.
- Those who fail CsA therapy may have excessive morbidity, particularly after surgery
- Primary treatment with CsA may be considered for those who are susceptible to steroid-induced psychosis.

Toxic megacolon

- Patients should be assessed and treated as for toxic colitis
- Many surgeons and gastroenterologists feel that the development of toxic megacolon (transverse colon >5.5cm or caecum >9cm) is an absolute indication for surgery
- It may be reasonable to consider a 24–48h trial of IV steroids in a stable patient who presents with a dilated colon
- There is little experience of ciclosporin in toxic megacolon and its use is not recommended
- Failure to respond or development of a megacolon in a patient already undergoing corticosteroid treatment for toxic colitis is an indication for surgery
- Although toxic megacolon complicates <10% of cases of fulminant colitis, it is the main diagnosis in 25% of patients undergoing surgery.

Predictors for failure of medical therapy and decision to proceed to surgery

Timing of colectomy for severe colitis remains one of the more difficult decisions that a gastroenterologist and colorectal surgeon must make. The increasing complexity of potential medical interventions can further complicate this process. The natural history of the disease process is that untreated patients have an ↑25% mortality compared with <1% in specialist centres. However, mortalities of up to 24% have been reported for severe colitis as recently as 2001.

Indications for immediate surgery
• Perforation/peritonitis
• Septic shock
• ↑ colonic dilatation
• Massive haemorrhage.

Although clinical decision-making is straightforward in the presence of complications, this represents a minority of patients. The decision to proceed to surgery is much more difficult when there has been some progress in the clinical condition. This is especially so in patients with a new diagnosis of IBD who may be having difficulty coming to terms with the diagnosis, not to mention the need for urgent surgery with the prospect of a stoma. A number of indices have been developed to assess the risk of a poor outcome (Table 4.8).

Further indications for surgery
• No real signs of improvement after an adequate trial with corticosteroids or second line therapy (IFX or ciclosporin). A trial is usually defined as 5–7 days of aggressive medical therapy although high risk patients can be identified at 3 days after starting therapy
• Toxic colitis with any sign of deterioration in the criteria outlined in Box 4.3, e.g. radiological signs such as small bowel or colonic dilatation, pyrexia when none was present at the start of treatment, failure of CRP to fall or development of localized abdominal tenderness, even in the absence of free gas on an erect abdominal film.

Choice of operation
• Surgical options are limited in the acute situation. For most patients, the procedure of choice is a subtotal colectomy and end ileostomy (Ⓔ Surgery for acute colitis p.556)
• Proctocolectomy may have a role in very selected cases such as rectal perforation, overwhelming haemorrhage or in less severely unwell patients who would not be a candidate for a future ileal pouch
• Some authors advocate emergency or 'urgent' restorative proctocolectomy and loop ileostomy for patients with acute colitis. This is associated with ↑ operative morbidity and ↑ anastomotic leak rate
• On very rare occasions, consideration may be given to fashioning a loop ileostomy and decompressive 'blowhole' colostomy in the very sick patient with a toxic megacolon.

Table 4.8 Risk stratification of severe acute ulcerative colitis

Swedish/Lindgren Index*
Risk factors for poor outcome
At presentation:
Short duration of disease
Steroid treatment before exacerbation
On day 3 after starting treatment:
Elevated temperature
Persistent diarrhoea
Passage of blood
Elevation in CRP
75% risk of colectomy if CRP of >25mg/l and >4 bowel movements/
day on day 3

Travers/Oxford Index†
Risk factors for poor outcome
Stool frequency of >8 stools
Stool frequency between 3 and 8 and CRP >45mg/l
85% risk of colectomy if either of these criteria were present
Parameter's measured on day 3 of treatment

Ho/Edinburgh Index‡

Mean stool frequency	Score	Total score	Risk of colectomy
<4	0	0-1	11%
4.5	1		
6.9	2	2-3	43%
>9	4	≥4	85%

Colonic dilatation	
Present	4
Not present	0

Hypoalbuminaemia <30g/l	
Present	1
Not present	0

Parameters measured within the first 3 days of treatment

*Adapted from Lindgren SC, Flood LM, Kilander AF et al. Early predictors of glucocorticosteroid treatment failure in severe and moderately severe attacks of ulcerative colitis. *Eur J Gastroenterol Hepatol* 1998;10:831–835.

†Adapted from Travis SPL, Farrant JM, Rickett C et al. Predicting outcome in severe ulcerative colitis. *Gut* 1996;38:905–910.

‡Adapted from Ho GT, Mowat C, Goddard CJR et al. Predicting the outcome of severe ulcerative colitis; development of a novel risk score to aid the early selection of patients for second-line medical therapy or surgery. *Aliment Pharmacol Ther* 2004;19:1079–1087.

Box 4.3 Factors associated with a poor outcome in severe ulcerative colitis

Mucosal islands on plain abdominal x-ray
Small bowel loops/dilatation
Temperature >38°C
Albumin <30g/l
Heart rate >100/min
Frequent stools (>8/day)
Elevation in CRP (>25mg/l)
Faecal calprotectin >1,922mcg/g

Subtotal colectomy and end ileostomy
- This is the preferred surgical option for the vast majority of patients
- Avoids mobilization of an oedematous inflamed rectum
- Risk of post-operative haemorrhage and injury to the nervi erigentes and hypogastric nerve plexus is substantially reduced
- Definitive surgery (e.g. completion proctectomy with IPAA) can be performed when the patient has fully recovered and is off immunosuppressive drugs (usually not less than 6 months)
- Such an approach is also helpful if the nature of the underlying disease process is uncertain. A diagnosis of UC or indeterminate colitis means a pouch can be considered. If CD is seen on histology, an ileorectal anastomosis or completion proctectomy can be considered.

Outcome
- Advances in the care of patients with toxic colitis have led to a dramatic reduction in mortality from ~50% before the introduction of steroids in the 1950s to ~30% in the 1960s and current mortality rates of <1% in specialist centres
- Mortality is much more likely in patients who have already become septic or developed a colonic perforation by the time of surgical intervention, a disastrous situation that can usually be avoided by close cooperation between gastroenterologist and surgeon
- Colonic dilatation complicated by perforation carries a mortality of up to 30%
- If patients decide not to undergo further surgery after subtotal colectomy and end ileostomy, they should be counselled on the need for rectal stump surveillance as malignancy may develop in up to 3% of cases
- Signs of colonic dilatation or perforation urgent laparotomy and subtotal colectomy with end ileostomy is indicated. If there is a failure to respond to medical therapy the same procedure should be performed.

References

Macken L, Blaker PA. Management of acute severe ulcerative colitis (NICE CG 166). *Clin Med (Lond)*. 2015;15(5):473–476. doi:10.7861/clinmedicine.15-5-473

Seah D, De Cruz P. Review article: the practical management of acute severe ulcerative colitis. *Ailment Pharmacol Ther* 2016;**43**:482–513

Lindgren SC, Flood LM, Kilander AF et al. Early predictors of glucocorticosteroid treatment failure in severe and moderately severe attacks of ulcerative colitis. *Eur J Gastroenterol Hepatol* 1998;**10**:831–835.

Ho GT, Mowat C, Goddard CJR et al. Predicting the outcome of severe ulcerative colitis; development of a novel risk score to aid the early selection of patients for second-line medical therapy or surgery. *Ailment Pharmacol Ther* 2004;**19**:1079–1087.

Travis SPL, Farrant JM, Rickett C et al. Predicting outcome in severe ulcerative colitis. *Gut* 1996;**38**:905–910.

Indeterminate colitis

Indeterminate colitis (IC) can be thought of as an uncertain or temporary diagnosis. There is evidence that some patients within this group may have a distinct phenotype of IBD.

IC was first described by Price in 1978 and was a purely histological diagnosis. It related to colectomy specimens usually from patients with severe colitis where, due to overlapping features, a clear diagnosis of UC or CD could not be reached. The major pathological features were as follows:

• Deep V-shaped or slit-like fissures
• Normal or minimally abnormal intervening mucosa
• No granulomas
• Appearances may be due to treatment effects or severity of disease.

The term is now more broadly used to describe patients where standard clinical, endoscopic, radiographic and histological findings do not allow a more specific diagnosis of either UC or CD. Although it has been proposed to use a new term IBD-Unclassified, the most recent ICD-11 classification (2016) continues to only use the term indeterminate colitis.

• Patients should have evidence of IBD on clinical and endoscopic grounds
• Definitive histological evidence of CD or UC may be lacking (colonic biopsies are diagnostic of CD or UC in ~70%)
• There should be no evidence of small bowel involvement (endoscopy, capsule endoscopy and enteroclysis may be helpful)
• Infection should be ruled out although 20% of IBD patients will have positive stool cultures
• Minimal histological changes are seen in early or inactive disease.

Natural history

• 10–15% of patients will be labelled IC at initial diagnosis. This is dependent on the experience of the supervising clinical team, the severity of inflammation at presentation, the extent of investigation, the ability to recognize unusual variants of CD and UC and interobserver variability in histological interpretation. Rates may also be higher in children
• Subsequently ~50% will be given a definitive diagnosis, the majority being UC. The remaining patients have a durable diagnosis of IC, which suggests that it is likely to be a true third IBD category
• A more severe clinical course is common in IC, with younger age at onset, more extensive disease and high rates of colectomy.

Serological markers and IC

• Anti-*Saccharomyces cerevisiae* antibody (ASCA) is more common in CD (80%)
• Perinuclear anti-neutrophil cytoplasmic antibodies (P-ANCAs) detected in UC in 60–80%
• Patients with negative serology and a diagnosis of IC are more likely to keep the diagnosis. This may suggest that these patients form a distinct subgroup or phenotype
• Serological markers currently have little use in the clinical setting.

Treatment

- There is little evidence to guide medical treatment in IC
- One small study of IFX showed response in 16/20 patients. Eight responders were eventually diagnosed as CD, but a similar clinical response was seen in the 8 who remained as IC
- It is common to treat IC patients as UC
- Patients with IC are appropriate candidates for ileoanal pouch anastomosis
- Long-term complications (20%) and pouch failure (up to 10%) following IPAA may be marginally worse in IC patients compared to those with a confirmed diagnosis of UC. However, outcomes after IPAA are definitely better than patients with CD who undergo IPAA. However, pre-operative counselling should discuss these issues
- Approximately 10% of patients will subsequently be diagnosed as CD.

References

Tremaine WJ. Review article: indeterminate colitis—definition, diagnosis and management. *Aliment Pharmacol Ther* 2007;25:13–17

Yu CS, Pemberton JH, Larson D. Ileal pouch–anal anastomosis in patients with indeterminate colitis: long-term results. *Dis Colon Rectum* 2000;**43**:1487–1496.

Extraintestinal manifestations

Up to 40% of patients with IBD develop EIMs (Fig. 4.26). This figure may be higher in the paediatric population. Certain symptoms may be a direct consequence of the disease such as anaemia from GI blood loss or renal oxalate stones 2° to fat malabsorption. Other EIMs tend to occur together, the triad of joint–eye–skin involvement being typical.

In CD, EIMs are strongly associated with colonic disease and occur more frequently than UC. The pathogenesis is unclear, but autoimmunity and genetic factors are thought to be important. Those EIMs associated with disease extent usually respond to therapy for disease control.

Musculoskeletal

Arthritis is the most common EIM of IBD, affecting ~20% of all patients. Many patients with IBD may also complain of musculoskeletal pain. Arthropathy may develop before, during or after the diagnosis of IBD. IBD-related spondyloarthropathies are seronegative and similar to psoriatic arthritis and ankylosing arthritis.

Type 1 peripheral arthritis
- No clear association with gender or age
- Pauciarticular affects <5 large joints and is asymmetrical
- Knees affected more than hips, ankles, wrists and elbows
- Episodes are usually short (5-10 weeks) and self-remitting related to disease activity

Type 2 peripheral arthritis
- Polyarticular affects >5 joints (typically small joints) and is disease independent.
- The metacarpophalangeal joint is most commonly affected. Knees, ankles and shoulders affected to a lesser degree

Axial arthropathy
- Consists of two syndromes
  - Spondylitis which is indistinguishable from ankylosing spondylitis (AS), other than the fact that it common in females (40%) and the male/female ratio for primary AS is 8:1
  - Isolated sacroiliitis
- Spondylitis affects 2–6% of patients with IBD
- Prevalence is 20–30 times higher than the general population
- More than 50% of patients with spondylitis are HLA-B27 positive
- Low back pain is worse in the morning, relieved by exercise and disappears as sacroiliitis progresses to AS
- Methotrexate is commonly used and anti-TNF agents may help in resistant cases
- Asymptomatic sacroiliitis is common (radiological abnormality in 15% and abnormalities in 70% on bone scan)
- Sacroiliitis alone is not associated with HLA-B27 and may not progress to spondylitis.

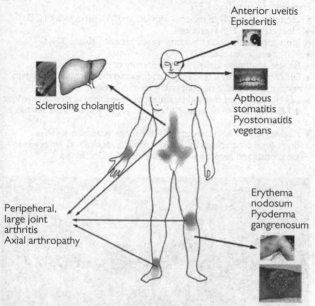

Fig. 4.26 Some of the more common sites of extraintestinal manifestations of inflammatory bowel disease.

Osteoporosis
- Fracture risk is only modestly increased by ~30% in chronic IBD
- Consider lifestyle factors including calcium and vitamin D intake
- Screening with dual energy x-ray absorptiometry (DEXA), steroid avoidance ± bisphosphonates in high risk patients (>65yrs, steroids >3 months, body mass index (BMI) <20).

Clubbing and hypertrophic osteoarthropathy
More common in CD than UC. Correlates with disease activity. Clubbing usually painless but periostosis with new bone formation may be painful.

Skin and mucous membranes

Aphthous stomatitis
- Superficial round ulcers indistinguishable from common aphthae
- Tend to mirror intestinal disease activity
- LA for symptom relief ± triamcinolone/NSAID paste
- Other oral manifestations include angular stomatitis, cobblestoning, pyostomatitis vegetans.

Erythema nodosum (Fig. 4.27)
- Occurs in up to 4% of patients with UC and 15% patients with CD
- Most common EIM in children
- Most commonly occurs in women aged between 20 and 30yrs
- May precede onset of IBD
- Related to disease activity but not severity or extent
- Sudden onset warm, tender, red nodules commonly on the shins with fever, malaise and joint pains lasting up to 6 weeks
- Leg elevation, bed rest and treatment of bowel disease is recommended ± NSAIDs (should be used with caution as they may induce a relapse in the IBD)
- Also associated with streptococcal infections, tuberculosis (TB), drugs (oral contraceptive pill, sulphonamides, penicillin's), lymphoma, sarcoidosis and autoimmune diseases including sarcoidosis.

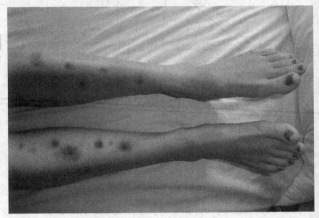

Fig. 4.27 Erythema nodosum.

Pyoderma gangrenosum (PG) (Fig. 4.28)
- Uncommon complication with an incidence of 2–5%
- Most common in UC affecting patients between 25 and 55yrs
- No clear correlation with disease activity and lesions may recur after colectomy
- Pain and pustules which rapidly ulcerate usually affecting the lower extremities and extensor surfaces, but can occur anywhere
- PG displays pathergy i.e. an exaggerated response to superficial trauma leading to PG developing at surgical wounds, stoma sites etc
- Differential diagnosis
  - Bacterial, mycobacterial or fungal infection
  - Malignancy
  - Vascular and autoimmune disease

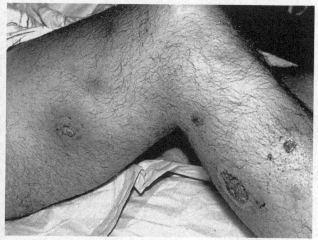

Fig. 4.28 Pyoderma gangrenosum.

- Some lesions run an independent clinical course remitting in <1yr but frequently recurs. In up to 50% of cases, activity may mirror intestinal disease activity
- Mild cases can be treated with moist wound dressing + sodium cromoglycate topically/systemically. Systemic corticosteroids ± ciclosporin for severe cases (once infection excluded). IFX may help.

Metastatic Crohn's disease
Non-caseating granulomas of the skin can occur. Erythematous nodules plaques and ulcers, combined with oedematous swelling can occur in the face, arms extremities and vulva (Fig. 4.22).

Other skin manifestations
Psoriasis, apthous ulcers, erythema multiforme, Sweet syndrome.

Ophthalmological

Ocular manifestation occur in up to 5% of all IBD patients. Tend to occur in association with peripheral arthritis and erythema nodosum.

Episcleritis
- Painless hyperaemia of sclera and conjunctiva without visual loss
- Most common ocular manifestation. Flares tends to mimic intestinal disease activity
- Oral NSAIDs or topical steroids are effective combined with treatment of intestinal disease.

Uveitis
- Painful red eye with blurred vision, photophobia and headache
- Rapid treatment with corticosteroids is essential to avoid visual loss
- Independent of bowel disease activity but frequently associated with skin and joint EIMs.

Hepatobiliary

Primary sclerosing cholangitis (PSC)

- Diffuse inflammation and fibrosis of intra- and extrahepatic bile ducts (Fig. 4.29)
- At least 75% of patient with PSC have UC and 5-10% have CD
- Complicates 5–10% of all patients with UC with 2:1 male: female ratio and 2% of patients with CD
- 1/3 patients will have ↑ antinuclear antibody and 80% have positive antineutrophil cytoplasmic antibodies
- Median diagnosis at 40yrs with jaundice, pruritus, fatigue and weight loss
- MRCP is the investigation of choice. It is important to exclude cholangiocarcinoma
- ERCP should be reserved for treating high grades strictures but is associated with ↑ risk of cholangitis due to poor biliary drainage
- Medical therapy does not appear to impact survival
- Randomised trials have shown no benefit with ursodeoxycholic acid
- Slow progression to cirrhosis. Liver transplant is the definitive treatment. Clinical course is independent of bowel disease activity
- Increased risk of cholangiocarcinoma and CRC (25% in 25yrs).

Other hepatobiliary conditions

Steatosis, cirrhosis may occur in IBD. Thiopurine induced hepatitis and pancreatitis may also occur.

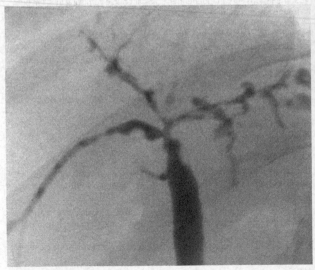

Fig. 4.29 Sclerosing cholangitis.

Miscellaneous

Anaemia

- Typically, iron deficiency or anaemia of chronic disease
- Multifactorial but may involve chronic blood loss, dietary deficiency, malabsorption of B12 (ileum) + folate (proximal small bowel) and haemolysis.

Growth retardation

- More common in CD
- Malabsorption, poor dietary intake, protein losing enteropathy, fistulae and intestinal resection can lead to a variety of nutritional deficiencies.

Stones

- ↑ Gallstones 2° to bile acid malabsorption in ileal disease/resection
- Renal calculus disease due to calcium oxalate or uric acid stones
- Management is the same as for non-IBD-related stone disease.

Thromboembolism

- Thromboembolic disease may be 4× greater in IBD patients.
- Portal vein thrombosis may also occur

Rare manifestations

These include myelodysplastic syndrome, amyloidosis, drug-induced lung disease, fibrosing alveolitis, bronchiectasis, abnormal pulmonary function, endocarditis, myocarditis, peripheral neuropathy and myopathy.

References

Levine JS, Burakoff R. Extraintestinal manifestations of inflammatory bowel disease. *Gastroenterol Hepatol (N Y)*. 2011;**7**(4):235–241.

Cancer risk in IBD

Chronic inflammation of the colonic mucosa increases the risk of colo-rectal carcinoma. Synchronous cancers are far more common in patients with IBD. In the setting of IBD-related CRC, the mean age at diagnosis is younger (40-50 yrs) versus 60 years for sporadic CRC. This led to the hypothesis that the development of cancer in the setting of chronic colitis may represent a field change.

Dysplasia

- Dysplasia is a histological abnormality which serves as a marker for risk of co-existing and future colonic cancer
- It is difficult to detect dysplasia accurately in the setting of actively inflamed colonic mucosa.
- All diagnoses of colonic dysplasia should be independently confirmed by 2 pathologists with a specialist gastrointestinal interest
- Most dysplasia in IBD is endoscopically visible
- Raised dysplastic lesions were previously described as dysplasia-associated lesion or mass (DALM). This term probably should be abandoned in favour of a detailed description to include
    - Morphology, size and Paris classification (→ Colonic polyps p.320)
    - Description of any colitis in adjacent mucosa
    - Description of the borders of the lesion (distinct or indistinct)
    - Features of submucosal invasion (e.g. failure to lift)
    - Kudo pit classification is not helpful in this setting as colitic changes can be mistaken for abnormalities in the pit pattern
- Management of dysplasia is complex and may benefit from MDT review. If circumscribed dysplasia is identified in a visible flat or raised lesion, consideration may be given to endoscopic removal if possible. Scarring however often precludes successful resection. Surgical resection should be considered in the event of an incomplete resection or development of recurrent dysplasia
- The finding of "invisible" dysplasia in random biopsies of flat/normal mucosa is a cause for concern
    - Up to 50% of patients with low grade dysplasia (LGD) will progress to high grade dysplasia (HGD)
    - The European Crohn's and Colitis Organisation (ECCO) recommends proceeding to surgical resection if "invisible" HGD is found in flat/normal mucosa

Polyps and polypoid dysplasia

- Sporadic adenomas can occur in the setting of IBD
- They are either sessile or pedunculated. Typically, biopsies of the surrounding mucosa shows no evidence of dysplasia
- Treatment should follow the standard guidelines for sporadic adenomas in the general population, assuming there is no evidence of flat dysplasia elsewhere in the colon

Pseudopolyps

- Pseudopolyps are irregularly shaped islands of colonic mucosa and occur at sites of previous severe colonic ulceration and subsequent regeneration
- They hamper colonoscopic surveillance as true dysplastic lesions can be easily missed
- They are not thought to be pre-malignant but do seem to confer an increased risk of bowel cancer. Dysplasia may be found in nearby mucosa, suggesting that the severity of the initial insult in those who go on to develop pseudopolyps is so great as to also initiate the dysplasia–carcinoma sequence.

Control of disease activity and reducing the risk of cancer

- There is reasonably strong epidemiological evidence that regular mesalazine therapy can reduce the risk of colon cancer in chronic IBD
- ECCO notes that 5-ASA drugs may reduce the incidence of CRC in UC and suggest administration to all UC patients
- Previously it was uncertain if this represented an anti-neoplastic effect of the therapy or whether it was due to a reduction in colonic inflammation was uncertain. However, recent data shows that long-term thiopurines have a similar effect in reducing the risk of CRC. This suggests their mode of action is mediated through a reduction in disease activity

Risk factors for colon cancer in IBD

Although the risk of CRC is increased in both CD and UC, the risk in UC has been more extensively investigated. It is likely that the risk in CD is similar to UC for pan-colonic disease. The risk in patients after ileal pouch surgery is discussed elsewhere (→ Ileal pouch complications p.176).

For patients with extensive disease, the risk of CRC becomes manifest 8-10 years after diagnosis. The most important risk factors are:
- Duration of disease. The cumulative risk of CRC is
  - 1% after 10 years
  - 2% after 20 years
  - 5% after > 20 years
  - 30% after 30 years
- Extent of colitis. Pancolitis i.e. disease proximal to splenic flexure is associated with greatest risk
  - The risk CRC in disease confined to the left colon increases around a decade later than those with pancolitis (ie after 15-20 yrs)
  - Patients with disease limited to rectum and sigmoid are probably not at increased risk of CRC
- Severity of inflammation
- Stricturing disease
- Co-existent primary sclerosing cholangitis (PSC)
- Pseudopolyp formation
- Male sex
- Young age at onset. It is not clear if this is an independent factor or simply relates to duration of disease
- Family history of sporadic colon cancer

Colonoscopic surveillance

- Colonoscopic surveillance to detect dysplasia in chronic IBD has never been proven in an RCT to improve survival. Nonetheless, it is almost universally recommended by gastroenterology societies worldwide
- A recent Cochrane review concluded that colonoscopic surveillance may reduce the risk of CRC and CRC-related mortality in patients with long-standing IBD, although the evidence was of low quality
- Most surveillance strategies recommend scheduled colonoscopies with random biopsies in the hope of detecting mucosal dysplasia. The technique is poorly sensitive and interval cancers are well documented
- Studies suggest that the yield of dysplasia surveillance can be increased up to 5-fold with the use of contrast dyes such as indigo–carmine, chromocolonoscopy.
- Current UK guidelines recommend screening should commence 10 years after diagnosis of colitis. Ideally, screening colonoscopy should be performed when disease is quiescent. Pancolonic dye-spray/chromoendoscopy should be performed to enable targeted and random biopsies (→ Flexible sigmoidoscopy and colonoscopy p.76)
  - Low-risk patients (pancolitis but no active inflammation or left sided colitis): 5 yearly colonoscopy
  - Intermediate risk (Mildly active pancolitis, post-inflammatory polyps or family history of CRC): 3 yearly colonoscopy
  - Higher risk (moderate/severe pancolitis, history of stricture, dysplasia, PSC or family history of CRC in first degree relatives < 50 years): annual colonoscopy

References

Lamb CL, Kennedy NA, Raine T., et al. British Society of Gastroenterology consensus guidelines on the management of inflammatory bowel disease in adults. *Gut* 2019;68:s1-s6

Bye WA, Nguyen TM, Parker CE, Jairath V, East JE. Strategies for detecting colon cancer in patients with inflammatory bowel disease. *Cochrane Database Syst Rev.* 2017;**9**:CD000279.

Cairns SR, Scholefield JH, Steele RJ et al. Guidelines for colorectal cancer screening and surveillance in moderate and high risk groups (update from 2002). *Gut* 2010;**59**:666–690

Annese V, Beaugerie L, Egan L, Biancone L et al. European Evidence-based Consensus: Inflammatory Bowel Disease and Malignancies. *J Crohns Colitis.* 2015;**9**(11):945

Reproduction and IBD

More than 50% of patients with UC and CD are <35yrs old at the time of diagnosis and 1/4 of them conceive for the first time after diagnosis.

Patients with active disease may be sexually inactive because of abdominal pain, diarrhoea, fear of incontinence or dyspareunia, which may be associated with perianal disease. These direct and treatment-related consequences of IBD can have a significant impact on quality of life, sexual function, fertility and pregnancy. Management of these issues is complicated by a lack of good quality evidence.

Male sexual dysfunction

Erectile dysfunction (ED) may manifest itself as impotence, failure of erection or retrograde ejaculation. Retrograde ejaculation may be a specific consequence of damage to the hypogastric nerve plexus during pelvic surgery. Although many studies have focused on these specific problems, only a small number have addressed wider issues such as sexual desire and intercourse satisfaction.

Medication
- ED has not been reported with most of the standard medications used to treat IBD
- Methotrexate can be associated with impotence
- Secondary medications including anti-depressants (e.g. Fluoxetine) and anxiolytics are frequently associated with ED including anorgasmia.

Surgery
- A recent meta-analysis found a pooled incidence of sexual dysfunction to be ~46% after IPAA for UC, with erectile dysfunction accounting for 1–2% and failure of ejaculation 3–4% (anorgasmia also reported)
- Similar results are seen after conventional proctocolectomy
- Sildenafil may be effective in up to 80% of men with post-operative ED.

Depression
- Rates of depression and anxiety are higher in patients with IBD compared with the general population and even those with newly diagnosed cancer
- Depression is the single most important determinant of ED in patients with IBD
- Drugs used to treat depression also play an important role in ED
- Men in remission or those with mildly active disease have rates of ED similar to a healthy population.

Male infertility

The precise infertility rate for men with IBD has been difficult to establish, but it seems clear that men have reduced fertility after diagnosis. One study suggested that 25% of men with IBD had no children compared with 15% of the general population, although many of these were taking sulphasalazine which is no longer used as first-line therapy. It also appears that many men with IBD decide not to have children.

Medications

See below under the heading 'Medication and impact on fertility'

Secondary causes of male infertility

- Poor nutritional status and zinc deficiency may contribute to male infertility
- Some studies have found anti-sperm antibodies in both men and women with IBD. There is no direct evidence however that this leads to a direct reduction in fertility.

Surgery

There are few data on the direct effect of surgery on male fertility although pelvic surgery does carry a small risk of ED which can lead to infertility (see above).

Female sexual function and fertility

- Although evidence is very limited, it has been reported that females with IBD have similar rates of sexual activity and dyspareunia compared to aged matched controls
- Females with quiescent IBD do not appear to have reduced fertility compared to age matched controls in the general population
- Lower birth rates in IBD patients may be due to following, often ungrounded concerns
  - impact of IBD on pregnancy and childbirth
  - potential for drug related teratogenicity
  - impact on disease activity
- Patients with longstanding active UC may have reduced fertility
- Females with active CD have reduced fertility, in part due to
  - dyspareunia
  - inflammation/adhesions involving the ovaries and fallopian tube
  - poor nutrition with consequent reduction in ovulation
  - patient behavior (decreased desire for intercourse, avoidance of pregnancy, etc.)

Medication & impact on fertility

- Sulphasalazine can have a profound effect on male fertility. It may produce oligospermia, secondary to the sulphapyridine component. There may also be an increased risk of congenital malformations and it should be stopped prior to attempts to conceive.
- Sulphasalazine does not have a negative effect on female fertility
- Other 5-ASA drugs do not appear to affect fertility
- Steroids, ciclosporin and azathioprine do not appear to affect male or female fertility and do not appear to be teratogenic
- Methotrexate should be avoided in females of child-bearing age due to its teratogenic and mutagenic actions.
- Methotrexate may produce oligospermia in men and is likely to impair male fertility. It should be stopped before men try to conceive
- Infliximab, adalimumab and certolizumab appear to compatible for use in men and women during conception and throughout pregnancy

Surgery and fertility in IBD

Ulcerative colitis
- Up to 30% of women will experience sexual dysfunction after proctectomy and dyspareunia is reported by up to 30%.
- In females, IPAA may be associated with less dysfunction compared to total proctectomy as the pouch maintains anatomic integrity and stops the vagina from becoming angulated posteriorly
- Sexual satisfaction, desire, ability to experience orgasm and frequency of sexual intercourse appear to be maintained or improved after IPAA. This may be secondary to an overall improvement in health.
- IPAA is, however, associated with an infertility rate of ~40-50% vs ~15% for age-matched controls. This 3-fold increase in infertility after IPAA is likely secondary to adhesions and tubal infertility
- After IPAA, up to 30% of children are born after IVF treatment, compared with 1-2% in the general population i.e. 1/3 of females who get pregnant after IPAA, do so only after IVF
- Although there is clearly a reduction in fertility, the lifetime chance of a female with an IPAA having at least one live birth is 80%
- Consideration should be given to delaying surgery in women of child-bearing age when it is safe to do so
- There is some evidence that laparoscopic surgery may have a lesser impact on fertility compared to open surgery
- One-third of patients with an ileal pouch will experience disturbed bowel function, especially towards the end of the pregnancy

Crohn's disease
- Colonic and small bowel surgery in females with CD does not appear to have a negative impact on fertility
- Proctectomy in CD is associated with a reduction in fertility, although many choose not to become pregnant
- If surgery for CD is necessary during pregnancy, there is an increased risk of miscarriage, foetal and maternal mortality. The main indications for surgery are obstruction, acute fulminating colitis, bleeding and free perforation

Disease activity and pregnancy

Ideally, women should try and get pregnant when their disease is in remission as pregnancy can have a beneficial effect on disease activity. In contrast, up to two-thirds of those who conceive when the IBD is active experience a further relapse/deterioration during the subsequent pregnancy.
- Overall, pregnant women with UC are more likely to have active disease compared to those with CD. Theoretically, cessation of smoking during pregnancy may have a role in these changes
- Most patients with IBD have a normal pregnancy. However, women with severe active disease appear to have an increased risk of preterm birth, spontaneous abortion and still birth
- Other than methotrexate, most medications for IBD should be continued during pregnancy

- The coating of some mesalamine preparations (e.g. Asacol) contain dibutyl phylate which can cause abnormalities in males. These should be switched to a different mesalamine preparation
- Biological drugs should be stopped, if disease is in remission in the final trimester as they cross the placenta; joint discussions between the GI & obstetric teams is required in such cases

Pregnancy and Crohn's disease

- Up to 25% of patients with quiescent CD at conception will relapse during pregnancy. Relapse is most common in the first trimester and the puerperium
- Little is known of the likely outcome following a new diagnosis of CD during pregnancy. However, the outcome is thought to be generally poor, with miscarriage or still birth a possibility
- Vaginal delivery is generally safe unless there is active perianal disease when a caesarian section is almost always indicated

Pregnancy and ulcerative colitis

- Up to 1/3 of patients with chronic UC in remission will relapse (most commonly in the 1st trimester) during pregnancy
- One-third of patients with active disease will go into remission during pregnancy
- ~50% of those with active UC at conception will experience a deterioration in their symptoms, although surgery is rarely necessary
- In patients who relapse, medical treatment should be pursued if possible, ideally over 34 weeks gestation. Colectomy may not be necessary, but each case must be assessed on an individual basis
- It is fortunately rare to develop a first attack during pregnancy. If surgery is required there is a risk of fetal and maternal death
- Although it is possible to develop severe acute colitis in the puerperium, fortunately this is a rare event. If an emergency colectomy is necessary, this can be technically difficult because of a large uterus and engorged pelvic veins. The rectal stump should be left long and dissection in the pelvis avoided
- Vaginal delivery in patients with an IPAA appears to be safe, but despite this, up to 50% of patients have a caesarean section
- A vaginal delivery or caesarean section does not usually have a deleterious impact on IPAA function

References

Palomba S, Sereni G, Beltrami M et al. Inflammatory bowel diseases and human reproduction: A comprehensive evidence-based review. *World J Gastroent* 2014; **20**(3): 7123–7136

Benign colonic conditions

Diverticular disease: background

- *Diverticulosis* (colonic diverticulae in the absence of symptoms) is common in the Western world, with a rising incidence over the last century and in increasingly younger age groups
- Prevalence increases with age from 10% at 40yrs to 60–80% at 80yrs
- Recent studies suggest that 4% of patients with diverticulosis develop symptoms (ie. *diverticular disease*) and of these 15% develop complications
- Recent population studies from the UK and America suggest that the incidence of acute cute presentations with diverticulitis is increasing, particularly in younger patients
- Diverticulae form at the point where the terminal arterial branches penetrate the circular muscle adjacent to the taeniae coli and hence do not have a muscle layer (Fig. 5.1)
- Diverticulae usually form in the sigmoid colon but can affect the whole colon.

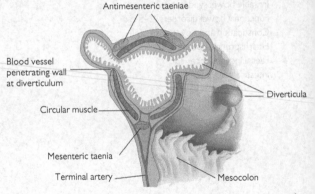

Fig. 5.1 Diverticulosis. Diverticulae form at the point where the terminal arterial branches penetrate the circular muscle adjacent to the taeniae coli.

Pathogenesis

- The pathogenesis has not yet been clearly defined
- The popular theory is that a low residue diet causes prolonged colonic transit and high segmental intraluminal pressures of up to 90mmHg
- High intraluminal pressure predisposes to herniation of mucosa at sites where the vasa recta passes through the muscle layer to supply the mucosa
- Diverticulae do not have a muscular covering which is consistent with an acquired process

- Diverticulae may be more common in the sigmoid colon as the narrower calibre predisposes to higher intraluminal segmental pressures (Laplace's Law)
- Hypertrophy of circular muscle and shortening of the longitudinal muscle with progressive accumulation of elastin causes bunching of the circular muscle and in-folding of the colonic wall giving a corrugated appearance. The cause for these wall abnormalities is unknown
- Pericolic inflammation may exaggerate wall thickening and luminal narrowing
- It has recently been postulated that a diet low in soluble fibre leads to altered intestinal microbiome and a change in bacterial flora, which in turn causes low grade inflammation of the mucosa, abnormal motility and a segmental colitis
- An increasing understanding that infection may not be the sole driver for diverticulitis. Inflammation may be driven by a proinflammatory cxytokine mediated response that may not always be best treated by antibiotic therapy
- The protective effect of fibre may be related to stool bulking reducing segmental pressures and maintaining luminal diameter.

Risk factors

- Diets low in fruit and vegetables and high in red meat ↑ symptoms
- NSAIDs, opioid analgesics and corticosteroids are associated with an increased risk of perforated colonic diverticular disease
- Hypertension, warfarin and aspirin are associated with a significantly increased risk of diverticular haemorrhage
- Central or visceral obesity is associated with a 2-fold increased risk of diverticulitis and 3-fold increased risk of diverticular haemorrhage
- Smoking is variably reported as a risk factor for complications.

References

Stollman N, Smalley W, Hirano I: American Gastroenterological Association Institute guideline on the management of acute diverticulitis. *Gastroenterology* 2015;**149**:1944–1949.

Morris AM, Regenbogen SE, Hardiman KM, Hendren S: Sigmoid diverticulitis: a systematic review. *JAMA* 2014;**311**:287–297.

Floch MH: A hypothesis: is diverticulitis a type of inflammatory bowel disease? *J Clin Gastroenterol* 2006;**40**(suppl 3):S121–S125.

Diverticular disease: presentation

Non-urgent presentation

- It is postulated that diverticular disease can be associated with pain without inflammation as a result of increased intraluminal pressure and reduced colonic wall compliance
- Diverticular disease can present at the clinic with lower abdominal pain, distension and altered bowel habit
- It will usually be diagnosed by colonoscopy in the process of trying to exclude neoplastic conditions
- It can cause similar symptoms to IBS and indeed there is overlap in theories of aetiology and conservative treatment
- Patients with symptomatic uncomplicated diverticular disease run a benign course with low incidence of subsequent complications (<2%).

Emergency presentation

Diverticulitis/abscess/peritonitis

- Infection of a diverticulum (*diverticulitis*) is thought to be caused by occlusion of its mouth with faecal material with subsequent bacterial proliferation in the closed space
- Acute diverticulitis generally presents with acute onset lower abdominal or left iliac fossa pain and fever
- Depending on the position and length of the sigmoid colon, diverticulitis can be confused with appendicitis, UTI and other infective conditions such as gastroenteritis and PID
- The degree of inflammation varies and there is a spectrum which ranges from cellulitis, localized perforation and pericolic abscess formation, generalized suppurative peritonitis through to faecal peritonitis which has been classified by Hinchey (Box 5.1)
- Rate of development of infection determines the sequelae, with slow-burning infection allowing time for adhesion of the inflamed bowel to surrounding structures which contains the infection locally or rapid development leading to perforation and generalized peritonitis
- Age-specific incidence of diverticular perforation has doubled in the past decade
- Small bowel may become involved in a diverticular inflammatory mass, resulting in enterocolic fistula or small bowel obstruction.

Box 5.1 Hinchey classification of diverticulitis

I Pericolic or mesenteric abscess/phlegmon
II Pelvic/remote intra-abdominal/retroperitoneal abscess
III Generalized purulent peritonitis
IV Generalized faeculent peritonitis

Fistula

- Fistula formation can occur between the inflamed diverticulum and any adjacent viscus. The most common fistulae are colovesical (usually posterior wall or dome of bladder) and colovaginal (vault of vagina, usually post-hysterectomy).

- Colovesical fistula presents with pneumaturia, recurrent UTI and faecaluria, while colovaginal fistulae present with faecal matter per vagina
- Fistula formation is relatively more common in young males
- Complex/multiple fistulae or recurrence after surgical treatment should raise the suspicion of co-existent CD.

Haemorrhage (➲ Acute colonic bleeding p.432)

- Haemorrhage can occur from a colonic diverticulum, presenting with dramatic PR bleeding
- Aetiology is unclear but thought to be due to rupture of vasa recta in apex of diverticulum possibly due to faecal trauma
- Bleeding is never into the abdominal cavity
- It is rarely associated with diverticulitis and hence is painless
- The colour of the bleeding depends on the location of the bleeding diverticulum (bright red if left sided, darker if right sided, the most commonly affected part).

Stricture

- Stricture formation can occur as a consequence of fibrosis following episodes of diverticulitis or pericolic abscess
- May present with lower abdominal pain and altered bowel habit, but can progress to acute LBO
- Colonoscopy may overestimate the severity of stricturing so contrast examination and correlation with symptoms is required before surgical intervention is considered.

Recurrence of complicated diverticulitis is estimated at 10–20% for patients who are admitted to hospital. The severity of attack and younger age increases the risk of recurrence.

Investigation

- Clinical assessment of patients with diverticulitis has a low sensitivity (50–70%) and thus most patients are diagnosed on CT
- Colonoscopy is usually only performed after a delayed interval to reduce the incidence of perforation and incomplete examination
- An elevated white cell count (WCC) and CRP will indicate the presence of infection
- Plain AXR and erect CXR may show bowel obstruction or a pneumoperitoneum from perforation
- Contrast studies have largely been superseded by CT. May be useful in defining fistulae or severity of strictures (Fig. 5.2)
- CT scan of the abdomen and pelvis is the most common imaging modality used to confirm the presence of acute diverticulitis. It is very sensitive and specific and can be used to grade severity. It contributes significantly to the management strategy including radiological drainage of abscesses. Air in the bladder on CT is diagnostic of fistula in the absence of instrumentation of the genitourinary tract (Fig. 5.3)
- US is occasionally used to identify collections, but its main use is as an assistant to radiological drainage of abscesses previously diagnosed on CT.

Differential diagnosis
- Differential diagnoses include appendicitis, IBD, ischaemic colitis, gastroenteritis, CRC, IBS and UTI.

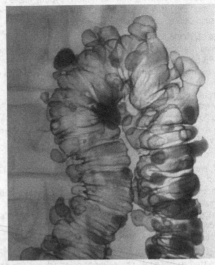

Fig. 5.2 Uncomplicated diverticular disease on barium enema.

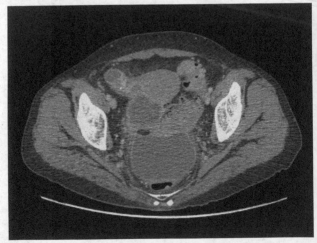

Fig. 5.3 Pelvic abscess. Loculated fluid-filled abscess with marked diverticular change in the adjacent sigmoid colon.

Diverticular disease: management

Diverticulosis

- High fibre diet or bulk laxatives prevent progression and may reduce development of diverticulitis, although strong evidence is lacking
- Resection for debilitating symptoms is occasionally indicated, but results are variable probably due to co-existent functional abnormalities. Patient selection is crucial to success.

Uncomplicated diverticulitis

- Mild symptoms and findings can be managed with oral antibiotics on an outpatient basis
- Outpatient treatment (+/- a short (< 24 hr) initial inpatient stay) and ongoing outpatient oral or IV antibiotics appears safe and has similar outcomes to inpatient treatment, but is less expensive
- More severe cases with pyrexia, peritonism and raised inflammatory markers require inpatient treatment with IV antibiotics
- Some studies report no benefit to antibiotic therapy in uncomplicated diverticulitis. A 2014 Cochrane review however concluded that there was insufficient evidence to recommend omitting antibiotics.
- In 2017, the American Gastroenterological Association recommended a selective individualised rather than routine use of antibiotics
- Although there is theoretical evidence that diverticulitis may be driven by inflammation rather than infection, there is no evidence that anti-inflammatory aminosalicyclate drugs (5 ASA) are superior to controls
- There is insufficient evidence to support the use of probiotics in preventing recurrent attacks
- Studies which have addressed alterations in the microbiome by treating with a combination of poorly absorbed antibiotics such as rifaximin fibre supplementation have reduced symptoms and complications for up to one year after the initial attack
- After recovery from an acute attack, long-term fibre supplementation may prevent recurrence in >70% of patients
- Colorectal cancer will be identified in ~1% of patients who undergo colonoscopy following an episode of uncomplicated diverticulitis and up to 11% of patients following complicated diverticulitis. The role of routine colonoscopy following uncomplicated diverticulitis is therefore debatable but should be considered for all following a complicated attack
- Following successful medical management of acute diverticulitis 1/3 will have a further attack, with 1/3 of these going on to have another attack. The decision to recommend elective surgery should be influenced by the general health of the patient, the frequency and severity of attacks and any persistent symptoms. Most patients who present with complicated diverticulitis do so during their first attack
- A laparoscopic approach is appropriate for elective sigmoid resection. A primary anastomosis is usually possible, although this may be combined with a defunctioning stoma.

Complicated diverticulitis

- Defined as diverticulitis associated with abscess, fistula, obstruction, bleeding or free intra-abdominal perforation.

Non-operative

- Abscesses 2–4cm in diameter usually resolve with IV antibiotics
- For larger abscesses CT- or US-guided drainage may prevent the need for surgery in the acute phase
- The majority of patients with complicated diverticulitis can be managed with non-operative or minimally invasive measures
- ASCRS (American Society of Colon and Rectal Surgeons) recommend elective resection of the affected colon after recovery from a conservatively managed diverticular abscess as 40% will otherwise develop severe recurrent sepsis.

Operative

- Emergency surgery is required in patients who fail to respond to conservative therapy or who have generalized peritonitis or obstruction
- Non randomised studies have reported that laparoscopy & washout for Hinchey grade 2 and 3 patients is successful in ~90% and avoids the need for resection or stoma. Recurrence of diverticulitis in the short term is low
- Randomised trials comparing laparoscopy & washout versus resection and stoma (Hartmann's procedure) have not shown a clear benefit for *either* strategy i.e. lower stoma rates but higher abscess and need for further surgery rates in the lavage & washout groups
- Hartmann's procedure is standard management for faecal peritonitis (➔ Hartmann's procedure p. 488)
- Operative mortality rate of Hartmann's procedure for diverticular perforation is >20% and up to 60% of patients who survive remain unfit for reversal of the colostomy because of advanced age and co-morbidity
- Primary anastomosis, with or without a diverting loop ileostomy, may be considered in selected fit patients with minimal peritoneal contamination, but it carries an increased risk of anastomotic leak
- Primary anastomosis is more commonly used for the treatment of fistulae and strictures. For fistulae to the bladder, bladder drainage for 5–7 days is all that is required. Vaginal defects should close spontaneously or can be closed primarily.

Natural history of diverticulitis

- ~85% of patients presenting with acute diverticulitis can be managed conservatively and do not have a further attack (although may have ongoing symptoms
- Contrary to previous thinking, those who present with 2 or more uncomplicated attacks are not thought to have a poorer long-term outcome
- Patients who present with complicated diverticulitis are at increased risk of further attacks, which may be of increased severity and as a consequence, up to 60% may ultimately require surgery

Elective surgery for diverticular disease

- 15–30% of patients will have recurrent attacks of diverticulitis and many will have ongoing low-grade diverticulitis
- Elective surgery is considered to either prevent further attacks to treat chronic symptoms
- Previous guidelines recommended resection after 2 attacks of diverticulitis or a single attack in younger patients. More recently, professional bodies have adopted an individual approach, in part because the disease does not tend to progress in severity of attacks and surgery is not without its complications
- Laparoscopic resection and primary anastomosis has been shown to significantly improve quality of life versus conservative management in patients with persistent symptoms or recurrent frequent episodes of diverticulitis

Diverticular haemorrhage

- Haemorrhage can be managed conservatively in the vast majority
- In persistent/exsanguinating haemorrhage, mesenteric angiography followed by superselective embolization/immediate resection can be used (➔ Acute colonic bleeding p. 390)
- Although colonoscopic adrenaline injection, endoclipping, band ligation and coagulation of bleeding points have been reported, it is difficult to obtain an adequate endoscopic view if bleeding is dramatic
- Colonoscopy is usually performed after bleeding has settled to exclude other causes of bleeding.

References

Morris AM, Regenbogen SE, Hardiman KM, Hendren S: Sigmoid diverticulitis: a systematic review. JAMA 2014;**311**:287–297.

Myers E, Hurley M, O'Sullivan GC, Kavanagh D, Wilson I, Winter DC. Laparoscopic peritoneal lavage for generalised peritonitis due to perforated diverticulitis. Br J Surg 2008;**95**:97–101.

Salem TA, Molloy RG, O'Dwyer PJ. Prospective, five-year follow-up study of patients with symptomatic uncomplicated diverticular disease. Dis Colon Rectum 2007;**50**:1–5.

Shah SD, Cifu AS: Management of acute diverticulitis. JAMA 2017; **318**:291–292.

Sharma PV, Eglinton T, Hider P, Frizelle F: Systematic review and meta-analysis of the role of routine colonic evaluation after radiologically confirmed acute diverticulitis. Ann Surg 2014;**259**:263–272.

Cirocchi R, Di Saverio S, Weber DG, Tabola R, Abraha I, Randolph J, et al: Laparoscopic lavage versus surgical resection for acute diverticulitis with generalised peritonitis: a systematic review and meta-analysis. Tech Coloproctol 2017;**21**:93–110.

Fozard JB, Armitage NC, Schofield JB, Jones OM: ACPGBI position statement on elective resection for diverticulitis. Colorectal Dis 2011; **13**:1–11.

Infectious diarrhoea

Introduction

Infections of the small bowel and colon form an important part of the differential diagnosis for acute or chronic diarrhoea ± rectal bleeding. This is particularly true in patients with a history of recent travel. Symptoms include fever, lower abdominal pain and tenesmus often relieved by a bowel movement/flatus.

The key to diagnosis is repeat stool cultures (shedding in certain infections is intermittent), microscopy of fresh stool specimens for ova, cysts and parasites, assays for toxins and serology (stool and serum) for specific pathogens. Despite investigation, in >30% of cases of infectious diarrhoea the pathogen will not be identified and the symptoms will be self-limiting.

Personal hygiene, clean water, sanitation, good housing and food hygiene for food-borne organisms are all important preventative measures.

Bacterial

Campylobacter

- Most common cause of diarrhoea in UK with *C. jejuni* and *C. coli*. the most common pathogenic subtypes
- Abdominal pain can be severe ± prodrome of fever, headache and nausea
- Usually affects small bowel but can cause colitis
- Major source is contaminated poultry, but unpasteurized milk and contaminated water have also been implicated
- Self-limiting, but erythromycin or ciprofloxacin can be used to reduce duration if severe disease.

E. coli

- Pathological strains are usually non-indigenous and include enteropathogenic (EPEC), enterotoxic (ETEC), enteroinvasive (EIEC), enteroaggregative and enterohaemorrhagic (*E. coli* O157:H7, EHEC)
- Incubation period is 1–3 days, with spread through contaminated food/water and person-person contact.
- EPEC/ETEC most common strains in infantile gastroenteritis
- ETEC strains are the most common cause of Travellers' diarrhoea on arrival in a country usually due to polluted water
- Certain toxin-producing strains, e.g. O157, produce haemorrhagic syndromes which can be life-threatening. Usually due to infected beef
  - Haemorrhagic colitis may affect children or adults
  - Haemolytic–uraemic syndrome (HUS) affects mainly children, leading to thrombocytopenia, haemolytic anaemia and renal failure (uraemia)
  - HUS develops in up to 10% of children infected with O157 preceded by diarrhoea which may be bloody
- EIEC shares similar pathogenesis with *Shigella* dysentery
- Rehydration and supportive management is the mainstay of treatment. with antibiotic therapy rarely required.

Salmonella

- Typically spread by faecal–oral route, outbreaks are associated with infected eggs, dairy products and meat
- Symptoms are often mild, but asymptomatic carriage possible
- *Salmonella typhi* and *paratyphi* cause enteric fever (*S. paratyphi* is the milder form)
- Antibiotics should be avoided if possible, to avoid drug resistance and prolonging carrier status. Rigorous food hygiene, cooking of potentially infected foods and good personal hygiene avoid spread.

Shigella

- *Shigella* species include *S. dysentriae* (severe dysentery in tropical countries), *S. sonnei* (70–90% cases in developed countries), *S. flexneri* (60% cases worldwide) and *S. boydii*
- Invasive organism leading to cell death, mucosal ulceration particularly in the distal colon and bleeding with toxin-mediated diarrhoea. Severe disease can cause obstruction, megacolon and perforation
- *Shigella* can produce toxins (Shiga toxin) similar to verotoxin of *E. coli* leading to HUS
- Sonné dysentery (90% UK cases) usually mild affecting children. Self-limiting, but ampicillin or ciprofloxacin can be used in severe cases.

Yersinia

- Includes *Y. enterocolitica* and *Y. pseudotuberculosis*
- Carriers include birds, domestic and wild animals with worldwide distribution, but particularly countries with cooler climates.
- Rarer cause of diarrhoea lasting up to 3 weeks but can cause symptoms which mimic appendicitis with mesenteric lymphadenopathy ± acute terminal ileitis
- Stool or blood culture may confirm diagnosis or mesenteric LN if laparotomy has been performed
- Post-infectious complications include erythema nodosum and reactive arthritis lasting months
- Usually self-limiting but if septicaemia develops (immunocompromised) mortality rates are high despite antibiotic therapy.

Staphylococcus aureus and Clostridium perfringens are also important causes of 'food poisoning'. For C. difficile, see ➔ Clostridium difficile p. 208.

Viral

The most common cause of acute GI infections, most viruses affect the upper GI tract and small intestine. These include norovirus, rotavirus, astrovirus, adenovirus and small round viruses. CMV and HSV colitis is rare and typically found in immunocompromised hosts (see later).

Parasitic

Entamoeba histolytica

- Most common cause of parasitic colitis, transmission is from contaminated water or person–person spread, with increased prevalence in developing countries
- Cysts are ingested, becoming trophozoites in the large bowel which multiply, encyst and pass in faeces. Can remain viable for months

- Invasion of organisms can occur years after the initial asymptomatic infection
- Symptoms include abdominal pain and bloody diarrhoea with flask-shaped mucosal ulceration affecting particularly the right colon
- Severe amoebic colitis can lead to fulminant necrotizing colitis and perforation
- Other complications include stricture, rectovaginal fistula, perianal ulceration, luminal mass (ameboma) and bowel obstruction
- Dissemination through portal system can lead to amoebic liver abscess usually in the right lobe (diarrhoea rarely concomitant)
- Treatment of asymptomatic disease is with paromomycin which is not absorbed from the intestinal tract. Invasive disease is treated with metronidazole followed by paromomycin to eradicate luminal carriage.

Giardia lamblia
- Flagellated protozoan with global distribution
- Usual source is contaminated fresh water or faecal–oral spread
- Parasite is confined to the small bowel, causing diarrhoea with fatty stools, abdominal cramps, bloating, flatulence and weight loss
- Metronidazole is the recommended treatment.

Strongyloides stercoralis (threadworm)
- Prevalence is highest in the tropics and subtropics and where sanitation is poor
- Larvae enter host through the skin, passing through the circulation to the lung where they are coughed up and swallowed, parasitizing the small intestine
- Symptoms include dermatitis, coughing, wheezing, abdominal discomfort and watery diarrhoea or can be asymptomatic in up to 50%
- In the immunocompromised host disease can be severe, with hyperinfection leading to ileus/obstruction, GI bleeding and superadded bacterial infection. Mortality in this condition is high
- Mebendazole or ivermectin are used for treatment.

Schistosomiasis
- Most prevalent in Asia, Africa and South America with ~200 million affected worldwide
- Infective species include *S. mansoni*, *S. japonicum* (intestinal) and *S. haematobium* (urinary)
- Infection is through fresh water contaminated by excreta of infected individuals. Eggs hatch and develop in snails then re-enter the water where they penetrate through the skin of the host. Eggs then travel through the circulation to the bladder or intestines via lungs and liver
- May be subclinical or cause anaemia, malnutrition, abdominal pain, diarrhoea, cough, fever and learning difficulties in children
- Chronic infection can lead to fibrosis of affected organ with portal/pulmonary hypertension, cystitis, glomerulonephritis
- Treatment is with praziquantel.

Diarrhoea in immunocompromised/HIV

A wide spectrum of bacterial, viral, parasitic and fungal pathogens can cause diarrhoea in the immunocompromised host. Some of the more important causes are listed below.

Cryptosporidium
- Caused by a coccidial parasite. *C. hominis* and *C. parvum* are most common in humans
- Infects domestic animals and livestock with transmission through contaminated water
- Diarrhoea in children or immunocompromised can last 2–8 weeks
- In HIV, disease can be severe and life-threatening with extreme weight loss
- Anti-retroviral treatment may reduce severity in HIV-infected patients but does not clear parasites. Evidence-based treatment is lacking.

CMV
- Infection is widespread (up to 90%) but asymptomatic in the immunocompetent
- Transmission is through contact with infected body fluids, making personal hygiene an important preventative measure
- Reactivation can cause repeated infection in transplant and HIV-infected patients
- Presentations include retinitis, hepatitis and pneumonia
- CMV colitis leads to diarrhoea and GI bleeding, with the caecum most commonly affected (can affect from mouth to anus)
- Ganciclovir is first-line treatment.

Mycobacterium avium-intracellulare
- Disseminated life-threatening infection can occur in immunocompromised patients
- Symptoms include fever, night sweats, weight loss, shortness of breath, diarrhoea, RUQ pain
- Incidence has declined with highly active anti-retroviral treatment (HAART)
- Treatment includes rifambutin, ethambutol and clarithromycin.

HIV enteropathy
- Functional and pathological changes with no identifiable infectious pathogen or malignancy
- Pathogenesis unclear but may be due to direct action of the virus itself.

Clostridium difficile

Background

Clostridium difficile is a Gram-positive spore-forming anaerobic bacillus. It is the most common cause of diarrhoea in the hospitalized patient, although it is not solely a hospital-acquired problem.

- 20% of cases of antibiotic-associated diarrhoea (AAD) are caused by *C. difficile* infection (CDI).
- The most important risk factors are recent antibiotic use and hospital admission, although 1/3 of patients have neither risk factor
- 20% of cases of CDI become recurrent (RCDI)
- Incidence, mortality and recurrence are increasing due to a hypervirulent strain ribotype 027 (BI/NAP1/027).
- Prevalence increases with duration of hospital admission
- Community sources include domestic and farm animals.

Pathogenesis

- Colonization due to exogenous infection with spores (faecal–oral spread) and alteration of normal bowel flora
- Altered bowel flora due to antibiotics (especially broad spectrum)
- Risk factors include GI surgery, immunosuppression and old age
- Possible link with increased PPI use due to increasing gastric pH
- Infection with a toxigenic strain causes either asymptomatic carriage or colonic symptoms
- *C. difficile* produces two protein exotoxins, (TcdA & TcdB) which disrupt epithelial tight junctions with loss of gut barrier function and cytokine induction, leading to cell death and apoptosis.

Presentation

- Mild symptoms consist of watery diarrhoea ± abdominal pain
- Severe symptoms include systemic upset: fever, malaise, nausea
- Toxic megacolon with paralytic ileus can present with abdominal distension and minimal diarrhoea
- Fulminant colitis develops in up to 5% with a mortality rate of >50%
- Inflammatory markers may be raised with a low albumin
- Perforation may present with generalized peritonitis
- If recurrent, symptoms usually recur within 1 week.

Investigations

- Enzyme immunoassay for toxins or DNA-based tests to identify microbial toxin genes in unformed stool establishes the diagnosis
- DNA-based tests are more sensitive and specific for toxigenic strains (but may over diagnose clinically insignificant infections)
- Endoscopy is rarely required but may help distinguish overlapping conditions such as inflammatory bowel disease
- Characteristic histological and endoscopic appearances with pseudomembrane (inflammatory exudates) and focal ulceration
- Plain radiology may be useful for the diagnosis and monitoring of patients with acute colitis

Management of CDI

- Rates can be reduced through antibiotic prescribing protocols
  - Use narrow-spectrum antibiotics where possible
  - Prophylaxis should be single dose
  - Limit the duration of antibiotics
- Pharmacy input at ward level to review prescribing
- Infection control policies should be in place and local guidelines followed
- Prompt isolation of cases with barrier nursing
- Strict hand hygiene with soap and water as spores are resistant to alcohol gel
- Cleaning of equipment/wards is difficult as spores are resistant to disinfectants
- Surveillance at local and national level (mandatory for over 65s in UK).

Treatment of CDI and RCDI

- Stopping antibiotics can lead to resolution in mild disease
- Although oral metronidazole has traditionally been used for first line therapy, a number of authors now suggest oral vancomycin as first line therapy
- If metronidazole is used first, switch to oral vancomycin if no response after 3 days
- Increased efficacy of vancomycin may be offset by cost and risk of vancomycin-resistant enterococci
- Avoid anti-motility agents which may reduce toxin clearance
- Resistant or recurrent cases may respond to higher doses, pulsed doses or fidaxomicin
- Antibiotic stewardship and local microbiology/infection control protocols are essential to control CDI
- *Lactobacillus GG* + *S. boulardii* found in probiotic yoghurt in combination with antibiotics can reduce rates of recurrent disease
- Faecal transplant via NG tube, enemas or at colonoscopy has been reported to reduce rates of recurrent disease
- Surgery is reserved for severe or uncontrolled disease manifest by toxic megacolon, perforation, haemodynamic compromise, immunosuppression, increasing leucocytosis and failure of medical therapy
- Total colectomy is the procedure of choice but associated with mortality rates of up to 80%.

Future strategies

- Newer cleaning methods/agents under investigation
- Newer antibiotics such as fidaxomicin, teicoplanin and rifaximin have shown efficacy
- Use of narrow spectrum antibiotics with high stool concentration to preserve normal flora
- Faecal microbial transplantation has a role, especially in recurrent infections and more recently in severe primary disease
- Oral/IV anti-toxin antibody preparations are being studied
- Vaccines containing toxin A + B may have a role

Mesenteric ischaemia

The GI tract receives 20% of cardiac output which increases 2-fold following a meal. Mesenteric ischaemia occurs when blood supply is insufficient to meet metabolic demand. Intracellular acidosis results in the release of free radicals and activated enzymes which cause cell death and tissue necrosis. Bacterial translocation and systemic inflammatory response syndrome (SIRS) can develop from loss of gut barrier function. Women in their 7th decade are most commonly affected.

Acute mesenteric ischaemia (AMI)

Embolic (~50%)

• Sudden severe abdominal pain with few clinical findings
• Associated with fever and faecal occult blood (FOB)+ve stools in a minority of cases
• Sources include left atrium (supraventricular arrhythmias), left ventricle (post-myocardial infarction), peripheral or coronary circulation (catheterization), thoracic aorta (following surgery)
• Most commonly affects the SMA territory.

Arterial thrombosis (~30%)

• May be preceded by chronic symptoms of atherosclerotic disease.

Venous thrombosis (~15%)

• Impedes arterial outflow leading to oedema and subsequent necrosis
• Causes include cirrhosis, intra-abdominal sepsis, pancreatitis, malignancy and clotting disorders, e.g. anti-thrombin III (ATIII), protein C/S deficiency and factor V Leiden

Non-occlusive

• 2° to low flow states including shock, cardiac failure, arrhythmias and vasopressor use
• Treatment should be directed to reversal of the low flow state.

Chronic mesenteric ischaemia (CMI)

• Presents with post-prandial pain and weight loss
• Occurs when atherosclerotic disease affects ≥2 vessels (Fig. 5.4)
• Single vessel disease can be symptomatic when vascular anatomy is altered (bowel resection/aneurysm repair)
• Asymptomatic disease (stenosis >50%) is present in at least 1/5 of those >65yrs and is not an indication for intervention
• Less common causes include vasculitides and fibromuscular dysplasia.

Investigations

• Diagnosis dependent on high index of suspicion and is often delayed
• ↑ WCC, amylase and lactate are non-specific late changes
• Duplex accurate for proximal stenoses/occlusion but limited by operator variability, body habitus and overlying bowel gas
• MR angiography and multislice CT increasingly used
• Selective angiography remains the gold standard and allows regional perfusion with vasodilator therapy
• A cut-off, usually in the SMA, without collateralization is diagnostic.

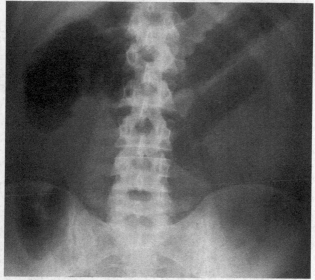

Fig. 5.4 Ischaemic colitis. Thumb printing of the wall of the transverse colon related to mucosal oedema in the watershed zone secondary to ischaemia.

Treatment

Medical

- Fluid resuscitation with broad-spectrum antibiotics
- Regional vasodilator infusion ± heparinization may improve survival if signs of bowel infarction are absent
- Papaverine (phosphodiesterase inhibitor) increases cAMP leading to vascular smooth muscle relaxation. 90% first-pass metabolism avoids systemic side effects
- Anti-coagulation with heparin/warfarin should commence 48h after surgery with the optimum duration a matter for debate
- Drugs to inhibit reperfusion injury are a focus of ongoing research.

Endoluminal

- Thrombolysis with tissue plaminogen activator (tPA), suction embolectomy and basket clot retrieval have all been described, following which angioplasty/stent insertion can be considered (Fig. 5.5)
- Outcomes are currently inferior to surgery but may be useful for high risk patients as procedural mortality is reduced
- Stent patency <70% at 5yrs with recurrent symptoms in ~50%
- Patency increased by use of anti-platelet therapy.

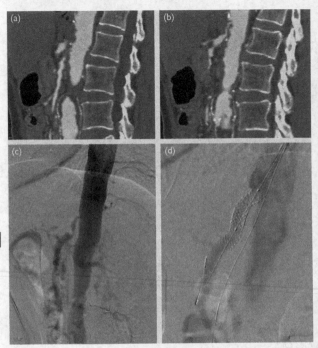

Fig. 5.5 Mesenteric artery stenting for ischaemia.

Surgery
- Surgery is focused on restoration of flow and limiting resection of non-viable bowel
- Testing viability is problematic. Visual assessment, palpation of pulses, fluorescein dye testing and Doppler assessment have all been proposed
- Revascularization should be attempted where there is reversible ischaemia and before any intestinal resection.
- By-pass (± embolectomy/endarterectomy) may be single or multiple, antegrade (supracoeliac aorta) or retrograde (iliac artery) by-pass with autologous or synthetic material (Fig. 5.6)
- No single strategy has been shown to be superior
- Second-look laparotomy may be required to reassess small bowel viability
- Graft patency of 80–90% and symptom recurrence in <30% reported
- Mortality from acute presentation still 60–90%, with many unsuitable for revascularization
- Extensive bowel resection may lead to short gut syndrome and permanent home parenteral nutrition (HPN) (➔ Intestinal failure p.264).

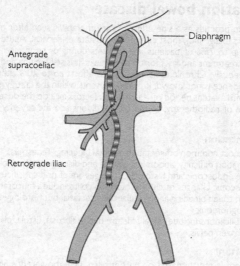

Fig. 5.6 By-pass for mesenteric ischaemia.

Radiation bowel disease

Radiation proctitis as a side effect of radiotherapy is seen after treatment for pelvic malignancy, most commonly prostate or cervical. Acute proctitis affects up to 75% of patients and presents during or soon after completion of treatment and lasts for up to 6 weeks. It is self-limiting and resolves spontaneously. Chronic radiation proctitis affects up to 20% although the true incidence is not known. It usually presents within the first 2yrs but can occur with a latent period of >10yrs. Risk factors include the dose and distribution of radiotherapy, co-morbid conditions and the severity of acute proctitis.

Presentation

- The most common presentation is rectal bleeding. Tenesmus, evacuation difficulty, abdominal cramps and diarrhoea may also feature
- Acute endoscopic and histological changes are of non-specific colitis
- Endoscopic changes of chronic radiation colitis include mucosal pallor, touch bleeding and vascular telangiectasia, but histology is not pathognomonic
- Complications include rectal stricture due to fibrosis, fistula, obstruction and frozen pelvis.

Treatment

Treatment is mostly based on uncontrolled, underpowered, single-centre studies. Minor symptoms may resolve spontaneously. Medical treatment is often unsatisfactory but may be used as first-line due to low risk of side effects and increased availability.

- Stool softeners, anti-diarrhoeals, anti-spasmodics and sitz baths may complement therapy
- 5-ASAs and hydrocortisone enemas are commonly used, but with equivocal results
- Sucralfate orally (2g tid) or by enema may be of benefit
- Metronidazole can be added if bacterial overgrowth is suspected
- Cholestyramine can be used for bile acid malabsorption where ileal involvement aggravates diarrhoea
- Short chain fatty acid (SCFA) enemas do not appear to be useful
- APC and heater probe thermocoagulation are less costly and with fewer side effects than laser. Repeated sessions are usually required (~3–5), with complications including stricture, fistula, ulceration and perforation
- Topical formalin causes chemical cauterization by direct application (4% solution for ~1 min) or instillation with response rates of 70–90%. Complications are reduced with direct application but include diarrhoea, tenesmus, incontinence to liquid and fever
- Hyperbaric oxygen promotes angiogenesis and has shown a disease-modulating effect. Treatment is expensive and cumbersome, with up to 40 sessions lasting 60–120 min
- Surgery is reserved for refractory or complicated cases. Morbidity is high, with options including stoma formation, coloanal resection/anastomosis.

Colitis—other

Microscopic colitis

The syndrome consists of chronic watery diarrhoea without abnormal colonoscopy findings. Symptoms may last >6 months but often relapse and remit over years. A chronic inflammatory cell infiltrate is seen in colonic mucosa but crypt architecture usually unchanged. TI may be affected.

Pathogenesis is unknown but thought to be due to an abnormal immune response to dietary or bacterial antigens. Bile acid malabsorption may be a 2° feature, with genetic factors thought to play a role.

10% of patients with non-bloody diarrhoea will have microscopic colitis on biopsy. Within this diagnosis 2 separate entities have been described.

Collagenous colitis

- Chronic inflammatory cell infiltrate in lamina propria & subepithelial collagen deposition forming a thickened band on microscopy (>10μm)
- Female to male ratio ~8:1 with median onset in the 6th decade
- 40% associated with other conditions including coeliac, thyroid disease, diabetes mellitus, rheumatoid arthritis, scleroderma and NSAID use
- Budesonide induces remission in ~85% with high relapse rate within 3 months and especially in patients <60yrs
- Mesalazine ± cholestyramine have also shown some efficacy.

Lymphocytic colitis

- Increased intraepithelial lymphocytes (>20/100 epithelial cells + predominantly T cells) with no increase in collagen deposition
- Stronger association with coeliac disease with 1/4 patients affected
- Randomized data lacking but budesonide/mesalazine used first-line
- Stronger immunosuppressives should be reserved for refractory cases.

Neutropenic enterocolitis (typhlitis/ileocaecal syndrome)

- Condition typically affecting patients undergoing chemotherapy for haematological malignancies but also recognized in patients having high dose chemotherapy for solid organ malignancies and with AIDS
- Incidence thought to be ~5% within this group
- Probably multifactorial due to mucosal injury from cytotoxic drugs, neutropenia and impaired host defense to colonizing bacteria
- Neutropenic patients present with fever, abdominal pain particularly in the right iliac fossa ± peritoneal signs
- Time delay following chemotherapy is often 10–14 days
- May present with signs of GI bleeding, obstruction or perforation
- Caecum is most commonly involved site, with CT showing bowel wall thickening, fluid-filled caecum and inflammatory changes in right lower quadrant. Features of complications may be present, e.g. free air or pneumatosis intestinales.
- Conservative management advised with broad-spectrum antibiotics and granulocyte colony-stimulating factor (G-CSF) to ↑ WCCs
- Two-stage right hemicolectomy is standard surgical management
- Mortality is >50% usually due to perforation and sepsis.

Diversion colitis

- Inflammation of the distal intestinal tract following surgical diversion of the faecal stream
- Probably related to deficiency of SCFAs which is the primary luminal cell nutrient source
- Diffuse mucosal chronic inflammatory infiltrate with lymphoid follicular hyperplasia seen in the majority of defunctioned patients
- Only 5–30% will experience symptoms of bleeding, mucus or pain
- Restoration of intestinal continuity leads to a rapid resolution of symptoms. Butyrate or SCFA enemas have no proven efficacy.

Collagen-vascular colitis

Chronic inflammatory autoimmune disorders lead to immune complex deposition in blood vessel walls affecting a range of different organs including the GI tract. Presentations range from constipation, incontinence and pseudo-obstruction to bleeding, ischaemia and perforation. Conservative management should be first-line treatment, with surgical intervention avoided where possible. Anastomosis is not advised following resection, with mortality rates >50%.

Scleroderma
- 50% of patients will have colonic involvement
- Smooth muscle is replaced by fibrotic tissue due to collagen deposition leading to chronic colonic dilatation.
- Laxatives can be effective. Incontinence may respond to biofeedback.

Systemic lupus erythematosus
- Patients with SLE present with pseudo-obstruction or ischaemic colitis
- Despite GI vasculitis, angiograms are usually normal and diagnosis often confirmed only after operation for complications of haemorrhage, infarction or perforation.

Dermatomyositis
- Dermatomyositis carries an increased risk of intestinal malignancy presenting in ~20% with the majority arising in the colon
- Screening should be offered.
- Colonic manifestations of constipation, dilatation and pneumatosis intestinales should be managed with immunosuppressives if possible.

Behcet's disease
- Presents as either mucosal ulceration/colitis or mesenteric ischaemia
- Patients usually are known to have Behcet's and present with vomiting, diarrhoea and right iliac fossa pain, with the ileocaecal region most commonly affected
- Immunosuppressives are the mainstay of treatment.

Polyarteritis nodosa
- GI involvement usually signifies poor prognosis with 50% developing an acute abdomen
- Rapidly progressive arteritis leads to infarction/perforation
- Aneurysmal dilation and rupture of mesenteric vessels can lead to massive intraperitoneal haemorrhage.

Colonic volvulus

This is a condition in which part of the colon becomes twisted on its mesenteric axis, resulting in partial or complete obstruction and a variable degree of impairment of the blood supply to the affected segment. The sigmoid colon is most frequently affected (70–75%) while other sites include caecum (25%) and, rarely, transverse colon (<5%).

In patients who develop sigmoid volvulus, the sigmoid colon appears elongated, with a long floppy mesentery and narrow parietal attachment. Caecal volvulus involves the ascending colon and ileum and is often associated with a mobile caecum.

Background

- Incidence 1–2 in 100,000 in developed world
- Accounts for <5% of intestinal obstruction in developed countries but up to 50% in developing countries
- Average age at presentation is 60–70yrs (younger for transverse colon).

Risk factors

- Chronic constipation
- Institutionalization
- Neuropsychiatric conditions (psychotropic drugs may affect intestinal motility)
- Adhesions/previous surgery
- Malrotation
- Other conditions include Chagas' disease, Hirchsprung's, pregnancy, distal obstruction or megacolon of any cause.

Clinical features

- May present as acute or intermittent obstruction and can be difficult to distinguish clinically from other causes of colonic obstruction
- Abdominal pain, vomiting and absolute constipation
- The abdomen is distended and tympanitic and in cachectic patients the volved segment may be visible through the abdominal wall (Fig. 5.7)
- Severe pain and peritonism with tachycardia and hypotension are ominous signs as they may represent colonic ischaemia with impending infarction and perforation
- A history of recurrent episodes is present in half of patients.

Diagnosis

- Plain AXR shows a grossly distended sigmoid loop extending towards the RUQ (or LUQ/midabdomen with caecal volvulus), taking the form of a 'bent inner tube' (Fig. 5.8)
- Contrast enema may show a 'bird's beak' deformity
- CT scan of the abdomen may show a characteristic mesenteric whorl The 'coffee bean' and 'bird's beak' signs can also be recognized
- When distension is massive radiology may be inconclusive
- A significant proportion of patients are diagnosed at laparotomy (Fig. 5.9).

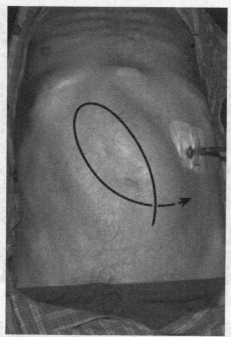

Fig. 5.7 Sigmoid volvulus.

Management

- The patient should be resuscitated, as necessary.

Non-operative decompression

- The sigmoid colon can be de-rotated by passing a rectal tube carefully and under vision through a proctoscope or rigid sigmoidoscope
- There should be a rush of gas and liquid faeces (usually within 20cm of the anal verge), with a rapid decrease in abdominal distension
- The flatus tube is taped to the thigh and left *in situ* for 24–48h
- Colonoscopic detorsion has the advantage of visualization of the point of rotation, an assessment of the viability of the volved segment and excludes stricturing pathology as the cause of the volvulus
- Success rates of ~80% are reported.

Emergency surgery

Indications

- Signs of peritonitis/perforation
- Ischaemia of the mucosa visible at colonoscopy
- Failed decompression by flatus tube or colonoscopy.

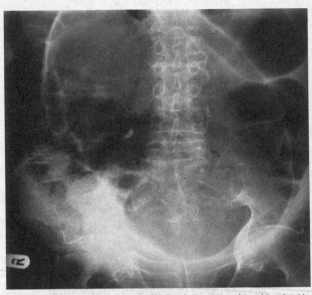

Fig. 5.8 Large bowel dilatation with 'coffee bean'-shaped viscus lying obliquely with its axis running from the left iliac fossa to RUQ in the line of the sigmoid mesentery.

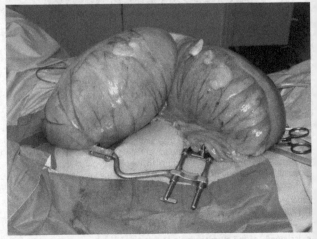

Fig. 5.9 Sigmoid volvulus operative view.

Procedure
- At laparotomy, the colon should be de-rotated if viable, decompressed and then resected
- If ischaemia is present early vascular isolation without detorsion avoids worsening bacteraemia
- The decision to perform a primary anastomosis or Hartmann's procedure is dictated by operative findings and the fitness of the patient
- In general, this is a frail population with significant co-morbidity and a Hartmann's procedure is recommended, particularly if there is ischaemia or peritoneal contamination
- Operative mortality ranges from 20-50%

Elective surgery
- If the volvulus can be decompressed by non-operative means consideration should be given to performing elective surgery as recurrence rates are high (up to 50%)
- An elective approach allows optimization of a frail patient
- Sigmoid colectomy can be performed through a midline laparotomy, small left transverse incision or using a laparoscopic-assisted technique
- A variety of fixation/pexy procedures have been described but recurrence rates are generally higher than for resection
- Percutaneous sigmoid fixation is also described. It has not entered mainstream practice because of complications causing significant morbidity, e.g. abdominal wall sepsis, persistent fistula, displacement.

References

Cartwright-Terry T. Phillips S. Greenslade GL. Dixon AR. Laparoscopy in the management of closed loop sigmoid volvulus. *Colorectal Dis* 2008;**10**:370–372.

Baraza W. Brown S. McAlindon M. Hurlstone P. Prospective analysis of percutaneous endoscopic colostomy at a tertiary referral centre. *Br J Surg* 2007;**94**:1415–1420.

Vascular malformations

Vascular malformations may present as an incidental finding or can be responsible for life-threatening haemorrhage.

Classification

Haemangiomas
- These are hamartomas rather than neoplastic lesions
- Vascular stroma is dilated with an increased volume
- Abnormal vessels are intramural and submucosal and may be described as capillary, cavernous or mixed
- They are non-progressive lesions
- In capillary haemangiomas, the vessels are not dilated and resemble normal capillaries. There may be a familial history
- Cavernous haemangiomas have large endothelial lined sinuses.

Angiomas
- These are true vascular neoplasms and are exceedingly rare
- They may be malignant or benign.

Arteriovenous malformations (AVMs)
- These are the most frequently identified lesion.

Type 1
- Angiodysplasia are acquired AVMs which appear with ageing
- They are more common in the right colon.

Type 2
- Congenital lesions.

Type 3
- Found in patients with a hereditary predisposition such as hereditary haemorrhagic telangectasia.

Colorectal varices
- These are permanently dilated tortuous veins in the submucosa
- 50% are due to portal hypertension.

Cavernous haemangioma

A rare, non-hereditary congenital anomaly. Most lesions consist of single mass of dilated vessels at the rectosigmoid junction, possibly extending out to the pelvic side wall. Can extend into the mesorectum or involve other organs, e.g. the bladder, vagina or uterus. Lesions are comprised of dilated vascular channels with endothelial lining, surrounded by smooth muscle and elastic fibres. May be thrombus formation or calcification.

Presentation
- Fresh red, painless rectal bleeding often beginning at an early age
- Investigation with colonoscopy/proctoscopy initially. Anal canal and distal rectum must be carefully viewed, as lesions can extend to anal canal
- Colonoscopy useful to define proximal extent/identify satellite lesions
- Plain AXR may show a cluster of phleboliths
- Appears as a compressible blue/purple lesion which may be polypoid or flat. Do not biopsy!

- Endoscopic US may show thickening of the bowel wall with hyperechoic tubular channels
- MRI appearances are diagnostic and important in defining the extent of the lesion when planning treatment.

Treatment

- Treatment is by resection. Low anterior resection may be necessary and can be difficult due to haemorrhage, fibrosis or organ involvement
- If the lesion is small and polypoid, endoscopic dissection by snare diathermy may be appropriate.

Angiodysplasia

- Incidence rises with age occurring in up to 25% by age 60yrs
- Thought to be the most common cause of major colorectal bleeding
- Majority of lesions in right colon but can occur anywhere in GI tract
- Lesions thought to develop 2° to obstruction of submucosal veins by contraction of colonic wall smooth muscle. Obstruction leads to dilation of the arterio-venous units in surrounding crypts
- Alternative theory suggests lesions 2° to repeated episodes of ischaemia
- Histologically difficult to identify unless specific specimen preparation performed. Consist of dilated thin-walled mucosal/submucosal veins.

Presentation

- Typical presentation is an elderly patient with profuse painless fresh/altered rectal bleeding. In the majority bleeding stops spontaneously
- Barium enema is unhelpful. It will either be normal or show coincidental diverticular change
- Colonoscopic appearances are of a small discrete raised lesion with visible vessels. They bleed easily
- Endoscopic ablation may be performed using electrocoagulation, laser or APC.

Colorectal varices

- Anorectal varices can cause severe life-threatening bleeding.
- Varices can also be present in the small bowel and colon
- Majority due to portal hypertension. Other predisposing conditions include congestive cardiac failure, mesenteric vein thrombosis and chronic pancreatitis with splenic vein thrombosis
- Appearances are similar to varices elsewhere in the GI tract
- Upper GI endoscopy is mandatory to exclude a proximal source of blood loss
- Lesions are best seen by inspection with a proctoscope or rigid sigmoidoscope. Insufflation of air at colonoscopy may make the diagnosis difficult by flattening the veins
- Treatment requires urgent correction of coagulopathy and pharmacological reduction of portal pressure. If varices are confined to the distal rectum, control by under-running is possible.

Irritable bowel syndrome

Introduction

IBS is a chronic, functional bowel disorder, characterized by chronic recurring abdominal pain or discomfort and altered bowel function not sustained by structural changes. The condition should be differentiated from functional abdominal pain syndrome (no alteration in bowel function) and from chronic functional constipation and chronic functional diarrhoea, which are not associated with pain and discomfort.

IBS has a prevalence of 10–15% and is one of the more common reasons for presentation to primary care, colorectal surgery and gastroenterology services. Symptoms frequently date back to childhood or teenage years and the female:male ratio is 2:1. Later onset symptoms may be related to the development of post-infectious IBS which affects 10% of patients after bacterial or viral enteric infections.

Pathophysiology

The aetiology of IBS has not been elucidated but is likely to be multifactorial. There is a strong association between symptoms of IBS and stress, both at initial presentation and with subsequent exacerbations. The incidence is higher in those who seek healthcare and in those with psychosocial factors including primary anxiety, somatization, depression and symptom-related anxiety. Around 50% of IBS patients who seek medical care are depressed or suffer from anxiety and there is a heightened association with suicidal attempts and ideation.

Although the pathophysiology remains unclear, increased perception of visceral stimuli may contribute to abdominal pain. In some, there may be an alteration in GI motility and the balance between secretion and absorption. This may be mediated by deregulation of the gut-based serotonin signaling system.

Post-infectious IBS may be secondary to the persistence of a mild inflammatory response (T cells and mast cells) and enterochromaffin cell hyperplasia, as well as increased mucosal permeability. Inflammatory cells release mediators (e.g. histamine, proteases and cytokines) and enterochromaffin cells release 5-HT. These affect the enteric nervous system and smooth muscle activity, leading to intestinal motor dysfunction. These mediators may also interact with sensory afferents to evoke increased sensory perception.

Evaluation

A diagnosis of IBS can be reached by taking a careful history, performing a general examination and performing routine blood tests in patients who satisfy the Rome criteria (Box 5.2) and who do not have any warning signs. Warning signs include rectal bleeding, weight loss, anaemia, family history of colon cancer, onset after 45yrs of age and a major change in symptoms. The differential diagnosis for those without warning signs includes coeliac disease, atypical CD and microscopic and collagenous colitis.

IBS may be characterized on the basis of predominant bowel habit into IBS with predominant constipation (IBS-C; more common in females), IBS with predominant diarrhoea (IBS-D; more common in males) and IBS with mixed bowel function. Each group accounts for ~1/3 of all patients. Pain and bloating may predominate in others.

Box 5.2 The Rome IV criteria for diagnosing IBS

Recurrent abdominal pain, on average, at least 1 day/week in the last 3 months, associated with two or more of the following criteria:
- Related to defecation
- Associated with a change in frequency of stool
- Associated with a change in form (appearance) of stool

Criteria fulfilled for the last 3 months with symptoms onset at least 6 months before diagnosis.

Source: Data from Drossman DA. Functional Gastrointestinal Disorders: History, Pathophysiology, Clinical Features and Rome IV. *Gastroenterology* 2016;150:1262–1279.

Management

Most patients with mild symptoms settle with sympathetic reassurance and symptomatic management aimed at reducing pain and regulating bowel function. Cognitive-behavioural therapy (CBT) and the use of other drugs including low dose tricyclics should be considered in patients with severe ongoing symptoms.

Constipation

- Osmotic laxatives (e.g. lactulose or polyethylene glycol) can be helpful
- Fibre and other bulking laxatives are not of benefit. They may exacerbate bloating and are frequently not well tolerated
- Probiotics may help symptoms of gas and bloating
- Lubiprostone, activates chloride channels in small bowel epithelium resulting in an increase in intestinal fluid secretion and intestinal motility. It has shown benefit in IBS-C
- Linaclotide & plecanatide are guanylate cyclase-C agonists which increases intestinal fluid secretion. Both have shown some benefit in IBS-C
- Prucalopride is a highly selective serotonin (5-hydroxytryptamine, 5HT)-4 receptor agonist and prokinetic. Around 30% of patients achieve 3 bowel movement/ week following 12 weeks of treatment in addition to improved quality of life. Long-term efficacy remains unproven.
- Rectal irrigation therapy may offer symptom relief in select patients

Diarrhoea

- Loperamide is the most commonly used anti-diarrhoeal agent and is generally effective
- Short courses of rifaximin, a non-absorbed antibiotic may be helpful in exacerbations of IBS-D
- Alosetron, a 5-HT$_3$ receptor antagonist has been approved for use in the USA for females with IBS-D. Use is restricted, however, due to rare but serious side effects including severe constipation with perforation and ischaemic colitis.
- Eluxadoline is a μ- and κ-opioid receptor agonist and δ-opioid receptor antagonist with preferential activity in the enteric nervous system. It may be of benefit in patients with IBS-D. Side-effects including pancreatitis have limited its widespread use.

Abdominal pain
- Anti-spasmodic agents are frequently used (hyoscyamine, mebeverine and slow release peppermint oil) and may be of some help
- Low dose tricyclic anti-depressant medication (e.g. amitriptyline 10–50mg) may have a beneficial effect in IBS, although data on efficacy are inconsistent
- Selective serotonin reuptake inhibitors (SSRIs) may also improve general well-being and abdominal pain
- Part of the effect of tricyclics and SSRIs may be to improve mood and treat concomitant depression and anxiety.

Dietary interventions
- Prebiotic carbohydrates may selectively facilitate growth of bifidobacteria and other bacteria that have a positive impact on gastrointestinal health
- Studies suggest that some fermentable carbohydrates increase ileal luminal water content and colonic hydrogen production
- Diets low in fermentable oligosaccharides, disaccharides, monosaccharides and polyols (FODMAPs) appear to induce to a change in the gut mirobiome, leading to a reduction in GI symptoms and abdominal pain and improved quality of life in IBS patients

Cognitive-behavioural therapy
- Cognitive techniques aim to change inappropriate and anxiety-producing thinking patterns underlying the perception of somatic symptoms
- Behavioral therapy modifies dysfunctional behaviour through relaxation techniques, rewards for positive behaviour and assertion training
- Patients undergoing CBT and hypnotherapy show a significant reduction in symptoms. The estimated number of patients to treat in order for one patient to have an improvement is two.

References

Drossman DA. Functional Gastrointestinal Disorders: History, Pathophysiology, Clinical Features and Rome IV. *Gastroenterology* 2016;**150**:1262–1279

Ford AC, Lacy BE, Talley NJ. Irritable bowel syndrome. *N Engl J Med* 2017;**376**:2566–2578.

Functional bowel disorders

Most colorectal surgeons would include colonic transit problems, IBS, solitary rectal ulcer syndrome and pelvic floor disorders in the rather diffuse category 'functional gastrointestinal (GI) disorders'. Functional dyspepsia may also be a feature. In their most recent edition, the Rome IV multiconsensus group (Box 5.3) provided the following definition "Functional GI disorders are disorders of gut–brain interaction. It is a group of disorders classified by GI symptoms related to any combination of the following: motility disturbance, visceral hypersensitivity, altered mucosal and immune function, altered gut microbiota and altered central nervous system processing" (Drossman 2016). The Rome IV criteria also stress the need to remove the term "functional" where possible as it is potentially stigmatizing and non-specific e.g. "functional abdominal pain" may be best referred to as "centrally mediated abdominal pain syndrome".

Many patients probably have several different aspects to their bowel problem and it is vital to treat the patient's symptoms rather than the abnormalities found on investigation in isolation.

- Psychological problems and illness behaviour appear to be common in these patients, but it is not always clear whether these are the cause or effect of the bowel problems
- Sexual abuse, family problems or toileting difficulties in childhood are sometimes revealed as investigation proceeds
- There is now evidence that in these patient's abnormal mast cell function may lead to a hypersensitivity reaction which upregulates serotonin release and so modulates the response of the enteric and central nervous system
- Musculoskeletal pain and analgesic use often compound the bowel problem
- In females, previous vaginal delivery may contribute to pelvic floor problems
- The symptoms are often extremely troublesome to the patient and they become frustrated by a succession of negative investigations
- Pathology should always be excluded before any surgical intervention is considered
- Careful selection is vital and multidisciplinary input and support is recommended
- Beware of pain-predominant symptoms as outcome in these patients following surgery is almost universally poor
- Irritable bowel has previously been described (→ Irritable bowel syndrome p.244)
- Surgery for constipation and slow transit is covered in detail elsewhere (→ Constipation and slow transit p.250)

References

Drossman DA. Functional Gastrointestinal Disorders: History, Pathophysiology, Clinical Features and Rome IV. *Gastroenterology* 2016;**150**:1262–1279

Lacy BE, Mearin F, Chang L et al. Bowel disorders. *Gastroenterology* 2016;**150**:1393–1407

Box 5.3 Rome IV classification of bowel GI disorders

C1 Irritable Bowel Syndrome
See Box 5.2

C2 Functional Constipation
Diagnostic criteria*
1. Must include two or more of the following:
   * Straining during more than 25% of defecations
   * Lumpy or hard stools more than 25% of defecations
   * Sensation of incomplete evacuation more than 25% of defecations
   * Sensation of anorectal obstruction/blockage more than 25% of defecations
   * Manual maneuvers to facilitate more than 25% of defecations (e.g. digital evacuation, support of the pelvic floor)
   * Fewer than three spontaneous bowel movements per week
2. Loose stools are rarely present without the use of laxatives
3. Does not meet Rome IV criteria for IBS

C3 Functional Diarrhoea
Diagnostic criteria*

Loose or watery stools without predominant abdominal pain or bothersome bloating, occurring in > 25% of stools

Patients meeting criteria for diarrhoea-predominant IBS should be excluded

C4 Functional Abdominal Bloating/Digestion
Diagnostic criterion*
* Recurrent bloating and/or distention occurring, on average, at least 1 day per week; abdominal bloating and/or distention predominates over other symptoms (mild pain related to bloating may be present as well as minor bowel movement abnormalities)
* There are insufficient criteria for a diagnosis of irritable bowel syndrome, function constipation, functional diarrhoea or postprandial distress syndrome

C5 Unspecified functional bowel disorder
Diagnostic criteria* Must include both of the following:

Bowel symptoms not attributable to an organic aetiology that do not meet criteria for IBS or functional constipation, diarrhea or abdominal bloating/distention disorders.

*Criterion fulfilled for the last 3 months with symptom onset at least 6 months prior to diagnosis.

Source: Data from Lacy BE, Mearin F, Chang L et al. Bowel disorders. *Gastroenterology* 2016;150:1393–1407.

Constipation and slow transit

Among the uncomplaining population the frequency of bowel habit varies between 3 times daily and 3 times weekly. The consistency of stool accepted as normal also varies widely. However, 'constipation' is a frequent complaint which may refer to the frequency of defecation, the consistency of the stool and/or difficulty in defecation. An accurate history is vital to further assessment.

Causes of constipation

- Poor diet and fluid intake
- Medication such as analgesics, anti-depressants and calcium channel blockers
- Lack of physical activity
- Metabolic disease such as hypothyroidism or hypercalcaemia
- Strictures of the colon or rectum whether benign or malignant
- Distal inflammation of the rectum (usually with rectal bleeding)
- Diseases affecting the nerves to large bowel varying from spinal cord injury to multiple sclerosis (MS)
- Diseases affecting smooth muscle such as connective tissue disease
- IBS
- Diverticular disease
- Pelvic floor dysfunction which produces difficulty in emptying the rectum.

Investigation of constipation

Constipation is a common complaint and may not require investigation if there are no worrying features and it responds to simple treatment. Concerning features include:
- New onset of symptoms in an older patient (>40yrs) with no obvious simple explanation
- New symptoms persistent for >4–6 weeks
- Accompanying rectal bleeding or weight loss.

Constipation is generally a less concerning change in bowel habit than looseness or increased frequency of stool. In general terms, the concern in older patient is to exclude malignancy while in the younger patient the most common disease to be excluded is distal IBD. It would be rare for this to present without bleeding and therefore in the younger patient constipation which appears to have no worrying features on history or examination can generally be treated without prior investigation.
- In patients <40yrs of age in whom distal IBD is considered possible, rigid or flexible sigmoidoscopy should demonstrate an obvious abnormality
- New or persistent constipation in an older patient particularly if accompanied by rectal bleeding is generally investigated by means of colonoscopy, barium enema or CT colonography.

Once malignancy has been excluded, consideration can be given to the other causes listed above. Many patients are content to manage their symptoms once serious disease has been excluded.
- Many of the causes listed above can be identified by an adequate history and examination

- If no serious cause has been identified, conservative treatment with attention to diet and fluid intake and bulk-forming or osmotic laxatives is usually tried before further investigation is undertaken.

If the patient has persistent troublesome symptoms despite this, investigation should aim to identify whether the constipation is due to a problem with colonic transit or a pelvic floor problem.
- Metabolic disease should be excluded by TFTs and serum calcium levels
- Colonic transit studies
- Defecating proctogram.

Colonic transit studies

Colon transit abnormalities can be identified by radiological marker studies or by radioisotope transit studies. Radiological marker studies may be performed in 2 ways:
- The patient swallows a fixed number of markers on a single occasion and plain abdominal films taken after 5–10 days are used to demonstrate the number of markers left behind. In the asymptomatic population, 80% of insoluble markers disappear by 5 days
- The patient swallows a fixed number of markers, but these are given as different shapes on successive days. An estimate of segmental transit time can thus be obtained.

Radioisotopes can be used in various forms of meal to examine gastric emptying, transit time to the caecum and colonic transit time. It is obvious that the patient must avoid the use of laxatives, suppositories or enemas during the time of the transit studies.

Defecating proctogram

- Imaging of pelvic floor activity can be achieved by fluoroscopy or MRI
- Some patients may have both rectal emptying problems and slow colonic transit
- Proctography is described in more detail with obstructed defecation (→ Obstructed defecation p. 274).

Interpretation of results of investigations for constipation

- Even in a specialized referral practice, the most common causes of constipation are poor diet and fluid intake and IBS
- Many patients have several different problems which contribute to their sluggish bowel habit, e.g. back pain requiring analgesics with depression and poor diet
- Once it is clear that there is no structural abnormality, e.g. stricture, if measured colonic transit and defecating proctogram are unremarkable, it is likely that treatment will be conservative
- If it appears that pelvic floor problems may contribute to the symptoms because rectal emptying is poor on proctogram, anorectal physiology is usually the next step in investigation (→ Anorectal physiology p.96)
- A careful history and examination must be interpreted along with the results of the investigations.

Slow transit

Classical slow transit constipation is rare. Relatively slow transit due to several external factors such as diet and drugs is much more common.

Arbuthnott–Lane disease

• More common in young to middle-aged women
• Lifelong history of constipation
• Cyclical symptoms
• Relatively little abdominal pain except when the bowel has not moved for several weeks
• Gradual onset of symptoms during each cycle—there is no call to stool and the abdomen gradually becomes distended
• If no laxatives are used, eventually colicky abdominal pain develops
• After a variable number of days, the bowels move, initially with constipated stool in large quantity and relieving the abdominal pain
• Most patient also have abnormal gastric emptying and biliary motility
• ↑ dietary fibre tends to worsen/have no effect on symptoms and some patients ultimately take large amounts of stimulant laxatives daily.

Treatment of slow transit constipation

Operative treatment is problematic, mainly because operating inappropriately on patients with constipation-predominant IBS is easy.

• Operation should not be considered without full investigation. Significantly slow colonic transit should be demonstrated objectively, probably on more than one occasion
• Colonic pressure measurements may assist decision-making. Patients with irritable bowel syndrome have increased but disorganized and ineffectual colonic contractions, while patients with true slow transit constipation have no high amplitude propagated contractions (HAPCs) and virtually no colonic pressure activity
• The classical operation for slow transit constipation is subtotal colectomy and ileorectal anastomosis
• Colectomy fails to relieve constipation in ~10% of patients and produces troublesome diarrhoea in a further 10%
• If abdominal pain is a major part of the symptom complex, colectomy should be avoided as it is unlikely that the pain will be relieved
• Antegrade colonic enema (ACE) procedures have been used and seem to help some patients. This can be carried out after formation of an appendicostomy.
• If there is doubt about pelvic floor function, then a loop colostomy may be helpful
  • if the constipation is due to the pelvic floor only, the stoma will function normally
  • if slow colonic transit is significant, the stoma will not work well
• If there is doubt as to the wisdom of bowel resection, a loop ileostomy may be helpful. Relief of symptoms after ileostomy provides some reassurance that the colon is the source
• If colectomy is considered it is wise to ensure that the anal sphincter can produce adequate pressures or incontinence of loose stool may result.

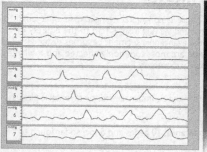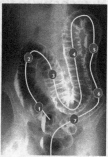

Fig. 5.10 HAPCs recorded at colonic manometry.

Reference

Wong SW, Lubowski DZ. Slow-transit constipation: evaluation and treatment. *ANZ J Surg* 2007;**77**:320–328.

Hirschsprung's disease

In Hirschsprung's disease there is congenital aganglionosis of a length of gut starting at the anal canal and varying from <1cm to the entirety of the bowel. The bowel above the aganglionic segment becomes distended. The rectum and part of the colon are most commonly affected and total intestinal involvement is fortunately extremely rare.

Pathophysiology

- Absence of ganglion cells in the submucosal and/or myenteric plexus over a variable length of bowel
- Incidence ~1 in 5,000 births
- Complex pattern of inheritance. 10 genes and 5 loci so far found to be involved
- Non-Mendelian, low sex-dependent penetrance with variable expression (male dominance)
- Long segment Hirschsprung's disease (5–10%) defined as involvement proximal to the midtransverse colon—may be difficult to diagnose There is a higher risk of enterocolitis, as they cannot be easily managed with rectal washouts (see below)
- Hypoganglionosis and neuronal intestinal dysplasia (hyperplasia) may also cause severe gut dysfunction.

Presentation

- Most Hirschsprung's disease presents in the neonate with delayed passage of meconium, abdominal distension and bile-stained vomiting
- Older infants may present with constipation and megacolon/rectum
- A very small number of patients with short segment Hirschsprung's present in teenage years or as young adults with megacolon ± rectum
- Hirschsprung's enterocolitis is the most feared complication in children under 5yrs and may occur before or after definitive surgery. Fever, abdominal distension and diarrhoea are characteristic. This may be the presenting feature. Mortality of up to 30%.

Diagnosis

- Plain abdominal film demonstrates dilatation of bowel proximal to the aganglionic segment and absence of gas in the rectum. Contrast enema may reveal the transition zone, but the level is frequently inaccurate
- Definitive diagnosis is by rectal biopsy which must include muscle in order to identify lack of ganglion cells and ↑ thickened nerve fibres on acetylcholinesterase staining. In infants this can be achieved by suction biopsy. In teenagers or adults more formal full-thickness biopsy is usually performed. This should be between 2 and 5cm from the dentate line in order to avoid the normal hypoganglionic area
- The rectoanal inhibitory reflex (RAIR) is absent in patients who present as adults with ultra-short Hirschsprung's. The anal sphincter fails to relax in response to rectal distension. In adult patients with megarectum this physiological test is generally used as a screening test before full-thickness biopsy is considered.

Management

Children

- In the past, loop stoma in an area of normal bowel proximal to the distended area was performed in the first instance and definitive surgery was then performed in the infant of 1–2yrs
- Current treatment usually involves daily or more frequent rectal washouts to decompress the colon. Where this is successful, definitive surgery can be planned for the first few months of life. If unsuccessful, a stoma may be necessary to avoid the development of enterocolitis
- Definitive surgery may be open, laparoscopically assisted or transanal
- Three main operations have been performed to bring normally innervated colon down to the anal canal (Fig. 5.11). Frozen section is used to ensure normal innervation of the colon used for anastomosis.

Newly diagnosed Hirchsprung's disease in adults

Hirschsprung's disease should be considered in all patients with constipation and megarectum or megacolon. Anorectal manometry is generally performed before rectal biopsy—if the rectoanal inhibitory reflex is present Hirschsprung's disease can be excluded. Interpretation can be difficult as the reflex may be blunted simply because of chronic rectal distension. Full-thickness rectal biopsy is needed if there is any doubt. It is said that in the rare ultra-short Hirschsprung's disease, full-thickness strip biopsy may be sufficient to relieve symptoms.

Management is by operation, most commonly either a Duhamel procedure or low stapled coloanal anastomosis.

Adults who have had surgery for Hirschsprung's disease in childhood

In contrast to patients who have had surgery for congenital anorectal atresias, these patients generally do well in adult life. Complications such as adhesive obstruction due to previous laparotomy may arise but in general bowel function is good. Presumably, this is because pelvic floor function is normal.

Reference

Masi P, Miele E, Staiano A. Pediatric anorectal disorders. *Gastroenterol Clin North Am* 2008;**37**:709–730.

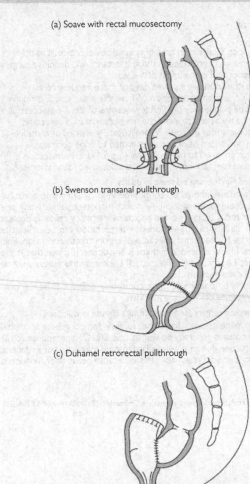

(a) Soave with rectal mucosectomy

(b) Swenson transanal pullthrough

(c) Duhamel retrorectal pullthrough

Fig. 5.11 Swenson, Duhamel and Soave anastomosis.

Faecal incontinence

Faecal incontinence (FI) is involuntary loss of stool with reported prevalence rates of 0.8-8% in the adult population. Prevalence is higher in women and increases with age to a prevalence of 16% in those >70yrs. FI can be either passive (loss without awareness) or urge (an inability to defer defecation until a socially appropriate time). The social and psychological costs are high.

FI often has a substantial negative impact on individuals by limiting social activity and leads to a reduction in their quality of life. It also has a significant financial impact on healthcare systems through diagnosis, treatment, ongoing care and a reduced ability to work.

Aetiology

Faecal continence is maintained by the interplay of complex activities relying upon sufficient rectal reservoir, normal colonic and rectal transit, adequate discriminatory anorectal sensation, coordinated inhibition of the puborectalis muscle during defecation, intact sphincter innervation and physical integrity and an appropriate stool consistency. Failure in any component can lead to incontinence.

Reduced stool consistency

Continent mechanisms are designed to handle the daily elimination of formed stool. The following may be associated with a reduction in continence due to loose stool.

- IBS
- IBD
- Malabsorption
- Laxative abuse
- Radiation enteritis.

Sphincter deficiency or injury

- Obstetric: 13–24% of patients will report new FI post-partum. Associated risk factors include:
  - Forceps delivery
  - Primiparous delivery
  - Previous sphincter injury
  - Episiotomy
  - Augmented labour
- Surgical
  - Fistula in ano
  - Lateral sphincterotomy
  - Haemorrhoidectomy
  - Anal stretch or dilatation
- Accidental or sexual trauma
- Congenital anorectal malformations
- Primary degeneration
- Systemic sclerosis
- Radiation injury.

Loss of rectal capacity and compliance

The non-diseased rectum has both viscous and elastic properties, which allow it to maintain a low intraluminal pressure despite a large volume. Decreased compliance is associated with FI in the following conditions.

* Proctitis
* Rectal surgery
* Intrinsic rectal disease
  * Prolapse
  * Tumour.

Neurological

* Stroke, dementia etc.
* Pudendal neuropathy
* Spinal cord injury
* Diabetic neuropathy.

Local reflex abnormalities

Transient external anal sphincter contraction and pronounced IAS reflex relaxation in response to rectal distension is a normal reflex allowing sampling of rectal contents. The reflex requires the rich profusion of nerve endings particularly in the vicinity of the anal valves. Defective sampling has been documented in patients with FI and is associated with childbirth, perineal descent syndrome and transanal mucosectomy.

History

* Risk factors for FI
* Continence history
  * Frequency and degree of incontinence
  * Passive vs urge incontinence.

Investigation

* Exclude other causes for symptoms including faecal impaction, treatable diarrhoeal states, lower GI cancer, rectal prolapse and acute disc prolapse or cauda equina syndrome
* Qualify, quantify and diagnose cause of FI.

Wexner incontinence/St Mark's incontinence score (Tables 5.1 and 5.2)

Examination

* Inspect for scars, fistulae, a patulous anus may indicate prolapse
* Rectal examination to exclude impaction or rectal pathology
* Palpation for resting anal pressure (RAP) and squeeze pressure (SP)
* Assess perineal sensation.

Flexible sigmoidoscopy

* To exclude intrinsic rectal pathology
* To exclude a treatable diarrhoeal state.

Endoanal ultrasound

EAUS allows direct visualization of IAS and EAS defects. 50–90% of women with post-partum incontinence will have a defect detected on US. Only 37-45% of women with an ultrasound detected defect will report symptoms of incontinence (➛ Endoanal and endorectal ultrasound p.92).

Table 5.1 Wexner incontinence score

	Never	Rarely	Sometimes	Usually	Always
Incontinence to solid	0	1	2	3	4
Incontinence to liquid	0	1	2	3	4
Incontinence to gas	0	1	2	3	4
Alteration in lifestyle	0	1	2	3	4
Wears pad	0	1	2	3	4

Never, 0; rarely, <1 episode/month; sometimes, <1/week, 1/month; usually, <1/day, 1/week; always 1/day. 0, perfect; 20, complete incontinence.

Reproduced with permission from Jorge JM, Wexner SD. Etiology and management of fecal incontinence. *Dis Colon Rectum*;36(1):77-97 (PubMed abstract). Copyright © 1993, Wolters Kluwer Health. doi: 10.1007/BF02050307

Table 5.2 St Mark's incontinence score

	Never	Rarely	Sometimes	Weekly	Daily
Incontinence for solid stool	0	1	2	3	4
Incontinence for liquid stool	0	1	2	3	4
Incontinence for gas	0	1	2	3	4
Alteration in lifestyle	0	1	2	3	4
				No	Yes
Need to wear a pad or plug				0	2
Taking constipating medicines				0	2
Lack of ability to defer defecation for 15 minutes				0	4

Never = no episodes in the past four weeks; Rarely = 1 episode in the past four weeks; Sometimes = >1 episode in the past four weeks but <1 per week; Weekly = 1 or more episodes a week but <1 per day; Daily = 1 or more episodes a day: Add one score from each row: minimum score = 0 perfect continence; maximum score 24 = totally incontinent

Source: Data from Vaizey CJ, Carapeti E, Cahill JA, et al. Prospective comparison of fecal incontinence grading systems, *Gut*; 1999, 44 (77-80).

Anorectal physiology

There is no standardized method of performing or interpreting this investigation (⊃ Anorectal physiology p.96). Reduced RAP can indicate IAS dysfunction. Reduced SP can indicate EAS dysfunction. Balloon distensibility enables assessment of the RAIR, rectal sensitivity, rectal capacity and compliance. Reduced urge and maximum tolerated balloon volumes are indicative of rectal hypersensitivity.

Normal parameters

- Resting anal pressure (RAP) 40–90cmH$_2$O
- Squeeze pressure (SP) 50–100% >RAP
- Balloon first sensation 40–70ml
- Urge volume 150–300ml
- Maximum tolerated volume 180–410ml

Pudendal nerve terminal motor latency

PNTML assesses pudendal nerve function. Normal latency does not exclude nerve injury as only the fastest remaining conducting fibres are recorded and there is a substantial anatomical overlap. Prolonged PNTML identifies pudendal neuropathy but not the level of injury.

Defecating proctogram

Dynamic MRI imaging or conventional cinedefecography allows assessment of the defecation process. They can be useful for identification of perineal descent, intussusception and obstructed defecation.

Treatment

Conservative

- Dietary modification. Avoid food/drinks that cause loose stool. Fibre and bulking agents augment stool consistency
- Pads
- Skin care products
  - Foam cleansers rather than soaps
  - Sudocrem or other zinc oxide-based products
- Anal plug. May be helpful for passive FI although poorly tolerated by most patients
- Biofeedback or operant conditioning therapy
  - Includes balloon training, EMG feedback, anal pressure training and counselling
  - Reported continence improvement in >60% of patients but a Cochrane review could not confirm that biofeedback was an effective treatment in a complex package of care, nor that any one form of biofeedback was better that the others
- Transanal irrigation
  - Patient self-administers transanal irrigation every 1-3 days, thereby emptying the bowel
  - up to 50% of patients have a successful outcome after more than 1 year

Neuromodulation

Chronic indirect or direct low-voltage stimulation of the sacral nerves can lead to a significant improvement in continence and quality of life in selected patients with faecal incontinence.

- Sacral nerve stimulation
  - indicated in patients with a sphincter defect of <180° sphincter defect who have failed medical therapy and biofeedback
  - trial stimulation period for 2 weeks using an external stimulator is performed. If successful, patients go on to have a permanent implanted stimulator wire and stimulator
  - following permanent implantation, 70-75% of patients report >50% continence improvement at 5yrs
  - reoperation rates of approx. 5% due to complications
  - 5% chance of serious complications requiring explantation
- Posterior Tibial Nerve Stimulation (TNS)
  - stimulation is delivered transcutaneously (TTNS) or percutaneously (PTNS) over a 4-12 week period
  - although it may be helpful, a recent meta-analysis reported that PTNS is not as effective as SNS in improving functional outcomes and quality of life
- Extracorporeal magnetic stimulation: non-invasive stimulation of pelvic floor muscles: case studies only.

Pharmacological

- Constipating agents
  - Loperamide: prolongs transit time leading to increased absorption, improved stool consistency and reduced stool weight. Furthermore, it increases RAP and reduces sensitivity of the RAIR
  - Codeine phosphate
- Evacuation aids: laxatives, enemas and suppositories can help post-defecatory soiling associated with incomplete emptying
- Amitriptyline: reported to reduce CNS activation to rectal distension in treatment of rectal hypersensitivity
- Topical sphincter stimulants
  - Phenylephrine: no impact on incontinence scores or RAP but has been shown to have some clinical effectiveness in ileoanal pouch patients.

Surgical

- Anterior sphincter repair
  - for patients with >120° sphincter defect
  - 60% of patients reported >50% continence improvement at 5yrs
- Injectable bulking agents
  - A wide variety of agents have been used including PTQ® (Uroplasty Ltd, Geleen, The Netherlands), Durasphere® (Carbon Medical Technologies, Minnesota, USA), Gatekeeper® (THD, Correggio Italy) and non-animal stabilized dextranomer in hyaluronic acid (NASHA Dx)
  - Evidence from trials is limited. NASHA Dx may be of sustained benefit in up to 50% of patients
- Radiofrequency energy (Secca therapy)

- Delivered transanally via a dedicated anoscope. It appears to be a safe intervention
- May be associated with an early improvement in continence scores for at least 6 months but benefits may not be sustained
- Post-anal repair
  - previously for intact sphincter FI
  - 30% of patients report 50% continence improvement at five years
- Neosphincters
  - Graciloplasty: 40–60% of patients report improved continence at 5yr follow-up but with a 30% morbidity
  - Artificial sphincters: 90% report solid continence but with 15% explantation rate
- Colostomy: once all conservative and surgical options considered
- Antegrade continent enema: for constipation or colonic motility disorders associated with FI.

References

Gordon PH. Anorectal anatomy and physiology. *Gastroenterol Clin North Am* 2001;**30**:1–13.

Ditah I, Devaki P, Luma H, *et al*. Prevalence, trends and risk factors for fecal incontinence in United States adults, 2005–2010. *Clin Gastroenterol Hepatol* 2014;**12**:636–43

Norton C, Whitehead WE, Bliss DZ, Tries J. Conservative and pharmacological management of faecal incontinence in adults. In: Abrams P, Cardozo L, Khoury S, Wein AS, eds, *Incontinence*, vol. 2. Plymouth: Health Publications, 2005:1521–1563.

Baig MK, Wexner SD. Factors predictive of outcome after surgery for faecal incontinence. *Br J Surg* 2000;**87**:1316–1330.

Simillis C, Lal N, Qiu S, *et al*. Sacral nerve stimulation versus percutaneous tibial nerve stimulation for faecal incontinence: a systematic review and meta-analysis. *Int J Colorectal Dis* 2018;**33**:645–648

Intestinal failure

Intestinal failure (IF) may be defined as the inability of the gut to absorb sufficient macronutrients (carbohydrates proteins and fat), micronutrients (electrolytes, vitamins and minerals) and/or water, resulting in the need for intravenous supplementation in order to maintain health and/or growth. It is estimated that 18/million adults require prolonged inpatient parenteral nutritional support annually and the prevalence of home parenteral nutrition (HPN) in the UK is 14.6/million adults.

Types of intestinal failure

- Type 1: short-term, self-limiting, often perioperative <14days
- Type 2: prolonged parenteral nutrition (PN) >14 days. Metabolic instability with sepsis ± renal impairment
- Type 3: long-term PN—stable HPN.

Some patients who have defunctioned bowel, often because of post-operative complications, will require HPN for a number of months until their general condition is good enough for further surgery and the abdomen has become less hostile. This is usually at least 6 months after the previous laparotomy and most surgeons who operate on intestinal failure patients prefer them to be as 'back to normal' as possible before embarking on what can be prolonged and difficult surgery to re-anastomose the bowel.

Causes of intestinal failure

- Crohn's disease
- Bowel ischaemia
- Post-operative complications
- Radiation enteritis
- Motility disorders such as chronic intestinal pseudo-obstruction or pseudo-obstruction due to connective tissue disease
- Many other rare small bowel diseases.

Short-term intestinal failure

Short-term intestinal failure is common on surgical wards. If post-operative ileus lasts only a few days, no specific nutritional support is needed in the well-nourished patient. However, if a patient cannot manage adequate oral intake for longer than 5 days for whatever reason, serious consideration should be given to nutritional support.

- If the failure is of the swallowing mechanism or due to oesophageal perforation or obstruction, it should be possible to by-pass this by the use of a fine-bore NG or NJ tube passed endoscopically if necessary. Longer term, a percutaneous gastrostomy, placed either endoscopically or radiologically, can be used
- If gastric emptying is a problem (e.g. in pancreatitis or the critically ill) an NJ tube should provide access to the GI tract for feeding.
- If there is true intestinal failure rather than merely difficulty with access to the gut, PN is needed. However, the risks of PN are relatively high, particularly if it is only used occasionally without the support of a nutrition team. PN should not be used for a few days only and should not be used because it is more convenient then enteral nutrition

- PN containing a relatively large amount of fat to reduce the osmolality can be given via a small peripheral cannula, inserted in a large vein away from a joint and with full sterile precautions. Despite this, phlebitis is generally troublesome and now that small diameter mid-lines (20cm long, inserted peripherally) and PICC lines (peripherally inserted central catheter) are available, PN via a peripheral cannula is used less often. Because the majority of patients who need PN have post-operative complications and poor venous access, it is most common to give PN via a central venous catheter. This should be inserted specifically for PN and only used for this
- Although pre-mixed standard PN bags made by commercial companies are convenient for short-term PN, it is important that an appropriate amount of fluid, electrolytes, protein and calories is supplied and that vitamins and trace elements are added to the bags in pharmacy. A dietitian should estimate the patient's protein and energy requirements. Overfeeding leads to an increase in septic complications and a higher chance of liver dysfunction.

Patterns of short bowel

If no colon is functioning, it is generally stated that 100cm of small bowel is needed to avoid parenteral supplementation. If at least half of the colon is functioning, then it is thought that 50cm of small bowel is needed. These figures depend on the remaining bowel being healthy. The distribution of small and large bowel which is left following surgery has a strong influence on the outcome and need for supplementation. Three main types can be distinguished:
- High jejunostomy
- Jejunocolic anastomosis
- Duodenoileal anastomosis.

In patients with motility disorders or obstruction, all of the small and large bowel may be present, but absorption is poor because of obstruction. Some patients with extensive small bowel disease may have the entire small and large bowel, but absorption is poor because of abnormal mucosa.

High jejunostomy

- Characterized by high fluid and electrolyte losses from stoma
- Magnesium, sodium and potassium are among the dominant electrolytes lost
- The upper jejunum secretes fluid and electrolytes into the lumen which is reabsorbed by the lower small bowel. Loss of the distal small bowel means that drinking hyper-osmolar fluids leads to an increase in stoma output and negative fluid balance.

Management of high jejunostomy

- Drugs to reduce gut motility such as loperamide, co-phenotrope and codeine phosphate may be needed in high dose. These drugs are most effective if taken about an hour before eating
- Loperamide is usually preferred because it has fewest side effects, but codeine phosphate may be added

- PPIs are the most effective drugs in reducing gastric acid secretion and should be used in high dose. Omeprazole has been studied most in these patients
- Omeprazole is best absorbed if the contents of the capsule are dissolved in bicarbonate
- In extremely short gut, IV PPI may be helpful
- In a small number of patients, octreotide helps to reduce output, but it is rarely sufficiently effective that it avoids the need for IV fluids
- A mixture of electrolyte solution containing at least 100mmol/l of sodium and some glucose is better absorbed than water and may be used orally instead of water
- If the above measures fail to achieve fluid balance, then either SC fluid (~1litre daily is the maximum amount practical) or IV fluid infusion is needed. Some patients are able to absorb sufficient nutrients but cannot maintain their fluid balance. This problem may be exacerbated if renal function is poor and they cannot concentrate their urine
- Dietary management centres on supplying high protein and calorie foods every few hours rather than 1 or 2 large meals a day. Snacking is encouraged. Fluids and food should be taken separately
- Multivitamin and trace element supplements will be required unless parenteral nutrition or a significant amount of enteral nutrition is used
- Remember to give vitamin B12
- Elemental feed is hyperosmolar and so is usually not helpful. Overnight enteral tube feeding with a polymeric or peptide feed is tolerated by some patients without excess stoma output and a fine-bore tube may also be used to give electrolyte solution (usually ~1litre daily to replace the same amount of water/hypo-osmolar drinks)
- If IV fluids or feed are needed, it is likely this will be needed 6 or 7 nights/week because of fluid balance problems. The amount of fluid necessary may be up to 5 or 6 litres daily, depending on the stoma output and the patient's ability to moderate their oral intake.

Jejunocolic anastomosis

- Characterized by gradual nutritional failure rather than fluid balance problems
- A common pattern of short bowel associated with CD
- Electrolyte imbalance is much less common.

Duodenoileal anastomosis

- Similar to jejunocolic anastomosis in that fluid balance problems are less dominant
- Less common than jejunocolic anastomosis
- Loss of jejunum is more easily compensated for than loss of ileum because ileum seems to adapt more easily.

Management of jejunocolic or duodenoileal anastomosis

- Encourage high calorie intake as mainly carbohydrate and protein
- Excessive fat intake will lead to steatorrhoea if the ileum has been removed
- Excess oxalate intake will lead to renal stones. It appears these patients absorb more oxalate from the colon than normal, perhaps due to bile acids and fat malabsorption leading to formation of calcium soaps

- Oxalate-containing foods include tea and rhubarb
- Vitamin B12 is needed parenterally but other multivitamin supplements may be well enough absorbed if given orally provided the gut length is not extremely short
- If weight loss and nutrient deficiencies continue despite oral supplements, enteral tube feeding overnight may be helpful
- Enteral feeds which are calorie dense may be more convenient for the patient
- If enteral feeding is insufficient, HPN may be necessary
- Since these patients do not generally have fluid balance problems, it may be possible to provide enough nutrition by feeding 4 or 5 nights/week which is more convenient for the patient.

Obstruction or motility problems

- Chronic intestinal pseudo-obstruction is characterized by long-standing functional bowel symptoms with grossly distended small bowel but no identifiable point of obstruction
- Pseudo-obstruction syndromes are more commonly seen in patients with connective tissue disease, though it may be difficult to prove unequivocally that this is the underlying diagnosis
- Patients with extensive peritoneal metastatic disease such as ovarian carcinoma may develop bowel obstruction which is difficult to relieve surgically. In the UK it is rarely considered appropriate to give these patients HPN because of the burden of treatment in a patient with a very poor prognosis.

Home parenteral nutrition

The prevalence of HPN varies throughout the UK, probably related to the availability of a service and the awareness of medical staff. The majority of patients in the UK manage their own HPN, but with the increasing age of the population this is likely to reduce in the future.

- Venous access is usually via a cuffed long-term IV catheter, but some patients use an SC port
- Teaching the patient about catheter care and management of HPN is key to successful treatment. This is done by the nutrition nurse specialist in hospital and takes several weeks, once the patient is fully mobile and well enough to concentrate on learning the techniques
- Commercial home care companies supply the patient with a fridge, pump, drip stand, ancillaries such as dressing packs and flushing solutions, as well as delivering feeds at 1- or 2-week intervals
- The nutrition multidisciplinary team plays a critical role in managing patients with IF
  - A dietitian calculates the patient's nutritional requirements and estimates the amount which is being absorbed from oral intake
  - A clinician typically prescribes the IV feed, consisting of fluid, electrolytes, protein, carbohydrate, fat, vitamins and trace elements. Particular attention is needed for patients with high output stomas.
  - It is important to avoid excess calorie intake, which leads to increased complications such as sepsis and liver dysfunction. Liver dysfunction is also associated with the amount of fat prescribed and is more likely in patients with extremely short gut or with other sources of liver damage
  - The pharmacist formulates a feed that is chemically stable

- HPN patients should be discharged with adequate plans for problem management, e.g. a reliable means of contacting an appropriate health professional for advice 24h a day and a straightforward means of ensuring rapid access to an appropriate hospital bed if unwell.

Monitoring and follow-up of patients with intestinal failure

- These patients have multiple problems and require MDT follow-up by a team which includes a dietitian, nutrition nurse specialist, pharmacist and clinician
- Weight, oedema and micronutrient levels should be measured, in addition to electrolytes, LFTs, protein and bone biochemistry and haematology including haematinics
- Review of the practicalities of enteral or parenteral access for feeding is needed as well as the arrangements for feed delivery, etc.
- These patients are at risk from metabolic bone disease. DEXA scans should be performed and referral to a mineral metabolism clinic is often needed.
- The underlying disease which caused the intestinal failure may require follow-up.

Evolving strategies

- A variety of hormone treatments (growth hormone, glucagon-like-peptide-1 (GLP-1) and GLP-2 agonists) have had varied success
- The recombinant analogue GLP-2 teduglutide has been shown to reduce PN requirements but the extremely high cost has limited use
- Intestinal lengthening procedures (e.g. Bianchi procedure) may have a role in highly selected children and adults with stable IF
- Intestinal transplant procedures are primarily used as a rescue procedure to prevent further complications associated with long-term HPN. Survival rates of up to 50% at 10 years have been reported

References

Nightingale J, ed. *Intestinal failure*. London: Greenwich Medical, 2001.
Klek S, Forbes A, Gabe S, et al. Management of acute intestinal failure: A position paper from the European Society for Clinical Nutrition and Metabolism (ESPEN) Special Interest Group. *Clin Nutr.* 2016;**35**(6):1209–18

Anorectal disorders

Rectal prolapse

Introduction

Rectal prolapse or procidentia is an intussusception of the rectum through the anal verge. It should be differentiated from occult rectal prolapse/intussusception, mucosal prolapse and SRUS (➔ Solitary rectal ulcer p. 260). There is controversy as to whether these form a spectrum of conditions with a similar pathogenesis.

Rectal prolapse is most common at the extremes of age. In the paediatric population it usually presents before the age of 4, with equal sex distribution until the peak incidence during the 7th decade when 90% of cases are in females.

Pathogenesis

The aetiology of rectal prolapse is a matter of debate, with several different theories proposed. The association with incontinence and constipation is clear. Difficulty arises determining whether related changes are primary or a consequence of the prolapsing rectum.

- Common anatomical changes include an abnormally deep pouch of Douglas and laxity of the anatomical fixation of the rectum including the mesorectum and lateral ligaments
- Redundancy and increased compliance of the sigmoid colon may be an important cause of post-operative constipation
- Weakness of the pelvic floor, internal and external anal sphincters with evidence of pudendal nerve neuropathy is described and may be more common in patients where incontinence is the predominant symptom
- Changes in the morphology of the anal canal–sphincter complex may be 2° to the physical stress from the prolapsing rectum
- Patient may have an impaired rectoanal inhibitory reflex with intermittent high-pressure rectal motor activity contributing to incontinence
- Rectal prolapse has been linked with both colonic dysmotility and defecatory disorders.

Presentation

- Symptoms include a lump at the anus which may reduce spontaneously or manually, as well as incontinence (50–80%), constipation (up to 50%), perineal heaviness, tenesmus and mucus leak
- The prolapse may only occur occasionally (e.g. during strained defecation), regularly post-defecation or on standing or may be continuously present
- Complications include pain, bleeding, incarceration and gangrene
- Symptoms of incontinence and constipation should be explored as they may affect treatment. Constipation pre-dating the prolapse might suggest delayed colonic transit
- Rectal prolapse can be associated with parity, connective tissue disorders, neurological/spinal abnormalities and psychiatric illness
- In children the most important association is with cystic fibrosis (affects ~20% CF patients). A sweat test should be considered as rectal prolapse may be the initial presentation in up to a third of cases.
- Paediatric rectal prolapse is also associated with chronic constipation, diarrhoea, coughing, malnutrition, Hirschsprung's disease, cloacal abnormalities and congenital hypothyroidism.

Diagnosis

- The main difficulty in diagnosis is differentiating rectal prolapse from mucosal or haemorrhoidal prolapse
- Concentric folds are seen on the surface of a full-thickness rectal prolapse compared with radial folds in mucosal prolapse (Fig. 6.1)
- The anus is in its normal position with a groove between it and the prolapsed rectum, while in mucosal prolapse the anoderm is everted with no such groove (Fig. 6.1)
- If more than a few centimetres of tissue is prolapsed it is almost certainly a rectal prolapse
- No external skin tags are visible, unlike haemorrhoidal disease
- Muscle should be palpable between the mucosal surfaces
- Pelvic floor weakness should be excluded. Signs of weakness include perineal descent, poor anal tone (IAS), poor SP (EAS) and reduced anorectal angle
- Genital prolapse may co-exist in 10–20% so vaginal examination should be carried out in females
- An EUA may be necessary if the prolapse cannot be reproduced on straining. A forceps may be used to apply traction to the mucosa or a swab inserted into the rectum and then withdrawn may demonstrate the prolapse
- Colonoscopy should be considered to exclude proximal pathology
- Anorectal physiology, transit studies and proctography may be considered as the results help to guide surgical management.

(a)   (b)

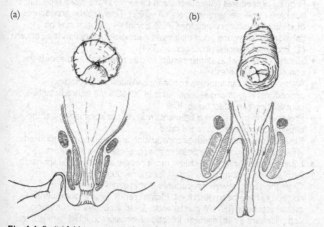

Fig. 6.1 Radial folds are seen on the surface of a mucosal/haemorrhoidal prolapse (a) compared with concentric folds in full-thickness rectal prolapse (b). When the anus is examined by inserting a finger between the prolapsed tissue and the perianal skin, in rectal prolapse the anus is in its normal position with a groove between it and the prolapsed rectum (b) while in mucosal prolapse the anoderm is everted with no such groove (a).

Treatment

More than 100 procedures for rectal prolapse have been described suggesting that the ideal procedure is yet to be found. It is important to remember that rectal prolapse is an anatomical abnormality associated with
functional problems which must be considered when deciding on the best
course of treatment. It may also be associated with other pelvic floor abnormalities including incontinence, cystocoele, vaginal vault prolapse and
enterocoele.

Operative procedures broadly fall into abdominal or perineal approaches
± resection of the rectum/sigmoid. Abdominal procedures include mobilization ± rectopexy using a variety of methods (⊃ Prolapse: rectopexy
p.570). Procedure selection should take into account patient age, co-
morbidity, previous surgery, concomitant symptoms (e.g. incontinence) and
surgeon preference.

Paediatric rectal prolapse

- Conservative treatment is the first choice for children under 4 as most
  will resolve spontaneously. If recurrent, then injection sclerotherapy has
  a high success rate (90–100%)
- Presentation after the age of 4 is less likely to resolve without surgery.

Elective treatment

- Adults gain little benefit from conservative therapy
- Although popular in Japan, anal encirclement (Thiersch wire) is now
  rarely used due to perceived high recurrence rates
- Perineal procedures (Altemeier's and Delorme's) are easily repeatable
  but have higher recurrence rates (10–30%). They are the procedures
  of choice for patients unfit for GA. A perineal approach may be
  considered for young adult males where sexual dysfunction is a concern
  (⊃ Prolapse: perineal procedures p.574)
- Suture rectopexy has similar results to other methods and avoids the
  complications of mesh
- All procedures can improve continence. Abdominal rectopexy
  procedures may improve continence in 30–60% but unpredictable
  constipation can affect up to 40%
- Preservation of the lateral ligaments may reduce constipation at the
  expense of higher recurrence rates
- Resection rectopexy reduces constipation and should be considered
  where constipation is the predominant pre-operative symptom
- Laparoscopic surgery may allow more people an abdominal approach
  with quicker recovery and similar functional outcomes
- Over the years, several procedures that use mesh to facilitate
  rectopexy have been described. Most recently, laparoscopic ventral
  mesh rectopexy (LVMR) gained widespread acceptance. However,
  complications including mesh infection & erosion coupled with general
  anxiety regarding the use of mesh in pelvic floor repairs has meant that
  it is no longer viewed as being an acceptable operation for primary
  repair of rectal prolapse
- In patients with concomitant FI, it may be best to wait for at least 6
  months to assess outcome after prolapse repair before considering
  surgical treatment of sphincter defects, etc.

Acute rectal prolapse
- Irreducible prolapse is treated by elevating the foot of the bed, analgesia, cold compress and gentle manual pressure
- Application of sugar has been suggested to reduce oedema
- Gangrenous prolapse can be treated by a perineal or abdominal approach.

Obstructed defecation

It can be difficult to be certain whether a patient is describing defecatory difficulty due to structural abnormality, slow transit or pelvic floor disorder. Investigation of the patient who complains that the bowel fails to move adequately therefore proceeds as already described (➔ Constipation and slow transit p.250).

Obstructed defecation

- Patients describe difficulty in emptying the rectum with straining at stool
- Frequency of defecation may not be reduced, in fact some bowel movement may be achieved many times daily
- The patient feels that the rectum is not empty and this is borne out on investigation by proctogram
- Digitation to aid rectal emptying is common.

Assessment

Because of the difficulty in achieving private and realistic investigation conditions, the results should be considered in the context of the history, examination and results of other investigations. Patients with IBS frequently complain of incomplete emptying but proctogram does not confirm this. If the history is characteristic and the rectum fails to empty on both proctogram and at anorectal physiology tests, then the conclusion that there is obstructed defecation is more certain.

- Examination most often reveals the characteristic findings of chronic straining at stool: a flat perineum with further descent on straining down, rectocele and an abnormal anal sphincter
- Anorectal physiology will allow objective assessment of rectal sensation, compliance and pressures, as well as sphincter pressures and perineal descent (➔ Anorectal physiology p.96)
- Some patients have a tight anal sphincter while others have a lax sphincter due to either previous vaginal delivery or occult rectal intussusception
- Proctography should be carried out in all patients prior to intervention (Fig. 6.2)
- The principal question to be answered by these examinations is whether the rectum empties normally or not. If the rectum does not empty this may be due to the difficult circumstances of the test, but paradoxical contraction of the puborectalis muscle may be demonstrably the cause of the patient's symptoms. Rectal prolapse may also be demonstrated unexpectedly. Other findings such as rectocele, intussusception and perineal descent are associated with prolonged straining so may be the result of long-standing symptoms rather than the cause.

Defecating proctogram

- Imaging of pelvic floor activity can be achieved by fluoroscopy or dynamic MRI
- In both methods the rectum is filled by thick contrast medium (barium or US gel) and the patient is asked to attempt defecation while either video fluoroscopy or dynamic MRI (image acquisition every 1–2s using either an endoanal coil or phased array imaging) is performed
- MR proctography may need to be performed supine, in which case it is less accurate in detecting intussusception

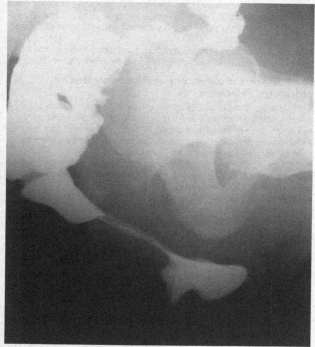

Fig. 6.2 Proctogram showing anterior rectocele.

- MR proctogram is advantageous in visualizing the entire pelvic floor, including the bladder and genital organs
- It is virtually impossible to make such examinations completely physiological, but it seems obvious that the results will be more likely to be helpful if the circumstances are as relaxed and private as possible.

Anismus, puborectalis paradox and obstructed defecation

- The term 'anismus' is used to describe failure of relaxation of the anal sphincter mechanism during attempted defecation
- 'Puborectalis paradox' implies contraction of the puborectalis muscle rather than relaxation as attempts to defecate are made
- These abnormalities are identified on investigation, either anorectal physiology or proctography
- In general, the term 'anismus' is used in association with physiological testing, whether using sphincter pressure measurement or EMG, while 'puborectalis paradox' is used to describe an abnormally contracting puborectalis on proctography
- Some patients seem to be unable to empty the rectum yet do not demonstrate these other measurable abnormalities

- Some patients who have pelvic floor damage, probably neurological and often after traumatic vaginal delivery, seem to be unable to empty the rectum because the pelvic floor is weak and unable to move adequately to empty the rectum
- In some patients no abnormality other than inability to empty can be identified and psychological difficulties have therefore been implicated.

Biofeedback and other conservative treatment for obstructed defecation

- Many patients are helped by advice and support which is a mix of information, advice on diet/fluids, reassurance and toilet positioning
- The influence of the advisor themselves is probably very significant
- Pelvic floor physiotherapy or biofeedback training may be of help to those with uncoordinated pelvic floor function
- If the pelvic floor is very weak and major abnormalities are identified on anorectal physiology testing, it is less likely that biofeedback or physiotherapy will be successful
- Some patients find that improving rectal emptying with stimulant suppositories such as glycerine or bisacodyl is of help
- Sacral nerve stimulation has been reported to be helpful, but the effect is less marked than in patients with incontinence (→ Sacral nerve stimulation p.600).

Rectocele repair

- A degree of rectocele, i.e. bulge between the rectum and vagina, is a common finding, especially in parous women
- Gynaecologists are often referred women who complain of the bulge of a large rectocele
- Some patients with rectocele complain of difficult defecation and they are generally referred to colorectal surgery
- The problem is whether the rectocele itself is the cause or whether it represents the result of a pelvic floor muscle dysfunction
- If the underlying problem is the pelvic floor, it is likely that symptoms and the rectocele will recur after repair
- Successful defecation after digitations of the vagina has been considered to imply that repair of a rectocele will be helpful, as has barium trapping in a rectocele at proctography. This is not always borne out in practice
- Rectocele repair may be carried out via the vagina by gynaecologists, transanally by colorectal surgeons or via the perineum. No significant difference is evident between the results from these approaches (→ Prolapse: perineal procedures p.574)
- Several procedures that incorporate mesh into the repair have been described. However, anxiety regarding the risks of mesh have led most surgeons to either abandon or severely curtail their use.

Rectopexy for intussusception

Some patients with difficult defecation have a rectal intussusception identified at proctography or EUA. The debate about operative treatment in these patients is similar to that in patients with similar symptoms who are found to have a rectocele.

- If the intussusception is a full-thickness rectal prolapse which comes out beyond the anal margin it seems logical that operative treatment will be beneficial in patients who are fit enough. Symptomatic prolapse is likely to develop and stretching of the sphincter may lead to incontinence
- If the intussusception does not come out through the anal canal and the main symptom is constipation or difficulty with defecation the outcome of operation is less certain
- The most certain means of abolishing the intussusception is abdominal rectopexy, which may be carried out laparoscopically. However, a significant number of patients have troublesome constipation after this procedure and do not feel that the operation has been beneficial.

Stapled transanal rectal resection (STARR)

STARR was introduced in early 2000 as a procedure to treat disordered and obstructed defecation. Although it gained widespread early acceptance, increasing concern regarding the risk of complications, coupled with poor longer-term outcome data has led to a substantial decline in its use.

References

Koh CE, Young CJ, Young JM, Solomon MJ. Systematic review of randomized controlled trials of the effectiveness of biofeedback for pelvic floor dysfunction. *Br J Surg* 2008;**95**:1079–1887.

Hirst GR, Hughes RJ, Morgan AR, Carr ND, Patel B, Beynon J. The role of rectocele repair in targeted patients with obstructed defaecation. *Colorectal Dis* 2005;**7**:159–163.

Brown AJ anderson JH, McKee RF, Finlay IG. Surgery for occult rectal prolapse. *Colorectal Dis* 2004;**6**:176–179.

Corman ML, Carriero A, Hager T et al. Consensus conference on the stapled transanal rectal resection (STARR) for disordered defaecation. *Colorectal Dis* 2006;**8**:98–101.

Chronic anorectal pain

Functional anorectal pain describes a group of conditions characterized by pain in the absence of any organic proctologic disease. In 2016, criteria for their diagnosis were agreed by the Rome IV international collaborative committee. Their true prevalence is unclear as they are probably under-reported, but it is suggested to be ~10%.

Functional anorectal pain can be divided into 3 categories
Levator ani syndrome
Unspecified anorectal pain
Proctalgia fugax

Levator ani syndrome

Possibly due to levator spasm or inflammation in the arcus tendon of le-vator. Many patients have dyssynergic defecation.

- Chronic or recurrent rectal pain.
- Often unilateral and females > males
- Episodes last >30min
- Symptoms must be for at least 3 months out of 12.
- Tenderness during traction on the puborectalis or levator ani
- Other causes of rectal pain such as infection, abscesses, IBD, haemorrhoids and fissures should be excluded
- Several treatments have been described, perhaps testament to the fact that no single intervention works in all patients
  - Electrogalvanic stimulation
  - Biofeedback training
  - Muscle relaxants e.g. diazepam
  - Direct digital massage of the levators

Unspecified anorectal pain

- As above without tenderness on posterior traction on the puborectalis.

Chronic proctalgia is described as a dull ache or pressure high in the rectum. It is often worse while sitting and during the day, particularly the afternoon. Suggested treatments include reassurance, muscle relaxants (benzodiazep-ines, baclofen), sitz baths, digital levator massage, electrogalvanic stimula-tion and biofeedback. Evidence base for treatment is lacking and surgery has no clear role.

Proctalgia fugax

- Recurrent episodes of sudden, severe pain localized to the anus or lower rectum
- Episodes last from seconds to minutes
- Pain may awaken patients from sleep
- Complete resolution of pain in between attacks
- Other causes of rectal pain such as infection, abscesses, IBD, haemorrhoids and fissures should be excluded

Pain may be caused by abnormal smooth muscle contractions. Attacks are infrequent and irregular (roughly monthly) and may be more common in women. Symptoms before puberty are rare. Stress and anxiety may precipi-tate attacks. Reassurance is often all that is required, although salbutamol (β-adrenergic agent) and calcium channel blockers have been reported to improve symptoms. Direct digital massage may also be helpful.

Coccygodynia

- Pain arising from the coccyx which can radiate to the sacral region
- Much more frequent in women (due to pelvic anatomy)
- The acute injury may be due to a fall or childbirth
- Manipulation of the coccyx may reproduce pain
- Sitting and standing lateral x-rays do not always show an abnormality
- Treatment is usually conservative—doughnut-shaped cushion, sitz baths, massage and infiltration of LA or steroid
- Coccygectomy can be helpful but requires careful patient selection.

Reference

Rao SS, Bharucha AE, Chiarioni G, *et al.* Functional Anorectal Disorders. *Gastroenterology* 2016;S0016-5085(16)00175–X

Solitary rectal ulcer

Solitary rectal ulcer syndrome (SRUS) is also referred to as mucosal pro-lapse solitary rectal ulcer syndrome (MPSRUS). The term SRUS is misleading as lesions may not be solitary or ulcerated or even confined to the rectum.

Presentation

- Rectal bleeding is the most common presentation (>90%)
- Mucous discharge, tenesmus, straining and rectal pain may feature.
- Lesions may be asymptomatic
- Reported in both children and elderly with equal sex distribution
- Can be found on prolapsing stomas, haemorrhoids, adjacent to polyps, in mucosal folds around diverticulae and in cap polyposis.

Pathophysiology

- White slough-covered base surrounded by swollen, erythematous mucosa
- Multiple ulcers can be confluent, giving a butterfly appearance
- Lesions can also be polypoid (25%) or flat (20%)
- Often misdiagnosed as a malignant ulcer
- In the early stages, the only endoscopic finding may be patchy rectal erythema lying 5–15cm from the anal margin
- The condition may progress to polypoid erythematous areas without associated ulceration
- Differential diagnosis includes CD and infectious ulceration
- EAUS, anorectal physiology and defecating proctogram may be useful.

Histological findings

- Histological features are the key to diagnosis
- Madigan and Morson first described the histological features of mucosal prolapse in 1969
- Thickening and disruption of the muscularis mucosae ('fibromuscular obliteration')
- The lamina propria is replaced with smooth muscle
- Displaced mucus glands are also found deep within the submucosa and muscularis mucosae, giving rise to the name 'localized colitis/proctitis cystica profunda'
- This histological appearance may be confused with a well-differentiated adenocarcinoma.

Treatment

- Because the condition is rare there is little evidence base to guide treatment
- Patients may improve spontaneously or with simple treatment of constipation
- Biofeedback aims to improve toileting habits and coordinate pelvic floor contraction
- Biofeedback can lead to symptomatic improvement in 50–75% and ulcer resolution in 30%
- Use of topical steroids, salicylates and sucralfate enemas has been described
- Surgical intervention should be reserved for patients with refractory symptoms
- Local ulcer excision has a high recurrence rate
- Rectopexy and resection rectopexy may be helpful for persistent ulceration with prolapse (➔ Prolapse rectopexy p.570)
- Anterior resection and proctocolectomy has been described.

Reference

Madigan MR, Morson BC. Solitary ulcer of the rectum. *Gut* 1969;**10**:871–881.

Haemorrhoids

Background

The anal cushions are submucosal fibrovascular structures which are suggested to play a role in fine continence. The 3 classical positions described are left lateral, right anterior and right posterior.

The cushions consist of arteriovenous communications involving the superior, middle and inferior haemorrhoidal arteries and veins anchored to the sphincter with a connective tissue matrix. Distension within these vascular cushions is thought to contribute 20% of the internal sphincter resting pressure (Fig. 6.3).

Aetiology

The most recent theory is that degeneration of the connective tissue matrix allows descent of the anal cushions possibly exacerbated by straining and passage of hard motion. Venous return is then impeded, leading to dilatation, venous stasis and inflammation. Direct trauma or ulceration of the overlying mucosa then leads to bleeding. A shared pathogenesis with mucosal prolapse is controversial.

A competing theory is that increased venous pressure leads to dilatation of the arteriovenous communications which then prolapse.

- Incidence of 4–40% is reported but difficult to assess as many patients do not present for treatment
- Straining, poor fibre intake, constipation, diarrhoea, prolonged standing, spicy foods, advancing age and increased intra-abdominal pressure (e.g. pregnancy) are commonly associated with haemorrhoids, although evidence is limited

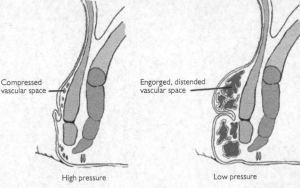

Compressed vascular space

Engorged, distended vascular space

High pressure   Low pressure

Fig. 6.3 When the resting anal pressure is high, the anal cushions which contain large vascular spaces empty of blood. When the anus relaxes these vascular spaces become engorged with blood and contribute to resting anal pressure and continence. Occasional impaired faecal continence after haemorrhoidectomy may be secondary to a loss of this continence mechanism

Reproduced with permission from Gibbons CP, Trowbridge EA, Bannister JJ, Read NW. Role of anal cushions in maintaining continence. *The Lancet*;1:886–888. Copyright © 1986 Published by Elsevier Ltd. doi: 10.1016/s0140-6736(86)90990-6.

- There is evidence to support a hereditary predisposition
- Haemorrhoids are not rectal varices and there is no evidence of increased incidence in portal hypertension.

Classification

- External haemorrhoids originate from the inferior haemorrhoidal plexus below the dentate line. Covered by modified squamous epithelium supplied by somatic pain fibres
- Internal haemorrhoids originate from the superior haemorrhoidal plexus above the dentate line. Covered by insensate columnar epithelium
- Patients may present with mixed internal and external component
- Goligher's classification of internal haemorrhoids:
  - Grade 1: bleeding but no prolapse
  - Grade 2: prolapsing but spontaneously reduce
  - Grade 3: prolapse requiring manual reduction
  - Grade 4: thrombosed prolapsed haemorrhoids[1]
- Skin tags are described separately
- Other classification systems have been described but are not in common use.

Presentation

- Symptoms include bleeding, prolapse, mucus discharge, perianal itch and pain
- Diagnosis is confirmed on examination with proctoscopy
- Colonoscopy is suggested for patients >50yrs or those >40yrs with risk factors for malignancy if no colonic assessment has been carried out in the last 3–5yrs
- Some patients also complain of incontinence, faecal soiling and difficulty with evacuation. These symptoms should be fully assessed as management may impact on treatment of the haemorrhoids
- Anorectal physiology and EAUS should be considered for patients with a history of incontinence (⊕ Endoanal and endorectal ultrasound and Anorectal physiology p.92 & p.96).

Treatment

Conservative

- Some patients will be satisfied with simple reassurance
- Initial treatment should include dietary advice with increased fibre and water intake. Constipation and straining should be avoided
- Fibre is proven to improve symptoms and reduce bleeding in ~50%
- Over the counter preparations include LAs, corticosteroids, astringents, antiseptics and barrier creams. They may give temporary relief of symptoms but evidence to support their use is lacking
- Oral flavonoids are plant extracts which may have anti-inflammatory activity and increase venous tone. May reduce pain, bleeding and itch but rarely used in the UK.

1 Reproduced from Goligher, JC. (1980). *Surgery of the Anus Rectum and Colon*, Fourth Edition. London, UK: Bailliere Tindall.

Rubber band ligation (RBL)
- Causes ischaemic necrosis with scarring and fibrosis
- RBL is the most effective non-surgical/outpatient procedure for haemorrhoids with cure in up to 80%. Repeat banding can be successful, with only a small proportion requiring surgical management
- Bands are placed at the base of the haemorrhoids, at least 1cm above the dentate line. Up to 3 bands are placed in one session
- Application too close to the dentate line may cause exquisite pain requiring removal
- Mild discomfort is experienced in 10–30%
- Secondary haemorrhage may occur 2-10 days after the procedure
- Pelvic sepsis/Fournier's gangrene is very rare but has been reported.

Injection sclerotherapy (IS)
- Method of action is fibrosis of submucosa ± intravascular thrombosis
- A variety of sclerosants have been used: 5% phenol in almond oil is the most popular
- IS is simple, cheap and painless but with a high failure rate (~70%)
- Inadvertent prostatic injection can cause prostatitis
- Contraindicated in the presence of other anorectal pathology

Photocoagulation
- Infrared beam leads to heat, intravascular coagulation and fibrosis
- Similar efficacy to RBL with less pain and few complications
- Use limited by requirement for repeated treatments and the expense of equipment.

Doppler-guided haemorrhoidal artery ligation
- A specially designed proctoscope incorporating a Doppler probe is used to identify branches of the superior haemorrhoidal artery which are sutured. A plicating suture may also be used to lift and anchor prolapsing haemorrhoidal cushions
- Up to 85% of patients have resolution of symptoms at 1 year.
- Patients have less pain compared to haemorrhoidectomy and few major complications but with increased recurrence rate
- Two proprietary devices are available, THD® (transanal haemorrhoidal devascularization) (THD S.p.a. Corregio, Italy) and HALO® (haemorrhoidal artery ligation operation) (AMI Feldrich Austria). Both systems incorporate a disposable proctoscope with integrated ultrasound, integrated light source and a design that allows for precise placement of sutures at point of focus of ultrasound (➔ Haemorrhoidectomy p.584).
- Superiority over RBL has not been proven

Haemorrhoidectomy
- Haemorrhoidectomy involves excision using scissors, diathermy, electrothermal sealing devices or ultrasonic dissectors while leaving adequate skin bridges to avoid anal stenosis (➔ Haemorrhoidectomy p.584)
- Wounds can be left open (Milligan–Morgan) or closed (Ferguson) with little evidence of difference in pain or wound healing
- Regional local anaesthetic techniques and restricted IV fluids reduce rates of urinary retention

- Post-operative metronidazole and stool softeners improve analgesia
- Topical glyceryl trinitrate (GTN)/calcium channel antagonists and botulinum toxin injection may improve post-operative pain control and wound healing
- Complications include pain, bleeding, urinary retention, anal fissure, anal stenosis and incontinence. Impaired continence may also occur although this is usually temporary.

Procedure for prolapse and haemorrhoids (PPH)/stapled anopexy

- Involves circumferential mucosal resection and stapling above the dentate line. This restores the relationship of haemorrhoids to the anal canal and disrupts the blood supply
- Reduced post-operative pain and faster return to normal activities compared with haemorrhoidectomy
- Increased rates of post-operative faecal urgency, chronic rectal pain and re-operation for recurrence and skin tags
- Small but definite risk of more serious complications including luminal occlusion, rectal perforation, anastomotic dehiscence, retroperitoneal sepsis and rectovaginal fistula
- Although still occasionally undertaken, concerns about complications and better outcomes with newer interventions such as the THD/ HALO operation mean that it's use is in sharp decline.

Direct current electrocautery (eXroid®)

- Recent renewed interest in a technique that was first described more than 30 years ago
- A direct current (DC) is applied the base of the internal haemorrhoid using a proprietary disposable probe and current generator (eXroid Technology Ltd).
- Thought to induce thrombosis in the haemorrhoid vascular pedicle
- Usually performed in an outpatient setting with no local anaesthesia
- Direct current up to 16 milliamps applied to each haemorrhoid for average of 10 minutes/haemorrhoid. 50% of patients require more than one treatment
- Appears to be well tolerated and good initial results but rather poor quality evidence on long-term outcomes

Radiofrequency treatment of haemorrhoids

- The **ra**dio **f**requency treatment of h**ae**morrhoids under **lo**cal anaesthesia (Rafaelo®) operation uses a proprietary probe (F care Systems, Antwerp) to treat haemorrhoids in an outpatient setting
- It appears to be well tolerated and with good initial results although long-term outcomes are not available

Outmoded procedures

- Anal stretch procedures (Lord's), internal sphincterotomy and cryotherapy and no longer recommended treatments.

Special circumstances

- Care should be taken with patients on anti-coagulants. Injection sclerotherapy/photocoagulation may be more appropriate than RBL to reduce risk of bleeding

- Haemorrhoids are not uncommon during pregnancy and conservative management should be followed
- Haemorrhoidal surgery should be avoided in CD if possible and certainly until perianal sepsis is controlled
- In HIV/AIDS wound healing and septic complications are increased and conservative measures are recommended as first line treatment.

Thrombosed acute haemorrhoids

- Conservative treatment involves analgesia, stool softeners, topical LAs and sitz baths
- Topical application of GTN, diltiazem or nifedipine has been shown to improve analgesia
- Botulinum toxin injection into the internal anal sphincter also gives rapid pain relief without significant side effects
- Conservative management is often associated with a long-term improvement in symptoms
- Haemorrhoidectomy may be considered within the first 48–72h for quicker resolution of symptoms
- Evacuation of thrombus is not advised due to haemorrhage and recurrent clot formation.

Skin tags

- Anal skin tags are most commonly idiopathic or primary
- May be secondary to haemorrhoids, chronic anal fissures, CD
- Skin tags are rarely symptomatic
- Trauma due to overenthusiastic cleaning can cause irritation with itch, discharge or blood noticed on the toilet paper
- Simple excision may be requested for cosmetic or hygiene reasons.

Perianal haematoma

- Acutely painful condition occurring typically after straining at stool
- A bluish/black acutely tender lump is visible at the anal verge
- Easily differentiated from a thrombosed haemorrhoid as the lump is continuous with anal verge
- These will resolve spontaneously (~5 days) with conservative management
- Instant pain relief can be achieved by clot evacuation under local anaesthesia.

Reference

Gibbons CP, Trowbridge EA, Bannister JJ, Read NW. Role of anal cushions in maintaining continence. *Lancet* 1986;**1**:886–888.

Anal fissure

Anal fissure

An anal fissure is a linear split in the mucosa of the anal canal. It is a common problem that presents with severe anal pain on defecation. Most heal spontaneously within a few days. A chronic fissure is defined as being present for at least 6 weeks and associated with other stigmata of chronicity such as visible fibres of the IAS within the fissure, induration, a sentinel pile and a hypertrophied anal papilla.

They occur most commonly in the first 4 decades of life. Most fissures are idiopathic although some may have a history of constipation or even diarrhoea. Most are sited in midline posteriorly (90%). Anterior fissures are more common in females and may occur post-partum. Other risk factors include CD, HIV, syphilis, sarcoid, TB and drugs (nicorandil) (Fig. 6.4). Fissures associated with these conditions may be deep, lateral and multiple.

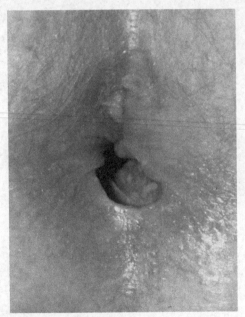

Fig. 6.4 Nicorandil-induced fissure/ulceration.

Pathophysiology

- Most anal fissures are associated with increased tone of the IAS
- High anal tone is associated with a reduction in blood flow to the anoderm rendering the posterior commissure of the anus ischaemic
- Normal pressure or low pressure fissures may occur in the elderly and in patients with CD, HIV, infection and post-partum
- Surgical or medical therapy is directed at reducing anal tone thereby inducing healing by restoring blood flow to the anoderm
- NO is the neurotransmitting agent in the noradrenergic nerves that mediates relaxation of the IAS. GTN promotes the release of NO and a reduction in resting anal pressure by relaxing the IAS.

Treatment

Conservative

- Avoid constipation. Dietary advice, laxatives and topical anesthetics.

Medical therapies

Topical GTN

- 0.2–0.4% ointment applied twice daily: healing rate 70%
- Side effects include transient headaches and pruritus
- Increased anal tone returns after cessation of therapy.

Botulinum toxin

- 15–30 units injected into the IAS or intersphincteric space
- Anterior IAS injection may be best location for injection
- Reduces resting anal pressure with full recovery by 3 months
- Healing rate 70%.

Calcium channel blockers

- Induce smooth muscle relaxation
- Oral and topical diltiazem and nifedipine are all effective
- 2% topical diltiazem has a healing rate of 65%.

Surgical therapies

Anal dilatation

- Variable finger or balloon dilatation of anal canal
- No longer viewed as appropriate due to high risk of sphincter damage (65%) and incontinence (12%).

Lateral internal sphincterotomy

- Procedure of choice after failure of conservative or medical therapy (➲ Lateral sphincterotomy p.598)
- Lateral site is preferred over posterior as it avoids a keyhole deformity
- May be performed as an open or SC procedure
- Long-term fissure healing in 95% of patients
- Minor incontinence/seepage in 2–20% of patients
- Should be avoided in normal pressure or low pressure fissures.

Fissurectomy and anal advancement flap
- May be appropriate in resistant fissures in patients at increased risk of incontinence (Box 6.1)
- Fissurectomy excises chronic scar tissue and stigmata of chronic disease, e.g. sentinel pile and hypertrophied papillae.
- V–Y advancement flap or anoplasty introduces a well vascularized pedicle flap into the chronically ischaemic fissure (Fig. 6.5)
- Variable healing and long-term results not certain, although these procedures appear most effective in patients with normal or low pressure anal fissures.

Box 6.1 Risk factors for incontinence following sphincterotomy
- Elderly patients
- Diabetics
- Multiparous women
- Irritable bowel patients
- Recurrent fissure following previous sphincterotomy
- Known normal or low pressure fissure

Anal stenosis

Anal stenosis is a disabling condition that is suggested by a history of consti-pation and difficulty in passing stool. Patients may volunteer that 'the anus is too tight' and that the stool is thin and elongated. The condition can be associated with rectal bleeding and anal pain which may be secondary to a concomitant anal fissure or neoplasm.

The diagnosis is confirmed by physical examination. Lichen sclerosis pre-sents with thickened whitish skin folds which may extend over the peri-neum. In the presence of anal pain, EUA may be necessary to confirm a true stenosis, as spasm or hypertrophy of the internal sphincter due to an anal fissure is readily identifiable under GA. EUA will also exclude anorectal neoplasia.

The stricture may be confined to a narrow band at the anal margin or may extend throughout the length of the anal canal with the upper margin at the level of the levators or anorectal ring. The condition and treatment should be differentiated from a rectal stricture which has a different patho-physiology and management.

The most common cause is scarring post-haemorrhoidectomy due to excision of excessive tissue or failure to maintain adequate mucosal bridges.

Causes

- Post-haemorrhoidectomy (incidence ~1%)
- Post-anal surgery (e.g. excessive diathermy ablation of anal warts, transanal excision of tumours, coloanal anastomosis)
- Anal fissure (rarely gives rise to a true stenosis)
- Inflammatory conditions associated with abscesses, fistulae and strictures (e.g. CD)
- Chronic diarrhoea or laxative use/abuse causing thin stools
- Chronic pruritus ani, especially if associated with lichen sclerosis
- Radiation therapy
- Congenital malformation (imperforate anus, stenosis or membrane)
- Neoplasia
- Trauma (lacerations, thermal or chemical injury)
- Infections (TB, lymphogranuloma venereum, syphilis).

Management

- Exclude anorectal pathology with an EUA if no obvious cause
- Punch skin biopsy if lichen sclerosis is considered
- Benign anal stenosis is initially treated with a bulk laxative and twice-daily use of an anal dilator
- Surgery is likely if an anal dilator cannot be easily passed
- Mild stenosis may respond to excision of eschar and sphincterotomy, but this may be associated with a risk of incontinence
- Moderate to severe stenosis will require an anoplasty
- Unilateral or bilateral V–Y or island advancement flaps are used if stenosis is <50% (Fig. 6.5)
- A rotation flap anoplasty is indicated for >50% stenosis.

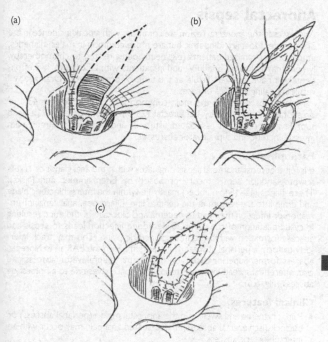

Fig. 6.5 (a) V–Y or Island advancement flap anoplasty. (b) The skin flap is mobilised and advanced. (c) Primary closure is completed.

Adapted with permission from Keighley M, Williams (Eds.) (2008). *Surgery of the Rectum and Colon*, 3rd Edition. Philadelphia, USA: Saunders, Elsevier.

Anorectal sepsis

Abscesses in the anorectal region are common, with a peak incidence in the 3rd decade. Most are idiopathic but are more common in males, diabetics, immunocompromised patients (e.g. neutropenia related to chemotherapy, lymphoma/leukaemia and HIV) and in patients with CD. Up to 1/3 of patients will have an overt fistula at the time of presentation. Drainage will result in healing in >50% of cases.

Perianal abscesses are the most common type, accounting for 43% of presentations, followed by ischiorectal (23%), intersphincteric (21%) and supralevator (7%). An associated fistula in ano is more common with intersphincteric and supralevator abscesses.

Pathophysiology

It is felt that most anorectal sepsis originates within the anal glands or crypts (cryptoglandular sepsis theory proposed by Eisenhammer and Parks). These glands (12–15 in number) mainly lie within the intersphincteric plane and drain into the rectum at the dentate line. Diarrhoea, anal canal inflammation or infection may lead to oedema and blockage of the duct, resulting in cystic dilatation of the glands. Superadded infection leads to sepsis and abscess formation within the intersphincteric plane. This may track inferiorly to form a perianal abscess. If it tracks through the EAS an ischiorectal abscess forms. Superior extension may form a supralevator abscess and circumferential spread in the posterior anal space gives rise to a horseshoe abscess (Fig. 6.6).

Clinical features

- Pain, erythema and swelling in the anorectal region (perianal abscess) or buttock (ischiorectal abscess). Deep-seated anal pain may occur with an intersphincteric abscess
- A supralevator abscess presents with pelvic pain and systemic upset
- Constipation or pain on sitting or defecation may occur
- An EUA may be necessary to establish the diagnosis if unclear
- Rarely imaging (e.g. MR or EAUS) may be necessary
- No external stigmata may be visible with an intersphincteric abscess but marked tenderness and swelling noted on rectal examination
- CD should be considered if multiple or recurrent abscesses.

Treatment

- The mainstay of management is the prompt drainage of the pus
- Incisions should be circum-anal rather than radial to minimize risk of damage to the sphincters
- Consider either a fistulotomy or Seton drain for concomitant fistula
- De-roof an intersphincteric abscesses via an internal sphincterotomy
- A pelvic source of sepsis should be considered with a supralevator abscess (e.g. diverticular disease or CD)
- Abscesses secondary to anorectal CD are often chronic and may require prolonged drainage and antibiotic therapy

- A horseshoe abscess is usually due to a posterior anal space abscess with bilateral ischiorectal anterolateral extensions
- Persistent discharge for >6 weeks after drainage suggests an underlying fistula in ano
- Debate surrounds the advisability of treating associated fistulae at the time of drainage of the abscess (Box 6.2).

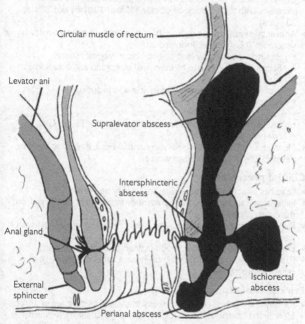

Circular muscle of rectum

Levator ani

Supralevator abscess

Intersphincteric abscess

Anal gland

External sphincter

Ischiorectal abscess

Perianal abscess

Fig. 6.6 Site and anatomical relationships of the most common anorectal abscesses.

Box 6.2 Should one treat associated fistulae when draining sepsis?

- Fistulae are present in most cases of anorectal sepsis
- Immediate treatment is associated with increased risk of incontinence (6% vs 0% for delayed treatment)
- Many fistulae will resolve following drainage of sepsis
- Aggressive early identification and treatment of associated fistulae is likely to lead to overtreatment and poorer outcomes, especially with respect to incontinence

Fistula in ano

A fistula in ano is an abnormal tract or cavity communicating between the skin and the rectum or anus. Most follow anorectal sepsis secondary to cryptoglandular infection (infection of an anal gland). The incidence of a fistula developing after drainage of an anorectal abscess is 15–40%. Other conditions may also give rise to fistulae

- Crohn's disease. More common with anorectal CD. The incidence increases with the duration of disease (15% at 10 years and 30% at 20 years)
- Anorectal sepsis secondary to HIV, tuberculosis, lymphogranuloma venereum (LGV) and actinomycosis
  - Obstetric trauma may lead to ano/ recto-vaginal fistulae
  - Nicorandil may give rise to deep anal ulceration and occasionally fistula in ano
- Several conditions may mimic a fistula in ano including
  - Hidradenitis suppurativa
  - Anal abscess or a Bartholin's abscess
  - Anal fissure or anal ulceration secondary to CD, TB or LGV
  - Low-lying pilonidal sinus
- Mean age at presentation is 40 years and males are twice as likely to develop a fistula compared to women.

Clinical presentation

- Features of active or old perianal sepsis may be present
- Patients will also complain of constant or intermittent discharge from the external opening.
- Pain, sometimes deep-seated, which may be less severe when fistula is freely discharging
- Discharge may be purulent, blood stained or frankly faeculent
- Patients may also complain of "non-healing" at site of drainage of a recent anorectal abscess

Principles of assessment

- Identify the external opening (usually at the site of drainage of abscess)
- Identify the internal opening (usually at the dentate line). If internal opening is above in rectum, this suggests an extrasphincteric fistula which may be iatrogenic or related to CD or pelvic abscess
- Outline the course of the primary track (can often be palpated as a thickened cord under skin). Note Goodsall's rule (Fig. 6.8).
- Extensions or secondary tracks may occur in the intersphincteric plane, the ischiorectal fossa and the supralevator space. The presence of such extensions may complicate management.
- Consider associated conditions such as CD or sphincter injury
- Try and determine the relationship to the sphincters in order to classify the fistula. Park's classification is the most widely accepted and used (Fig. 6.7). However, this classification ignores superficial/submucosal fistulae which are not uncommon but may have a different aetiology e.g. undermined residual track after an anal fissure, ulcer or anal operation wound had healed.

- Alternatively, fistulae may be classified according to complexity. A **complex fistula** might include the following
  - Suprasphincteric, extrasphincteric and transsphincteric fistulas that encompass ≥30% of the external sphincter
  - Horseshoe fistula
  - Fistulas associated with CD & other medical conditions
  - Fistula in association with diarrhoea and or incontinence
  - Any anterior fistula in a female
  - Recurrent fistulas
  - Fistulas with multiple or secondary tracks
- A **simple fistula** does not have any of the features of a complex fistula. They include superficial, intersphincteric and low transsphincteric fistulae that encompass < 30% of the external fistula

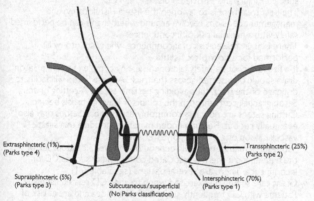

Extrasphincteric (1%)
(Parks type 4)

Suprasphincteric (5%)
(Parks type 3)

Subcutaneous/susperficial
(No Parks classification)

Transsphincteric (25%)
(Parks type 2)

Intersphincteric (70%)
(Parks type 1)

Fig. 6.7 Modified Park's classification of types of anal fistulae.

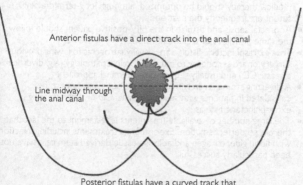

Anterior fistulas have a direct track into the anal canal

Line midway through
the anal canal

Posterior fistulas have a curved track that
terminates in midline posteriorly

Fig. 6.8 Goodsall's rule.

Imaging and other assessments
- Most simple/low fistulae do not require imaging
- EAUS is a useful adjunct to EUA. Hydrogen peroxide helps to highlight tracks. Associated sphincter defects may be seen.
- MRI is used to assess complex, recurrent and Crohn's related fistulae (Fig. 6.9)
- Fistulography has been superseded by MRI is assessment of fistulae
- Manometry may be used to assess anal sphincter function.

Management
- Management must be individualized and depends on the sex of the patient, the amount of external sphincter that the fistula encompasses, the location (e.g. anterior or posterior), previous anorectal surgery or sphincter injury and associated disease, e.g. CD.
- The best treatment is to lay open the fistula (fistulotomy) and management decisions revolve around whether this can be performed safely with a minimal risk of incontinence.
- There is an increased risk of incontinence when fistulotomy is performed for a **complex fistula**
- If a fistula cannot be safely laid open (ie. any complex fistula), a Seton drain should be inserted across the track. A loose Seton will facilitate drainage of the tract, thus avoiding perianal sepsis. A cutting or snug Seton gradually cuts through the sphincter leaving fibrosis behind. Cutting setons are now less commonly used. Loose Setons may also eventually cut out. Recommended materials include a thin silastic vascular sloop or a braided polyester suture.
- Subsequent management will depend on the type, location, sex of the patient and if there is associated co-morbidity such as CD or incontinence. There are several options (see Table 6.1)
- Great care should be exercised when treating CD related fistulae. Patients with CD frequently suffer from diarrhoea and are at risk of developing recurrent fistulae. Laying open even relatively superficial fistulae can be associated with immediate or subsequent incontinence. Medical therapy should be optimized, although long-term draining setons are frequently the best option.
- Anorectal sepsis and fistulae in the HIV-positive patient should follow the same principles of treatment for CD
- True extrasphincteric fistulae are usually iatrogenic following previous surgery or are secondary to intra-abdominal pathology (e.g. diverticular disease, CD) and usually require an abdominal approach.
- A diverting stoma is rarely necessary although may have to be considered in patients with severe perianal CD or when treating extrasphincteric fistulas
- The large number of available treatments is testament to the fact that there is no perfect solution. Experimental treatments including injection with fibrin glue, collagen and adipose tissue derived stem cells have not been particularly successful

Table 6.1. Treatment options for fistula in ano

Technique	Indication	Notes
Lay open fistula (fistolotomy)	Simple fistulae only	Very high success rate with low incontinence in selected patients
Draining/ loose Seton suture	Excellent initial treatment to allow sepsis to settle and enable more accurate subsequent assessment	Not designed to cure fistula. Some will work through sphincter in time. May be appropriate long-term in CD and other complex fistulas
Cutting Seton drain	May considered in simple fistula and some complex fistulae e.g. transsphincteric fistulae encompassing 30-50% of external sphincter in males with no other co-morbidity.	Fistula cure rates of 80-100% but incontinence rates of up to 30%. Post-operative pain an issue. Chemical impregnated Setons have also been used
Endorectal & endoanal advancment flaps	Suitable for many complex fistulas although technically difficult where there is a high internal opening (e.g. extrasphincteric) and when there is a lot of scarring within the anal canal	Fistula cure rates of 60-70%. Higher risk of recurrence in patients with CD. May have a negative impact on continence for some, but most patients find an improvement in continence.
Fistula plug (porcine collagen based)	Suitable for most fistulas other than those with a very short tract e.g. rectovaginal fistulae. Technically easy to perform	Long-term cure rates of 30-50%. Little impact on continence.
Ligation of the Intersphincteric fistula tract (LIFT)	Used to treat both simple and complex fistulae	Long term healing in up to 75%. Change in continence in up to 5% of patients.
Video assisted anal fistula treatment (VAAFT) & Fistula laser closure (FiLac®)	These 2 new techniques are suitable for most fistulae. Both require specialist (expensive) equipment	Long-term data is lacking but both techniques appear to have minimal impact on continence and cure rates of up to 70-80%

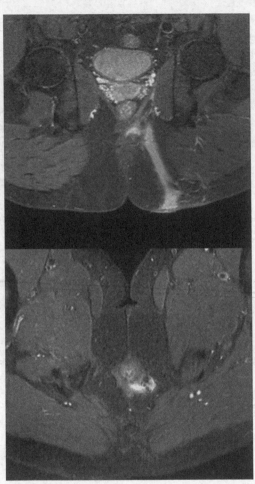

Fig. 6.9 T2-weighted sequences (fluid bright) showing relationship of fluid-filled fistula to anal canal.

Pruritus ani

A common condition characterized by intense perianal irritation which is temporarily relieved by cutaneous stimulation. Itching can damage the perianal skin, worsening the condition. Symptom severity is variable, with exacerbations and remissions. Incidence is uncertain but thought to be high. It is more common in the 2nd/3rd decade but can affect any age.

Pruritis ani may be $2°$ to numerous conditions, but for the majority the condition is idiopathic. In such patients, anal seepage may occur at lower rectal pressure than normal patients, possibly secondary to an exaggerated RAIR. Excess moisture, sweating and an irritant loose stool may also play a role.

Predisposing factors

Anatomical factors
- Obesity, deep natal cleft, hirsutism, tight-fitting clothing.

Anorectal disorders
- Haemorrhoids
- Anal fissure
- Anorectal sepsis and fistulae
- Anal skin tags and warts
- Prolapse (rectal/vaginal, full-thickness/mucosal)
- Tumours (tubulovillous adenomas and cancers)
- Faecal incontinence.

Skin conditions
- Psoriasis, eczema, lichen planus, leucoplakia, seborrhoeic dermatitis, contact dermatitis.

Infections and infestations
- Bacterial infections
  - Anal syphilis, TB, impetigo
- Fungal infections
  - *Candida albicans* is common especially if the skin is damaged by trauma, hypersensitivity or steroid use
- Viral infections
  - Condylomata accuminata, anogenital herpes, CMV, molluscum contagiosum
- Parasites
  - *Enterobius vermicularis* infection or threadworms (common in children), scabies, pediculosis pubis, spirochetes.

Diarrhoea
- Any cause including IBD, IBS, infectious diarrhoea and diverticular disease.

Systemic disease
- Diabetes, uraemia, jaundice, thyroid disease, iron-deficiency, polycythaemia, lymphoma.

Gynaecological
- Pruritus vulvae, vaginitis.

Psychological causes
- Anxiety, neuroses, dermatitis artifacta, localized neurodermatitis.

Clinical assessment

A careful history should assess duration and severity of symptoms, bowel function and will identify any underlying predisposing factors. The history should include details of previous anal surgery and any history of anoreceptive intercourse.

Clinical examination should exclude systemic skin disorders. Examination of the perianal skin and natal cleft may show the skin to be erythematous, excoriated or moist and stained with stool. Most commonly the skin will be pale and thickened, consistent with hyperkeratinization (lichen simplex chronicus). A proctoscopy and rigid sigmoidoscopy will exclude anorectal pathology. It may be possible to perform skin scrapings for mycology.

Management

The aim is to treat any associated medical conditions and to keep the perianal skin clean and dry.

General measures

- The importance of careful hygiene must be emphasized
  - Wash with plain water after defecation (over-washing can exacerbate the problem)
  - Use a soft dry or moist toilet paper
  - Skin should be padded dry (not rubbed)
  - A hairdryer can be used on a low setting
  - Avoid astringents, scented soaps, talc or baby wipes
- Scratching should be discouraged. Pinching skin can relieve irritation
- If nocturnal itching is a problem, consider cotton gloves. Sedating antihistamines may also be helpful
- Avoid food which may precipitate irritation (citrus fruits and juices, spicy foods, coffee, colas, chocolate and tomatoes)
- Limit activities that give rise to excessive sweating
- Use natural fabrics, e.g. loose cotton underwear
- A non-biological washing powder should be used, with clothes rinsed well to avoid residual detergent
- The use of topical over the counter creams should be discouraged.

Medical intervention

- Any underlying systemic condition should be treated
- Co-existing anal disease should be treated
- If diarrhoea is a dominant feature this should be controlled if possible, e.g. Loperamide.
- Bulking agent (e.g. ispaghula husk) may help aiming for 1–2 formed stools/day
- Conversely a low fibre diet to make stools firmer with less leakage may improve symptoms
- Short-term use of a mild steroid and anti-fungal cream (hydrocortisone 1% and clotrimazole 1%) can be used to treat exacerbations.

Pilonidal sinus

The term pilonidal sinus arises from 'pilus' meaning hair and 'nidus' meaning nest. It was first described in 1880 by Hodges.

Epidemiology

- Estimated incidence is 26/100,000 with 2:1 male: female ratio
- Rare before the age of 15yrs and almost never before puberty
- Uncommon aged >40yrs
- Many patients are hirsute or overweight.

Aetiology

'Pilonidal disease' is a chronic inflammatory disorder arising in the skin of the sacrococcygeal region and natal cleft. Tracts or 'pits' are lined with stratified squamous epithelium. The majority of the subcutaneous portion is lined with granulation tissue and contains loose hairs and debris.

Although it was originally thought to be a congenital condition, recent evidence suggests it is acquired. There is an occupational incidence in barbers (interdigital pilonidal sinus) and jeep drivers (it was known as 'Jeep Disease' in the Second World War). Pilonidal disease may also affect incisions remote from the perianal area.

Two aetiological mechanisms have been suggested:
- Obstruction of the hair follicle leads to follicle enlargement. This eventually ruptures into the subcutaneous tissues initially causing an abscess followed by chronic sinus formation
- Broken hair can become abnormally inserted into skin of natal cleft. This induces a foreign body reaction and infection leading to cyst or sinus formation
- There is little direct evidence available regarding the aetiology.

Presentation

Asymptomatic

The typical appearance is of tiny pits in the midline in the presacral area which are painless and may or may not contain hair. They are often associated with secondary tracts which tend to emerge laterally and caudally. It is possible for a tract to emerge distally in the perianal area.

Acute abscess

The patient presents with an acutely tender, inflamed hot red swelling slightly to one side of the midline in the natal cleft. Midline pits may or may not be visible. The abscess may discharge spontaneously or require formal incision and drainage. Bacteriology shows mainly S. aureus and S. epidermidis but can contain mixed anaerobes.

Chronic sepsis

A significant proportion of patients present with chronic symptoms of low grade discomfort and repeated discharge from the lateral 2° tracts. On examination midline pits are visible in association with 2° tracts and openings which discharge purulent material if compressed.

Differential diagnosis

Hidradenitis suppurativa
Unlike pilonidal disease this is not confined to the natal cleft. It is more common in women than men and tends to be progressive. Tracts are more superficial and do not contain hair. There may be evidence of sepsis elsewhere, particularly groins and axillae.

Fistula in ano
In the rare patient in whom the 2° tract emerges close to the anal canal differentiation between the two conditions can be difficult.

Congenital anomalies
A saccrococcygeal sinus is a remnant of the medullary canal. It may be continuous with the sacral canal or the central canal of the spinal cord. If there is a communication with the cord, the lesion is obvious at birth and may be associated with spinal bifida.

Management

Non-surgical
- Patients with minimal disease and no lateral complicating tracts can be healed by rigorous attention to hygiene and keeping the area hair free, by shaving, hair removal creams or laser depilation
- Ablation of the tracts by injection with phenol has been described but is painful and may be complicated by skin burns and fat necrosis. The recurrence rate is high and it has no place in modern management.

Surgical

Abscess
- Abscesses should be drained with a longitudinal incision just off the midline and lightly packed to keep the skin edges apart.

Definitive surgery
- The most commonly performed procedure is midline excision ± primary closure
- Due to prolonged healing times, wound infection, intensive dressing care and significant recurrence rates, a number of alternative procedures have been proposed
- Most procedures aim for asymmetric closure off the midline ± flattening of the natal cleft
- Karydakis flap, Bascom I + II, Limberg flap, V–Y advancement and Z-plasty are described in detail later (⊃ Pilonidal surgery p.592)
- For simple, localized disease, midline excision or Bascom's I is recommended
- For more diffuse or recurrent disease, a cleft-lift or rhomboid flap should be considered.

Colorectal malignancy

Colorectal cancer

Adenocarcinoma of the colon and rectum is the fourth most common cancer in the UK accounting for 11% of new cancer cases. It is also the second most common cause of cancer-related mortality. Peak incidence occurs in the 85–89 age group. 1 in 15 males and 1 in 18 females in the UK will be diagnosed with colorectal cancer in their lifetime.

In the UK, 44% of new cases are diagnosed in people ≥75yrs. The vast majority of cases are thought to arise from colonic adenomas and serrated lesions (➔ Molecular genetics of colorectal cancer, discussed later in this chapter, p.310).

- Incidence rates ♂: 84/100,000 and ♀: 56/100,000
- Since early 1990s, incidence rates have been stable for ♀ with a ↓ 3% in ♂ (in the last decade, ↓ 2% in ♀ and a ↓ 6% in ♂)
- Relative 5yr survival is 58% (has more than doubled in last 40 yrs)
- Survival is inversely proportional to age
- Rates of CRC are 10 times higher in developed countries, with Western diets thought to account for the majority of the effect.

Risk factors

CRC has a multifactorial aetiology where

- Sporadic cancers account for at least 70% of cases. Advancing age, dietary, and environmental factors play a pivotal role in these sporadic cancers
- Specific cancer syndromes with a defined inherited germline mutation (e.g. hereditary non-polyposis colon cancer (HNPCC)) account for 5–10% of cases
- Around 25% of patients will have a family history although the genetic basis and mode of inheritance is not well understood.

Dietary factors

- Countries with diets high in processed and red meat have highest rates of CRC. Red meat consumption has been linked to distal tumours.
  - Most studies pointing to this association have been observational
  - Studies which assessed the impact of reducing dietary and animal fat did not show any change in the risk of CRC
  - Overall, it seems that there may be a small increased risk with regular/daily consumption of processed meats which may be modified by genetic susceptibility
- High fat content in the diet has also been implicated, but the evidence is observational and not robust
- Low dietary folate is associated with adenoma recurrence and CRC risk possibly through DNA methylation interactions. However, folic acid supplementation does not clearly ↓ risk of adenomas or CRC
- Calcium and vitamin D deficiency linked with ↑ rates of CRC. Calcium action is possibly through binding of bile acids or inhibition of cell growth. Supplements may be protective in deficiency
- Low dietary selenium is linked to ↑ risk. Selenium is thought to protect colonic cells from reactive oxygen species, inhibit malignant cell growth, and aid apoptosis
- Epidemiological evidence for most dietary factors is fairly weak.

Lifestyle
- High BMI increases risk, which may be improved by weight reduction
- Physical exercise is protective
- High alcohol intake associated with ↑ risk, particularly beer and spirits
- Smoking clearly linked, with up to 40% increased mortality
- Deprivation increases both incidence and mortality.

Diseases and miscellaneous other conditions
- IBD is associated with increased risk of CRC (➔ Inflammatory bowel disease, Chapter 4, p.117)
- Primary sclerosing cholangitis is an independent risk factor
- Patients who have received abdominal or pelvic radiation (usually for another malignancy) are at increased risk of developing CRC This is especially relevant for survivors of paediatric cancer
- Ureterocolic anastomoses after cystectomy
- Patients with cystic fibrosis have significant increased risk of CRC
- Changes in the intestinal microbiota have been postulated as a potential link between ↑ risk and dietary factors. Several studies have suggested an association between infection/colonization with *S. bovis*, *H. pylori*, human papilloma virus (HPV), and other infective agents and ↑ risk of CRC
- Other conditions that have been shown to be associated with increased risk include acromegaly, renal transplantation, and diabetes mellitus.

Protective factors
- Regular physical activity associated with a ↓ 25% risk of CRC
- Aspirin, NSAIDs, and COX-2 inhibitors may reduce rates of CRC by up to 50% and improve cancer-specific mortality. The putative mechanism may involve reduced metabolism of arachidonic acid which induces apoptosis. Concern regarding side effects of GI haemorrhage, haemorrhagic stroke, and cardiac toxicity (COX-2) have limited widespread use of aspirin and NSAIDs as preventative medication
- Exogenous oestrogen (e.g. hormone replacement therapy (HRT)) appears to protect against CRC but effect reduces on cessation
- Starch and carbohydrate intake appear to be protective
- The effect of fruit, vegetables, and fibre is equivocal. It certainly seems that fibre supplementation has little impact on reducing risk of adenomas or CRC.

Reference

Jacobs ET, Thompson PA, Martinez ME (2007) Diet, gender and colorectal neoplasia. *J Clin Gastroenterol* **41**: 731–46.

Molecular genetics of colorectal cancer

It is thought that all CRC develops as a result of a series of genetic mutations which can be inherited or acquired.

- Germline mutations are present in the sperm/ovum and the cancer
  phenotype is passed from parent to offspring in a predictable pattern
  (➔ Genetic disorders and polyposis syndromes, discussed later in this
  chapter, p.328)
- Rarely, a new spontaneous mutation occurs in sperm/ovum which is
  responsible for a specific cancer phenotype. The new genetic mutation
  is then passed on to subsequent generations
- By far the most common pathway is that genetic mutations are acquired
  within individual cells at some point after fertilization of the ovum.
  These somatic mutations may confer a survival/growth advantage
  which promotes clonal growth of the mutated cell
- Additional somatic mutations within this clonal population may confer
  additional growth advantage at the expense of further loss of normal
  cellular control mechanisms, e.g. this equates to the transformation of
  normal colonic mucosa into a benign adenoma at the first mutation. If
  cells within this polyp acquire additional somatic mutations, the polyp
  may ultimately transform into an invasive cancer
- Three distinct pathways of genomic instability have been identified that
  account for the majority of cases of colorectal cancer:
  - Chromosomal instability (CIN)/adenoma–carcinoma sequence
  - Microsatellite instability (MSI)
  - CpG island methylator phenotype (CIMP) pathways
- The CIN/adenoma–carcinoma sequence accounts for 75% of CRC
- Germline mutations means that every cell of an affected individual
  has one of the mutations required for malignant transformation, thus
  expediting movement along a specific pathway
- The MSI and CIMP pathways account for around 25% of cases of CRC.
  These pathways appear to play an important role in the development of
  interval cancers as they do not necessarily progress from adenoma to
  carcinoma. Rather they may develop from non-adenomatous serrated
  lesions. This is termed the serrated pathway. The molecular-genetic
  basis for this progression includes the mutator phenotype/mismatch
  repair pathway and the hypermethylation (CIMP+) pathway
- CIN, MSI, and CIMP often overlap in molecular tumour subtypes.

Chromosomal instability/adenoma–carcinoma sequence

According to the Vogelstein-Fearon adenoma–carcinoma model, CRC
develops by progression of tissue from adenoma to invasive cancer by
sequential accumulation of multiple genetic mutations and chromosomal
instability causing microsatellite stable (MSS) cancers (Fig. 7.1). The
sequence in which an individual acquires these mutations is not critical.

Epidemiological evidence

- Prevalence of adenomas and carcinomas increases with age. Adenomas
  peak 10–15yrs earlier
- Geographical distribution of adenomas mirror CRC
- Many risk factors for cancer are also risk factors for adenomas.

Chromosomal Instability Pathway (CIN)

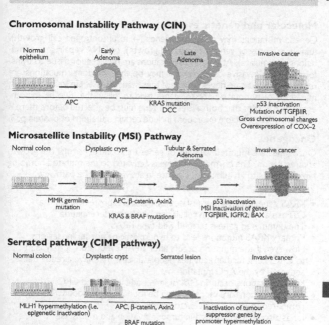

Fig. 7.1 Pathways for development of CRC.

Clinical evidence
- Adenomas have similar distribution to cancer within the colon (predominantly the rectosigmoid region)
- Removal of adenomas significantly reduces the risk of CRC
- Patients with cancer and co-existent adenomas are at increased risk of synchronous and metachronous lesions
- Cancer can develop at the site of previous adenomatous polyps
- In FAP, the development of cancer is almost inevitable.

Histological
- Rates of dysplasia and malignant foci are related to size of adenoma
- Adenomatous remnants often found alongside carcinoma in resection specimens, particularly in small lesions
- Early cancers are often seen within large adenomatous polyps.

Genetic
- Similar molecular and genetic changes have been demonstrated in adenomas and cancers.

Molecular and genetic events

Genetic mutations may affect oncogenes (→ to uncontrolled cell growth), tumour suppressor genes (uninhibited growth), or DNA repair genes (mutations accumulate). At least 5–10 mutations are required for tissue to transform into an invasive cancer and it may be that additional mutations are required that facilitate development of metastatic disease. Unlike oncogenes, mutations of tumour suppressor genes tend to follow the 'two-hit hypothesis' which implies that both alleles of a gene must be affected before there is an overt effect. Notable exceptions include certain mutations of protein p53.

Oncogenes

Oncogenes are mutated versions of genes that control normal cell growth and regulation. The normal/wild gene is activated so the mutated homolog typically leads to an additional increase in activation of the pathway.

KRAS

- KRAS gene/oncogene translates for the K-Ras protein which is a GTPase and is involved in cellular growth and differentiation
- The unmutated gene is termed wild-type KRAS
- Primary KRAS mutations lead to hyperplastic or borderline lesions. However, if the mutation occurs after an APC mutation, it may lead to CRC, i.e. it further activates neoplastic cells that have already been activated by the APC mutation
- KRAS mutations occur in 50% of larger adenomas and CRC
- KRAS mutations are more likely to be found in right sided CRC compared to left sided or rectosigmoid cancers
- It has also been implicated in tumour invasion and metastasis
- Identification of RAS mutations in faeces implies the presence of an advanced polyp or CRC. When combined with other markers, it can be used as part of a multi-target stool DNA testing for CRC
- KRAS mutation in a tumour is predictive of a poor response to anti-EGFR drugs such as cetuximab and panitumumab (Fig. 7.17)
- The RAS status of a tumour or a metastasis may change from wild-type KRAS to the mutated gene. It is thought that such a change might herald tumour progression as a result of acquired resistance to cetuximab.

Tumour suppressor genes

In contrast to oncogenes, tumour suppressor genes code for proteins that usually inhibit various aspects of the cell growth. If the defect is present in only one allele of the gene, the relevant protein will continue to be produced. Both copies of the gene therefore need to be mutated before the relevant phenotype is expressed, i.e. the two-hit hypothesis.

Adenomatous polyposis coli

- This important tumour suppressor gene is located at chromosome 5q21
- Somatic mutations in both alleles of the gene are found in up to 80% of sporadic CRC
- Germline mutations in one allele of the gene are found in FAP and familial CRC in Ashkenazi Jews. When such individuals lose the second allele within a cell (through somatic mutation or deletion), they develop a small adenomatous polyp. This suggests that mutation or loss of both alleles of the gene is an important early event in the adenoma–carcinoma sequence.

TP53

- The tumour suppressor gene TP53 (p53) on chromosome 17p plays an important role in carcinogenesis of 50–70% of CRC
- Somatic mutations and loss of the gene from both alleles occurs in 50–70% of cases of CRC but only 25% of adenomas
- A germline mutation in the TP53 gene occurs in Li Fraumeni syndrome, which is associated with carcinoma, sarcomas, and leukaemias
- The gene codes for the DNA-binding protein p53, which is produced in response to cell stressors such as hypoxia which damage DNA
- The activated gene produces the p53 protein which then activates several growth inhibitory genes. These genes induce cell arrest, which facilitates DNA repair. Ultimately the aim is to stop division and propagation of cells with damaged DNA
- Research is focused both on targeting TP53 mutant cells and gene therapy to correct TP53 gene function.

Other tumour suppressor genes

Several other tumour suppressor genes have been identified and play a potential role in CRC tumourigenesis. It is beyond the scope of this text to discuss in detail, but some are listed here:

- Chromosome 18q: DCC (deleted in colorectal carcinoma) gene
- SMAD4 and SMAD2 genes
- BRCA1 and BRCA2 genes.

DNA Mismatch repair (MMR) genes and the microsatellite instability pathway (MSI)

- The DNA-MMR genes code for a highly conserved pathway to recognize and repair base-pair mismatches and insertion/deletion and mis-incorporation during DNA replication and recombination
- Defects in several genes (MSH2, MLH1, PSM1, PMS2, MSH6, and MLH3) play a role in CRC tumourigenesis
- Defects in the MMR pathway lead to defects in microsatellites (tracts of repetitive DNA comprised of short sequences of nucleotide base-pairs) which are scattered throughout the genome (termed microsatellite instability (MSI)).
- Analysis for MSI can give three outcomes:
  - Microsatellite stable (MSS). 85% of sporadic cancers
  - Microsatellite instability—high (MSI-H). 15% of sporadic CRC and the majority of Lynch syndrome-associated CRC
  - Microsatellite instability—low (MSI-L). Of uncertain significance but may be important in the serrated neoplasia pathway and is associated with a poor prognosis in stage II and III CRC
- Although defects in microsatellites themselves may not be of direct importance, it may result in frameshift mutations in promoter regions of adjacent genes which are critical to regulation of cellular growth (e.g. TGFRB2, IGF2)
- Lynch syndrome-related cancers are secondary to a germline mutation in one of the MMR genes, most commonly in the homolog hMLH1 or hMSH2

- Methylation at gene promoter regions is a physiologic mechanism to regulate gene function
- MSI-H sporadic cancers show a failure of expression of the MLH1 gene which is blocked following aberrant hypermethylation of the promoter regions of both alleles of the gene (termed epigenetic alteration)
- Epigenetic alterations including DNA hypermethylation may also occur in the second allele of an MMR gene where a germline mutation has already inactivated the first allele, thus completely silencing gene expression
- MSI-H tumours (both sporadic and Lynch syndrome-related) are more likely to be poorly differentiated, right sided, mucinous cancers with lymphocytic infiltration. However, this does not appear to translate into a worse outcome.

Hypermethylation (CIMP+) pathway and serrated neoplasms

- Aberrant cystine methylation within the dinucleotide CpG (cytosine—phosphate—guanine) may result in silencing of tumour suppressor genes and is thought to play a pivotal role in the serrated pathway
- This epigenetic alteration is termed CIMP
- It may also give rise to MSI-H tumours through epigenetic inactivation of MLH1
- CIMP+ tumours account for 25–30% of all CRC
- It is now recognized that many colorectal sessile lesions (SL), which were previously called hyperplastic polyps, harbour BRAF mutations and are CIMP+. Occasionally KRAS mutations are also seen
- The serrated neoplasia pathway postulates that SL start with a BRAF or KRAS mutation, leading to epigenetic gene silencing and formation of sessile serrated lesions (SSL)
- Inactivation of tumour suppressor genes leads to dysplasia, i.e. SSL with dysplasia and ultimately cancer
- For uncertain reasons, BRAF mutant CIMP+ tumours that develop on this pathway are more common in the right colon.

MUTYH defects and familial colorectal cancer

- Germline mutations in the base excision repair gene mutY homolog (MUTYH) may have a recessive inheritance pattern and can predispose to formation of multiple colonic polyps, i.e. MUTYH-associated polyposis (MAP)
- Affected individuals may have biallelic germline mutations, i.e. carriers may have a mutation (not necessarily the same mutation) in both copies of the MUTYH gene
- The mutation often appears in association with a somatic mutation in the APC gene, expressing a phenotype of 10–100s of colonic polyps
- The recessive inheritance pattern may 'miss' out a generation and differs for the autosomal dominant pattern of inheritance in FAP
- It is thought to account for many cases of 'familial CRC'
- Heterozygotes may have a slight increased risk of CRC
- Stage for stage, the prognosis for MAP-associated cancers appears to be better than sporadic cancers that arise in the general population. (➲ Genetic disorders and polyposis syndromes, discussed later in this chapter, p.328).

Modifier genes

Several genes are known to have an ill-defined role in colorectal carcinogenesis, thus providing additional pathways to target therapy.

* There is good evidence that aspirin and other COX inhibitors may reduce polyp formation and may even induce polyp regression
* The COX-2 gene is upregulated in 80–85% of CRCs. Drugs such as aspirin and NSAIDs block this gene and may therefore have a beneficial impact ((⊖ Adjuvant therapy with aspirin, discussed later in this chapter, p.362)
* The peroxisome proliferator-activating receptor (PPAR) gene appears to have a role in colorectal carcinogenesis and loss of function in the gene is seen in sporadic CRC and patients with acromegaly.

Impact of molecular changes on clinical course of CRC

* Molecular and genetic assessments of tissue from individual CRC can be used to identify some of the specific genetic and epigenetic abnormalities that have led to the development of the cancer. This information also carries important prognostic and therapeutic implications
* The most common markers that are assessed include MSI, CIMP, BRAF mutation, and KRAS mutation status
* In a study of more than 2,000 cancers, Phipps et al. showed that MSI-H tumours tend to have the best prognosis, followed by MSI-H tumours with a BRAF mutation. BRAF mutated, CIMP+ tumours had the worst prognosis. Disease-specific 5yr survival rates were
  * 93%: MSI-H, BRAF and KRAS wild (i.e. no mutation), non-CIMP (4% of group)
  * 90%: MSI-H, BRAF mutated, KRAS wild, CIMP+ (7% of group)
  * 83%: MSS/MSI-L, BRAF and KRAS wild, non-CIMP (47% of group)
  * 72%: MSS/MSI-L, BRAF wild and KRAS mutated, non-CIMP (26% of group)
  * 49%: MSS/MSI-L, BRAF mutated, KRAS wild, CIMP+ (4% of group)
* CIMP+ and BRAF mutated tumours have the poorest prognosis
* CIMP+ has been shown in several studies to have a poor prognosis irrespective of MSI status
* Anti-EGFR drugs are contra-indicated in KRAS mutated disease
* BRAF V600E mutated cancers are associated with a worse prognosis and also confer resistance to anti-EGFR therapy, even if wild-type KRAS (non-mutated). BRAF is downstream of KRAS in signalling pathway (Fig. 7.17)
* 5-fluorouracil (5-FU) therapy does not appear to be as effective in MSI-H tumours compared with MSS tumours, although MSI-H have a good prognosis in any event.

References

Armaghany T, Wilson JD, Chu Q, Mills G (2012) Genetic alterations in colorectal cancer. *Gastrointest Cancer Res* **5**(1): 19–27.

Tariq K, Ghias K (2016) Colorectal cancer carcinogenesis: a review of mechanisms. *Cancer Biol Med* **13**(1): 120–35.

Phipps AI, Limburg PJ, Baron JA et al. (2015) Association between molecular subtypes of colorectal cancer and patient survival. *Gastroenterology* **148**(1): 77–87.e2.

Screening and family history

Introduction

CRC is the second most common cause of cancer-related mortality in the UK. It frequently presents at an advanced stage causing major morbidity and a high cost for healthcare systems. Treatment in the early stages of the disease often leads to a cure with improved surgical technique and better understanding of the natural history (→ Chromosomal instability/adenoma—carcinoma sequence, discussed earlier in this chapter, p.310). It is for these reasons, along with growing evidence for a variety of screening modalities, that CRC screening is being adopted by an increasing number of developed countries. While the case for screening has been accepted, the best method is still a matter of debate.

Screening modalities

Faecal testing

Guaiac-based faecal occult blood testing (FOBT)

- Guaiac-based tests use peroxidase effect of Hb on guaiac to give a blue colour change
- Large scale RCTs using a guaiac-based test showed that screening for bowel cancer was possible and cost-effective
- Compliance with screening 30–60%, population positivity ~1%, predictive value ~15%, and mortality reduction 15–30%
- At colonoscopy 15–20% diagnosed cancers and ~40% adenomas (20% 'high risk' adenomas)
- Sensitivity for detection of CRC is 30–80%, which increases with regular screening
- Incidence of CRC reduced probably due to polyp clearance
- ~1% of patients with CRC diagnosed with screening have disseminated disease at diagnosis vs 25% in symptomatic population
- Although guaiac-based tests are cheap and easy to use, they have been superseded by faecal immunological testing (FIT) which is more sensitive and specific.

Faecal immunological testing (FIT)

- FIT can detect human Hb with higher sensitivity than FOBT. See → Quantitative faecal immunochemical test (qFIT) Chapter 2, p.38 for a more detailed discussion on how the test works
- Test is easy to perform and only a single, tiny stool sample is required
- No dietary or drug restriction. Aspirin does not affect results
- Compared to FOBT, FIT is more sensitive and has higher screening participation rates as it is easier to perform
- FIT is a quantitative test; sensitivity for a positive result can be adjusted to limit impact on endoscopy services.
- A single FIT test has a sensitivity of ~80% for detection of CRC with a specificity of 95%. The sensitivity for detecting advanced adenomas is less at 25–55% with a 70–95% sensitivity
- When performed every two years as part of a bowel screening programme, successive testing increases the sensitivity to detect CRC, but there is a concomitant reduction in sensitivity and positive predictive value (as most cancers will have been detected in the index round of screening)

- FIT may be less sensitive in the detection of right sided cancers
- FIT is equally effective when performed every one, two, or three years. In the UK, most screening programmes are performed every two years and annually in the USA.

Faecal DNA/Multitarget stool DNA(MT-sDNA)/FIT-DNA

- Faecal DNA tests measure a combination of molecular markers including a FIT test for human globin, mutant and methylated DNA markers, and assay for mutated KRAS
- Shedding of cells from cancers is increased compared with normal mucosa and not intermittent like occult blood loss
- Initial results suggest ↑ sensitivity for detection of both CRC (92%) and advanced adenomas compared with FIT alone, at the expense of reduced specificity (87 versus 95%)
- It is expensive (currently up to 20 times the cost of FIT)
- Its role remains uncertain given the additional cost and the increased requirement for colonoscopy due to lower specificity.

CT colonography

- Modelling studies suggest CT colonography may be effective
- Sensitivity much higher than FOBT with similar specificity
- Radiation exposure risk difficult to estimate but likely to be significant if repeated examinations used
- Extracolonic findings in up to 20% lead to ↑ investigations which are often unnecessary.

Sigmoidoscopy/colonoscopy

- Screening sigmoidoscopy is associated with a 28% reduction in risk of dying from CRC versus no screening in the intention-to-treat group and a 50% reduction in mortality in those who participated per protocol
- UK trial showed compliance of 70%; distal adenomas in 12%; distal cancers in 0.3%. 5% were referred for colonoscopy with 18% proximal adenomas and 0.4% proximal cancers
- Flexible sigmoidoscopy is safer, quicker, and more acceptable than colonoscopy but only ~70% of the sensitivity. Colonoscopy rates 3–5 times that of FOBT screening
- No RCTs of colonoscopy as a screening tool in average risk population due to concern over compliance and risk of the procedure
- Colonoscopy, however, remains the standard of care for screening in high risk individuals e.g. those with germline mutations.

UK screening protocol

- Screening offered to people aged 50–74yrs in Scotland and 60–69yrs in the rest of UK. However, NHS England recently agreed to reduce the starting age to 50 years in line with Scotland
- Self-referral available to those older than the screening population
- FIT sent in post at 2yrly intervals from regional centre with referral as appropriate to local endoscopy screening centre
- In the UK 50–60% of people who are invited to participate in screening actually return their sample
- 2–3% who participate will have a positive result
- CRC is found in 12–15% of ♂ and 8% of ♀ who undergo colonoscopy due to a positive result.

Family history of colorectal cancer (FHCC)

- ~30% of the UK population will have a first-degree (FDR) or second-degree relative affected by CRC. Most do not have evidence of an inherited CRC syndrome. Personal risk increases with the number of affected relatives and younger age at presentation, e.g. individuals with two affected FDR or one affected FDR aged <45yrs have a less than 1 in 10 chance of developing CRC. Additional screening may be indicated in this group. Current UK guidelines suggest that individuals should be categorized as follows:
- Average risk of CRC:
  - No FHCC or FHCC that does not fulfil moderate or high risk categories below
  - Individuals should participate in bowel screening programme
- Moderate risk FHCC:
  - One FDR with CRC aged <50 yrs or
  - Two FDRs with CRC, any age. Individual being assessed is a FDR of at least one affected individual
  - Referral to a regional genetics service
  - A one-off colonoscopy at age 55yrs is recommended, with subsequent discharge to national screening programme or adenoma surveillance scheme as appropriate
- High risk FHCC:
  - Families with a cluster of at least three FDRs with CRC, diagnosed at any age, across at least two generations. Individual being assessed is an FDR of at least one affected individual
  - Referral to a regional genetics service
  - 5-yrly colonoscopies from 40–75yrs is recommended.

These guidelines do not apply to patients with an identifiable genetic mutation or who are members of a known polyposis family (➲ Genetic disorders and polyposis syndromes, discussed later in this chapter, p.328).

References

Hardcastle JD, Chamberlain JO, Robinson MHE et al. (1996) Randomised controlled trial of faecal-occult blood screening for colorectal cancer. *Lancet* **348**: 1472–7.

Elmunzer BJ, Hayward RA, Schoenfeld PS et al. (2012) Effect of flexible sigmoidoscopy-based screening on incidence and mortality of colorectal cancer: a systematic review and meta-analysis of randomised controlled trials. *PLoS Med* **9**(12): e1001352.

Monahan KJ, Bradshaw N, Dolwani S et al. (2019) Guidelines for the management of hereditary colorectal cancer from the British Society of Gastroenterology (BSG)/Association of Coloproctology of Great Britain and Ireland (ACPGBI)/United Kingdom Cancer Genetics Group (UKCGG). *Gut* **0**: 1–34.

Colonic polyps

The term 'polyp' refers to a projection above the level of the normal intestinal epithelium. Types include adenomas, sessile serrated lesions, hamartomas, inflammatory, hyperplastic, and a miscellaneous collection of other lesions including submucosal lesions.

Adenomas

- Benign neoplasms of glandular epithelium which may be pedunculated (on a stalk), sessile (broad based), flat, or depressed
- Risk factors for development include:
  - Advancing age: prevalence of adenomas is ~30% at 50yrs and 50% at 70yrs
  - Increasing body mass index and abdominal obesity
  - Family or personal history of adenomas
- Multiple in ~50% and most common in the rectum and distal colon
- Usually asymptomatic but may cause bleeding, anaemia, diarrhoea, obstruction, and intussusception
- Histologically classified as tubular, villous, or mixed depending on glandular structure
- They are pre-malignant but <5% progress to CRC over 7–10 yrs
- ~6% have high grade dysplasia (HGD). HGD is noted in
  - 1–2% of adenomas <5mm
  - 7–10% of adenomas 5–10mm
  - 20–30% of adenomas >1cm in size
- ~4% have invasive adenocarcinoma
- Risk of malignancy correlates with size: 90% of adenomas <1cm (1% risk malignancy); 10% >1cm (~10% malignant + ↑ HGD)
- Multiple polyps may occur as part of an inherited syndrome with significantly increased risk of malignancy (◐ Genetic disorders and polyposis syndromes, discussed later in this chapter, p.328)
- Morphologically, most polyps can be divided as follows:
  - Sessile: May be elevated. Base is same diameter as top of lesion
  - Pedunculated: Narrow base with mucosal stalk/pedicle
  - Flat: Height is < half the diameter of lesion. Up to 30% of adenomas. Easily missed at colonoscopy and these may account for many 'missed' or interval cancers
  - Depressed: Account for ~1% of lesions but have higher chance of harboring HGD or invasive cancer
- The Paris classification is used to classify lesions into polypoid and nonpolypoid lesions (Fig. 7.2)
- Flat lesions >10mm and depressed lesions are twice as likely as protruding lesions of similar size to contain areas of HGD or foci of invasive cancer
- Features suggestive of malignancy
  - Hard/indurated
  - Friable/touch bleeding
  - Ulceration
  - Among sessile polyps, a smooth velvety surface (i.e. a non-granular, laterally spreading tumour (NG-LST))
  - Non-lifting with submucosal injection
  - Paris classification II a+c or Kudo pit pattern V (Figs 7.2 and 7.3).

Type	Subclass	Notes
0–I: Polypoid	0–Ip: Protruded, pedunculated	
	0–Is: Protruded, sessile	
0–II: Nonpolypoid	0–IIa: Slightly elevated	
	0–IIb: Flat	
	0–IIc: Slightly depressed	
0–III: Excavated		

Fig. 7.2 Paris classification of superficial gastrointestinal neoplastic lesions.

Source: Data from The Paris endoscopic classification of superficial neoplastic lesions: esophagus, stomach, and colon: November 30 to December 1, 2002. *Gastrointest Endosc*, 2003, 58(6 Suppl):S3–43.

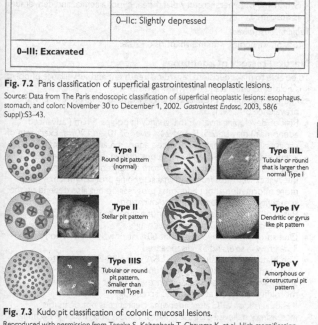

Fig. 7.3 Kudo pit classification of colonic mucosal lesions.

Reproduced with permission from Tanaka S, Kaltenbach T, Chayama K, et al. High-magnification colonoscopy (with videos). *Gastrointest Endosc*;64:604–13. Copyright © 2006, Elsevier

Histological classification of adenomas

Adenomas are classified according to the ratio of villous to tubular tissue. They are also assessed for dysplasia which is graded as LGD or HGD.

Tubular
- Defined by <25% villous morphology
- 75% of neoplastic polyps with overall malignancy rate 5%.

Villous
- >75% villous architecture; they account for ~10% of adenomas
- Larger than other types and most common in the rectum
- Up to 40% rate of malignancy
- Sessile, velvety with finger-like projections, and ill-defined borders
- Syndrome of hypersecretory diarrhoea, hypokalaemia, and dehydration is described.

Tubulovillous (mixed)
~15% of adenomas with malignant risk ~20%.

Natural history of adenomas

To be able to make decisions regarding treatment and surveillance of polyps it is helpful to understand their natural history.
- Although adenoma prevalence ranges from 30–40% (10% >1cm) the prevalence of CRC is 5%
- Risk of developing invasive malignancy in polyps >1cm ('advanced adenomas') may be 2.5, 8, and 24% over 5, 10, and 20yrs. Exact rate of progression from small to advanced adenoma and then from advanced adenoma to invasive malignancy is not known. One study suggests an annual progression rate of 3–6% from advanced adenoma to cancer. Interval cancer rates from national screening programmes may give more information about adenoma progression but also depend on the sensitivity of the colonoscopic examination
- Rates of advanced adenomas do not appear to increase with age despite rates of CRC increasing with age
- One study showed over 5yrs that 60% of polyps showed no growth, 35% grew in size, and 5% disappeared
- The National Polyp Study in the USA saw a 70–90% lower than expected rate of CRC in patients undergoing colonoscopic surveillance, adding weight to adenoma clearance as a major reason for the morbidity reduction attributed to screening
- Residual risk of CRC after adenoma clearance is not clear. It is increasingly believed that the greatest benefit in terms of preventing CRC is derived from the index polypectomy, rather than subsequent surveillance
- 20–50% of patients with distal polyps at sigmoidoscopy will have proximal polyps.

Adenoma surveillance post-polypectomy

30–50% of patients will develop polyps during follow-up, but to date no RCTs have proven benefit for colonoscopic surveillance after initial adenoma clearance. Guidelines on surveillance have been produced relying on expert opinion and current understanding of the natural history. The sensitivity of current guidelines is limited, but the addition of patient factors and molecular markers in the future may improve risk stratification. Updated UK guidelines for frequency of colonoscopy post-polypectomy were published in 2020. The most important recommendations are as follows:

- A good high-quality index colonoscopy and clearance of polyps is the keystone to effective CRC prevention. It is understood that subsequent surveillance has a minimal impact in preventing CRC and most patients do not derive benefit from this
- High risk findings defined as either of the following:
  - ≥2 premalignant polyps (serrated or adenomatous) to include ≥1 advanced polyp (i.e. serrated lesion ≥10mm, any serrated lesion with dysplasia, adenoma ≥10mm, any adenoma with HGD)
  - ≥5 premalignant polyps
- Patients with high risk findings should be considered for repeat colonoscopy in 3yrs
- Patients who do not have high risk findings do not need to undergo planned surveillance (but they should continue to participate in bowel screening programme)
- Patients undergoing excision of large (≥20mm) non-pedunculated colorectal polyps ([L]NPCP) are placed in a special category
  - If a LNPCP is removed *en bloc* with clear margins, follow-up as per high risk findings, i.e. colonoscopy in 3yrs
  - Patients who undergo piecemeal or histologically incomplete excision of a LNPCP should be considered for a site-check colonoscopy in 2–6 months and a further colonoscopy 12 months later
  - Patients who undergo piecemeal or histologically incomplete excision of a NPCP (10–19mm) should also be considered for a site-check colonoscopy in 2–6 months
- Patients older than 75yrs and those with a life expectancy <10 years should not be considered for routine surveillance
- Findings at 3yr colonoscopy determine the need if any, for subsequent surveillance
- CT colonoscopy may be considered for surveillance if it is not possible to perform a complete colonoscopy. However FIT testing or videocapsule colonoscopy are not viewed as acceptable alternatives.

Management of adenomatous polyps

Most adenomas can be dealt with endoscopically, with EMR for large or sessile polyps (Fig. 7.2). Elevation and cold snare can be used for polyps up to 7mm. Tattooing can help recognition of the polypectomy site for further follow-up or for laparoscopic surgery. Colotomy + polypectomy or segmental resection may still be required in some cases. It is important to attempt a complete clearance at initial polypectomy as subsequent attempts to remove remaining/recurrent polyp can be more difficult with increased risk of complications.

Management of LNPCP can be difficult. ESD techniques have enabled many colonic and rectal lesions to be removed *en bloc*. Surgical techniques to deal with large, villous, rectal lesions include transanal excision and rectal resection with or without restoration of intestinal continuity. Transanal excision is preferred, with a variety of methods including traditional transanal endoscopic microsurgery (TEM) and transanal minimally invasive surgery (TAMIS) (→ Transanal endoscopic microsurgery, Chapter 11, p.580).

Chemoprevention with agents such as aspirin and COX-2 inhibitors has been shown to reduce recurrent adenomas by up to 20% but is currently not recommended due to side effects (→ Colorectal cancer, discussed earlier in this chapter, p.308).

Malignant polyps

Invasive malignancy is present when neoplastic cells penetrate through the muscularis mucosae into the submucosa (which contains lymphatics and thus risk of nodal spread). The management of polyps found to harbour invasive malignancy is controversial. Factors associated with an increased likelihood of residual local or LN disease include:

- Carcinoma ≤1 mm from the resection margin
- Lymphovascular invasion
- Poorly differentiated tumours

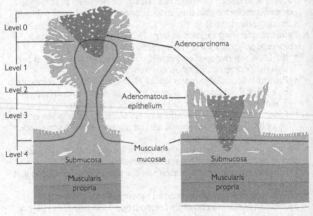

Fig. 7.4 Haggitt classification of malignant colonic polyps.

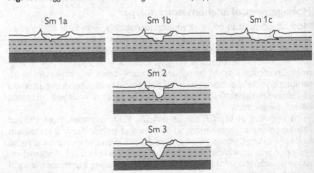

Fig. 7.5 Kikuchi levels.

- Invasion into the muscularis propria (T2 lesion)
- Flat or sessile lesions versus pedunculated lesions
- SM3 penetration or >1mm
- Staging systems for malignant polyps include the Haggitt and Kikuchi classifications (Figs 7.4, 7.5 and Boxes 7.1 and 7.2)
- The risk of LN metastasis is increased in sessile (10%) vs pedunculated (5%) lesions
- The risk of LN metastases is negligible for pedunculated lesions with invasion less than Haggitt level 4
- For sessile lesions LN metastasis rate for Kikuchi level sm1, sm2, and sm3 is 2, 8, and 23% respectively. It is not often possible to assess the full depth of the submucosal layer which may not be included in the specimen. A depth >1 mm is therefore used as a surrogate for sm3 invasion
- If one or more of the previously noted risks are present, formal surgical resection should be considered
- Early endoscopic follow-up is required following removal of a malignant polyp. Thereafter, patients can return to standard follow-up according to local guidelines
- There is no clear consensus on the need for a staging CT after removal of a malignant polyp. However, many perform a one-off CT chest, abdomen, pelvis (CAP).

Box 7.1 Haggitt classification

Used to grade pedunculated polyps containing invasive malignancy

Level 1:   Carcinoma through the muscularis mucosa into submucosa limited to the head of the polyp

Level 2:   Carcinoma invading to junction of adenoma and stalk

Level 3:   Carcinoma invading the stalk

Level 4:   Carcinoma invading the submucosal of bowel wall but not through the muscularis propria. By definition, this includes all sessile polyps

Adapted with permission from Haggitt, RC, Glotzbach, RE, Soffer, EE, Wruble, LD. Prognostic factors in colorectal carcinomas arising in adenomas: implications for lesions removed by endoscopic polypectomy. *Gastroenterology*;89(2):328–336. Copyright © 1985 Published by Elsevier Inc.

Box 7.2 Kikuchi levels

The submucosa is divided into thirds to describe the depth of invasion for sessile lesions

Sm1:   Invasion through mucosa to the upper 1/3 submucosa

a.   Invading front <1/4 width of lesion

b.   Invading front 1/4–1/2 width of lesion

c.   Invading front >1/2 width of lesion

Sm2:   Invasion to the middle 1/3 of submucosa

Sm3:   Invasion to the lower 1/3 submucosa approaching muscularis propria

Serrated polyps/sessile serrated lesion

The term serrated polyp is often interchanged with SL. SL of the colon is an umbrella term that refers to a diverse group of lesions, some of which carry significant neoplastic potential. Typically, it includes the following:
- Hyperplastic polyp
- SSL
- SSL with dysplasia
- Traditional serrated adenoma
- Mixed polyp.

Hyperplastic polyps (HP)
- Most common non-neoplastic colonic polyp. Most are small <0.5cm
- Multiple in ~50% and most common in the rectum and distal colon
- Characterized by long, serrated crypts lined by hyperproliferative epithelium in the base and large goblet cells in the upper portion
- Difficult to differentiate from adenomas without biopsy, but advances in chromoendoscopy and narrow band imaging may prove useful
- Proximal lesions may harbor BRAF mutations and they are increasingly thought to be an early intermediary in the serrated neoplasia pathway
- Some authors have also reported an increased risk of finding a proximal cancer if there was a distal HP
- Biopsy/excision may be helpful to confirm diagnosis and exclude a true SSL. All HP outside the rectum should probably be excised.
- Those with multiple small HP or those >10mm should be followed up.

Sessile serrated lesion
- SSL are also referred to as sessile serrated polyps and sessile serrated adenomas. They are typically flat or slightly elevated. They are more common in the right colon. They may appear dark/brown as faeces adheres to a mucus cap. The edges of these lesions are serpiginous. Close inspection often reveals dark spots in the crypts. Narrow band imaging may be helpful if differentiating SSLs from hyperplastic polyps
- HGD is found in 10–40% of these lesions. They may progress rapidly to invasive cancer. Rather than following the more common adenoma–carcinoma/chromosomal instability pathway, SSLs may be an important intermediary in the development of sporadic MSI-H CRC by the hypermethylation (CIMP+) pathway (➲ Genetic disorders and polyposis syndromes, see next heading in this chapter, p.328)
- The finding of a right sided SSL >10mm with dysplasia increases the risk of finding a synchronous advanced adenoma
- These lesions may account for many interval cancers, in part because of rapid progression to CRC and also given the difficulty in detecting them at screening colonoscopy.

Traditional serrated adenoma (TSA)
- Typically, these are exophytic villiform polyps containing eosinophilic cells and ectopic crypt foci
- TSA do not consistently show molecular changes, although KRAS and BRAF mutations and CIMP+ is seen in some lesions. However, they do not consistently display MSI-H or CIMP+. These lesions appear less likely to progress to CRC compared with SSL and SSLs with dysplasia.

Serrated polyposis syndrome (SPS)/Hyperplastic polyposis syndrome (HPS)
- The rare syndrome is associated with an increased risk of CRC. It is likely to have a genetic basis, but a single genetic abnormality has yet to be defined (➔ Genetic disorders and polyposis syndromes, see next heading in this chapter, p.328).

Other polyps

Inflammatory polyps
- Non-neoplastic polyps may occur in relation to inflammatory bowel disease (pseudopolyps) or 2° to mucosal prolapse
- IBD-associated pseudopolyps may occur in areas of dysplasia, although the polyps themselves do not have malignant potential, but care should be taken not to miss associated colonic dysplasia
- Prolapse inflammatory polyps may occur in the rectum with rectal prolapse/SRUS and in the sigmoid in association with diverticular disease. Normally, they do not require any specific treatment.

Hamartomatous polyps
- Hamartomatous polyps are lesions consisting of many tissue elements, normally found at that site, i.e. bowel wall. Most are benign but may cause symptoms due to bleeding or prolapse
- Juvenile polyps are hamartomatous lesions that occur in 2% of children aged <10yrs. Most are asymptomatic but some prolapse and bleed
- Similar polyps occur in the autosomal dominant condition juvenile polyposis syndrome which is associated with an increased risk of gastric and colorectal cancer (➔ Genetic disorders and polyposis syndromes, see next heading in this chapter, p.328).
- Peutz-Jeghers polyps usually occur in relation to Peutz-Jeghers syndrome, an autosomal dominant condition associated with an increased risk of gastric, small bowel, colon, and pancreatic cancer (➔ Genetic disorders and polyposis syndromes, see next heading, p.328)

References

(2003) The Paris endoscopic classification of superficial neoplastic lesions: Esophagus, stomach and colon: November 30 to December 1, 2002. *Gastrointest Endosc* **58**(6 suppl): S3.

Rutter MD, East J, Rees CJ et al. (2020) British Society of Gastroenterology/Association of Coloproctology of Great Britain and Ireland/Public Health England post-polypectomy and post-colorectal cancer resection surveillance guidelines. *Gut* **69**: 201–23.

East JE, Atkin WS, Bateman AC et al. (2017) British Society of Gastroenterology position statement on serrated polyps in the colon and rectum. *Gut* **66**: 1181–96.

Aarons CB, Shanmugan S, Bleier JI (2014) Management of malignant colon polyps: current status and controversies. *World J Gastroenterol* **20**(43): 16178–83.

Genetic disorders and polyposis syndromes

It is estimated that 85% of colorectal cancers are sporadic and the remainder have a genetic basis. Familial adenomatous polyposis coli (FAP) and Lynch syndrome (hereditary non-polyposis colorectal cancer: HNPCC) are the two best known colorectal cancer syndromes but together account for less than 5% of all colorectal cancers.

Lynch syndrome (HNPCC)

Lynch syndrome is an autosomal dominant condition with high penetrance. It can be divided into Lynch syndrome I (familial colon cancer) and Lynch syndrome II (associated with extraintestinal tumours). It occurs as a result of germline mutations in one of the mismatch repair (MMR) genes MLH1, MSH2, MSH6, PSM, and PSM2, which leads to micro-satellite instability (MSI).

Presentation

- HNPCC accounts for 3–5% of all CRCs
- Increases lifetime risk of colorectal (25–75%), endometrial (~40%), gastric (<12%), urinary(<6%), hepato pancreatico biliary (HPB) (<5%), brain (<5%), and small bowel (<5%) malignancy (Fig. 7.6)
- Colorectal and endometrial cancers present early around 4th decade
- Amsterdam/Bethesda criteria can select ~70–90% of cases (Box 7.3)
- Adenomas are few with increased numbers of flat lesions, high grade dysplasia, and villous component

---

Box 7.3 Criteria for diagnosis of HNPCC

Amsterdam criteria

- ≥3 family members with CRC or an HNPCC-related tumour with at least one in a first-degree relative of the other two
- Two successive generations affected
- One or more cancers diagnosed before the age of 50
- FAP excluded

Revised Bethesda criteria

- Colorectal cancer diagnosed before the age of 50
- Presence of synchronous or metachronous colorectal or HNPCC-related tumour regardless of age
- Colorectal cancer with MSI-H histology diagnosed under the age of 60
- Colorectal cancer with ≥1 first-degree relative with CRC or an HNPCC-related tumour with one diagnosed under the age of 50
- Colorectal cancer with ≥2 first- or second-degree relatives with CRC and an HNPCC-related tumour regardless of age

Reproduced from Omar A, Boland CR, Terdiman JP, et al. (2004). Revised Bethesda Guidelines for hereditary nonpolyposis colorectal cancer (Lynch syndrome) and microsatellite instability. *J Natl Cancer Inst*;96(4): 261–268. doi: 10.1093/jnci/djh034

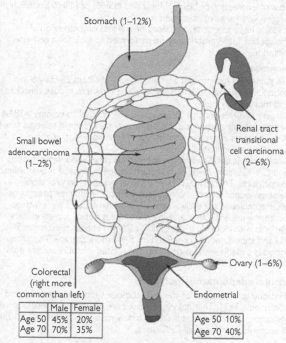

Stomach (1–12%)

Renal tract transitional cell carcinoma (2–6%)

Small bowel adenocarcinoma (1–2%)

Ovary (1–6%)

Colorectal (right more common than left)

	Male	Female
Age 50	45%	20%
Age 70	70%	35%

Endometrial

Age 50 10%
Age 70 40%

Fig. 7.6 Extracolonic malignancy in HNPCC.

- Transformation from adenoma to cancer is more rapid (<3yrs) but outcome is better than sporadic CRC
- CRCs can be synchronous (~45%) or metachronous (15% at 10yrs)
- Most cancers (~70%) are proximal to the splenic flexure
- Muir–Torre syndrome describes HNPCC associated with skin lesions (epitheliomas, epidermoid cysts, carcinoma, keratoacanthomas)
- Turcot's syndrome describes HNPCC or FAP with CNS lesions (medulloblastomas).

Genetic testing
- Genetic testing is carried out only after thorough counselling and family history review ideally by a clinical genetics service
- Testing should be guided by the Amsterdam/Bethesda criteria
- MSI is the cellular endpoint of defective MMR activity and can be detected by MSI profiling and immunohistochemistry (IHC) of tumour tissue from the patient or affected relative if available
- More than 90% of HNPCC-related cancers will demonstrate MSI. It is important to remember that up to 15% of sporadic cancers are also MSI-H.

- Loss of expression of MSH2, MSH2 and MSH6, or MSH6 alone is highly suggestive of a germline mutation
- If MSI is high, genetic testing based on the loss of expression of the specific MMR protein may be performed to look for a germline mutation.

Management
- UK guidelines recommend annual colonoscopy from 25–35 yrs and continuing 2yrly until 75yrs. This has been shown to reduce cancer risk and mortality by ~50%
- Surgery involves subtotal colectomy + IRA or total colectomy + IPAA
- Segmental colectomy and surveillance may be chosen in selected cases
- Risk of cancer in rectum after IRA is ~1%/yr so annual stump surveillance is indicated
- Annual pelvic examination, transvaginal US scan, endometrial biopsy, and CA-125 from 25–35yrs is recommended but not of proven efficacy
- Prophylactic TAH/BSO (total abdominal hysterectomy/bilateral salpingo-oophorectomy) considered in post-menopausal patients or after completion of family where endometrial cancers are a feature
- Screening upper GI and capsule endoscopy is not of proven efficacy
- Patients with MSI-H/deficient MMR (dMMR) appear resistant to 5-FU and should not be considered for 5-FU monotherapy. This group includes patients with Lynch syndrome-related tumours and the 15% sporadic CRC that are MSI-H.

Familial adenomatous polyposis

FAP is due to a mutation of the APC tumour suppressor gene located on chromosome 5q21. The majority of cases are due to autosomal dominant inheritance, with 20% of cases due to a new mutation. It affects 1 in 10,000 and accounts for <1% of all CRC cases.

Presentation
- Colonic polyposis (>100 adenomas) occurs with lifetime cancer risk approaching 100% (Figs 7.7 and 7.8)
- Polyposis in FAP is associated with EIMs
- Polyps develop at mean age of 15yrs (mainly left colon and rectum)
- Cancer develops at a mean age of 40yrs (multifocal in 50%) with similar outcomes to sporadic CRC
- An attenuated variant AFAP (8% of cases) presents later (mean age of cancer 55yrs) with fewer polyps (~25) predominantly right sided
- Gardner's syndrome describes a variant with increased extraintestinal tumours especially desmoids.

Extraintestinal manifestations
- Partly dependent on family history, location, and type of gene mutation
- Duodenal adenomas occur in 90% with 5% lifetime cancer risk
- Desmoid tumours (fibromatosis) present in up to 20% and although benign may lead to significant complications. More common around pregnancy and after surgery. Mean age of presentation is 30yrs.

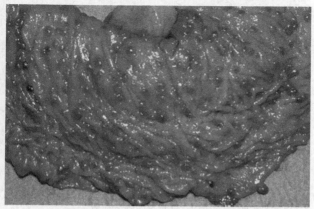

Fig. 7.7 FAP colectomy specimen.

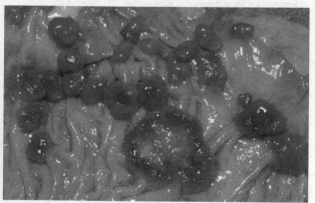

Fig. 7.8 FAP with synchronous cancers.

- Gastric fundic gland hamartomas in 50% with minimal malignant potential. Gastric adenocarcinoma risk not ↑ in Western population
- Osteomas in up to 80% but rarely symptomatic
- Hepatoblastoma presents in early childhood in 1%
- Link to adrenal adenomas, ileal carcinoid, bile duct, and thyroid cancer
- Congenital hypertrophy of the retinal pigment epithelium (CHRPE) can be useful for screening (present in 75%)
- Unerupted or supernumerary teeth in 20%.

Screening and surveillance
- Gene testing identifies the mutation in up to 90%. Results are only truly negative in the presence of an affected FDR with a positive test. Genetic counselling is essential
- In mutation-positive patients, surveillance should be lifelong with colonoscopy 1–3yrly starting at 12–14 years. Upper GI endoscopy starting at 25yrs and frequency dependent on Spigelman classification
- Individuals with an FDR with a clinical diagnosis of FAP are viewed as 'at risk' and screening should also be considered
- Dye spray may be utilized at colonoscopy to identify 'aberrant crypt focus' precursor of adenomas.

Management
- Prophylactic total colectomy + IPAA before 20yrs is recommended
- Subtotal colectomy + IRA is appropriate for some patients
- IPAA has a higher post-operative morbidity but avoids ~10% risk of cancer in rectal stump
- Pouch/stump surveillance is recommended at 6 month–1yr intervals
- Patients are ideally managed by a polyposis registry
- Management of desmoid tumours is controversial and in particular the requirement for and timing of intervention
- Sulindac combined with Tamoxifen may have efficacy.

MUTYH-associated polyposis (MAP)
- For MUTYH pathogenic variant gene carriers, UK guidelines recommend annual colonoscopy from 18–20yrs and upper GI endoscopy starting at 35yrs and frequency dependent on Spigelman classification.

Peutz–Jeghers syndrome (PJS)
PJS is a rare autosomal dominant condition (~1 in 200,000) causing multiple hamartomatous intestinal polyps and mucocutaneous pigmentation. The gene defect (STK11) is located on chromosome 19p.
- Polyps most common in the proximal small bowel but also found in colon and stomach
- Polyps cause abdominal pain, obstruction, bleeding, and intussusception
- Hamartomas have a muscular branching framework (arborization) originating from the muscularis mucosae
- Black/brown pigmented lesions affect the lips, buccal mucosa, palms, soles, and perianal region, but often fade after puberty
- Increased risk of GI, breast, pancreas, cervical, testicular, lung, and thyroid malignancies
- Lifetime risk of malignancy thought to approach 90%
- UK guidelines recommend initial assessment of the entire GI tract at 8yrs of age with ongoing small bowel assessment 3yrly thereafter. If no upper/lower GI lesions seen at initial assessment, defer further assessment of upper GI endoscopy/colonoscopy until 18yrs of age and then 3yrly thereafter.

Juvenile polyposis syndrome (JPS)

- Rare (1 in 100,00) autosomal dominant condition characterized by hamartomatous polyposis affecting predominantly the colon
- Usually presents in the first decade with pain, bleeding, and anaemia
- Extraintestinal sites are not affected
- Lifetime risk of CRC is ~40–50% and screening with biennial colonoscopy should be carried out
- Prophylactic surgery may be considered in some patients
- UK guidelines recommend 1–3yrly colonoscopy starting at 15yrs and 1–3yrly upper GI endoscopy starting at 18yrs.

Serrated polyposis syndrome(SPS)/Hyperplastic polyposis syndrome (HPS)

- A rare condition associated with an increased risk of CRC
- Criteria include:
  - ≥20 serrated polyps of any size distributed throughout the colon
  - At least five serrated polyps proximal to the rectum >5mm, of which two are ≥10mm
- Risk of CRC may be >50%
- Patients should be closely followed up. Ideally all serrated polyps should be removed. If this is not possible due to the number, those lesions ≥1cm should be removed. Associated advanced polyps should also be removed
- UK guidelines recommend 1–2yrly colonoscopy until 75yrs for affected individuals and 5yrly colonoscopy for FDRs starting at 40yrs of age.

References

Peltomaki P, Vason HF (1997) Mutations predisposing to hereditary nonpolyposis colorectal cancer: database and results of a collaborative study. The International Collaborative Group on Hereditary Nonpolyposis Colorectal Cancer. *Gastroenterology* **113**: 1146–58.

Monahan KJ, Bradshaw N, Dolwani S et al. (2019) Guidelines for the management of hereditary colorectal cancer from the British Society of Gastroenterology (BSG)/Association of Coloproctology of Great Britain and Ireland (ACPGBI)/United Kingdom Cancer Genetics Group (UKCGG). *Gut* **0**: 1–34.

Staging and prognosis

Staging of CRC is based on detailed pathological examination of the operative specimen. In 1932 British pathologist Cuthbert Dukes devised the first widely accepted classification, which was originally intended for rectal cancer. The importance of staging is to allow prediction of outcome and to help guide treatment decisions. The Dukes' classification is no longer used internationally but continues to be used in the UK.

Dukes' classification

Dukes A Tumour confined to the wall of the rectum
Dukes B Tumour invading through wall into perirectal tissues but without nodal involvement
Dukes C Lymph node involvement
In 1935 the system was modified to take account of apical node involvement
Dukes C1 Regional nodes involved but not the apical node
Dukes C2 Apical node involvement*

The Astler–Coller modification (1954) recognizes the fact that mural penetration is an independent prognostic factor for nodal involvement. It also added a fourth stage for advanced disease.
Stage B1 Incomplete penetration of the muscularis propria
Stage B2 Complete penetration of the muscularis propria
Stage D Distant metastasis.

TNM classification

The American Joint Committee on Cancer (AJCC) TNM system is the preferred international staging system. A summary of the 8th edition (2017) is seen below (Box 7.3). The TNM staging is also used to divide patients into prognostic stage groups (I–IV), with subgroups. These are roughly equivalent to Dukes' stage A–D.

Histological prognostic factors

Nodal involvement

LN involvement is probably the single most important prognostic factor in CRC and is used to select patients for adjuvant therapy. Both apical node involvement and >3 involved nodes correlate with reduced survival. A minimum of 12 nodes is required for accurate staging of node-negative tumours.

Tumour grade

- Grade 1 Well differentiated
- Grade 2 Moderately differentiated
- Grade 3 Poorly differentiated

Differentiation is a subjective assessment comparing nuclear and architectural features with the tissue of origin. Degree of differentiation within a lesion can vary and is therefore described by the predominant area. Poorly differentiated tumours have a worse prognosis than those with better differentiation.

* Reproduced from Dukes CE. The classification of cancer of the rectum. *Journal of Pathological Bacteriology;35*:323. Copyright © 1932 The Pathological Society of Great Britain and Ireland

Vascular invasion

Vascular invasion refers predominantly to venous invasion. Intra- and extramural veins may be involved. Extramural vascular invasion (present in ~30%) is a marker of poor prognosis ↑ likelihood of metastatic disease (25% ↓ 5yr survival). It may be used as a marker of high risk disease in node-negative patients to select for adjuvant chemotherapy.

Perineural invasion

Perineural invasion is an independent predictor of poor prognosis.

Mucin production

Mucinous adenocarcinoma (≥50% mucin production) accounts for 10–15% of CRC and carries a poorer prognosis with ↑ LN + peritoneal metastasis.

Signet ring cell carcinoma (SRC)

Signet ring appearance is due to mucin pushing the nucleus to one side in the cell. SRC is associated with younger age at onset, advanced stage at presentation, ↑ ovarian and peritoneal metastases, and poorer survival.

Tumour margin

The character of the tumour margin correlates with survival. Those with well-defined borders have a better prognosis than those with a poorly defined border where cells infiltrate normal tissue or budding appears.

Tumour-infiltrating lymphocytes

Tumours with a pushing margin, surrounded by an inflammatory infiltrate of plasma cells and lymphocytes metastasize less frequently than those with no inflammatory response. Improved prognosis may be due to host immune recognition of the tumour.

There is now a defined minimum data set to standardize reporting of CRC by pathologists in the UK.

Molecular prognostic factors

DNA content

Patients with aneuploid lesions have a poorer prognosis than those with diploid lesions. Although this has a bearing on prognosis it is not an independent variable and is no better than Dukes classification in predicting outcome.

Microsatellite instability (MSI)

Many centres routinely check for MSI in tumours from younger patients (<50yrs). However, European Society for Medical Oncology (ESMO) and other oncology societies now recommend MSI assessment of all colorectal tumours. Although more than 90% of HNPCC-related tumours will show MSI (◆ Genetic disorders and polyposis syndromes, p.328), it is important to remember that 15% of sporadic cancers also show MSI and fail to express an MMR protein.

- Absence of MSI and normal expression of all four MMR proteins using IHC excludes HNPCC/Lynch syndrome
- IHC for MMR protein expression may be unreliable when performed on rectal cancer tissue that has previously been treated with chemo-radiotherapy (CRT)
- Colorectal cancers that are deficient in MMR proteins (MSI-H) carry a better prognosis but may be less responsive to 5-fluorouracil

- Lesions tend to be right sided, mucinous, poorly differentiated, and with a significant inflammatory response
- Patients with MSI-H (i.e. MMR deficient) tumours are more likely to respond to immunotherapy with immune checkpoint inhibitors when treating metastatic disease.

Biochemical prognostic factors

Carcinoembryonic antigen (CEA)

CEA has been shown to reflect extent of tumour spread either locally or with metastases. Pre-operative CEA >5ng/ml may indicate poorer survival.

C-reactive protein (CRP)

The presence of a systemic inflammatory response indicated by an elevated CRP is a marker of poor prognosis. The Glasgow Prognostic score combines CRP and albumin to predict prognosis.

Clinical prognostic factors

Age

Age of patient at presentation has a bearing on outcome. CRC in younger patients carries a poorer prognosis due to more advanced stage at presentation. Stage for stage prognosis is similar.

Mode of presentation

Patients presenting as an emergency with perforation or obstruction have a poorer prognosis than those who present electively. This is due at least in part to more advanced stage and increased operative mortality.

Blood transfusion

There has been concern that immunosuppression related to transfusion may lead to recurrence, although data are equivocal. The use of leucocyte-depleted blood means it is unlikely to be a contributory factor.

Box 7.4 TNM staging of colorectal cancer

T—Primary Tumour	
Tx	Primary tumour cannot be assessed
T0	No evidence of primary tumour
Tis	Carcinoma in situ: invasion of lamina propria[a]
T1	Tumour invades submucosa
T2	Tumor invades muscularis propria
T3	Tumour invades subserosa or into non-peritonealised pericolic or perirectal tissues
T4	Tumour directly invades other organs or structures [b, c, d] and/or perforates visceral peritoneum • T4a: Tumour perforates visceral peritoneum • T4b: Tumour directly invades other organs or structures

Notes

[a] Tis includes cancer cells confined within the mucosal lamina propria (intramucosal) with no extension through the muscularis mucosae into the submucosa.

[b] Invades through to visceral peritoneum to involve the surface

[c] Direct invasion in T4b includes invasion of other organs or segments of the colorectum by way of the serosa, as confirmed on microscopic examination, or for tumours in a retroperitoneal or subperiotoneal location, direct invasion of other organs or structures by virtue of extension beyond the muscularis propria.

[d] Tumour that is adherent to other organs or structures, macroscopically, is classified cT4b. However, if no other tumour is present in the adhesion, microscopically, the classification should be pT1-3, depending on the anatomical depth of wall invasion.

N—Regional Lymph Nodes

Nx	Regional lymph nodes cannot be assessed
N0	No regional lymph node metastasis
N1	Metastasis in 1 to 3 regional lymph

- N1a: Metastasis in 1 regional lymph node
- N1b: Metastasis in 2 to 3 regional lymph nodes
- N1c: Tumour deposit(s), i.e. satellites*, in the subserosa, or in non-peritonealised pericolic or perirectal soft tissue without regional lymph node metastasis

N2	Metastasis in 4 or more regional lymph nodes

- N2a: Metastasis in 4 to 6 regional lymph nodes
- N2b: Metastasis in 7 or more regional lymph nodes

Note

*Tumour deposits (satellites) are discrete macroscopic or microscopic nodules of cancer in the pericolorectal adipose tissue's lymph drainage area of a primary carcinoma that are discontinuous from the primary and without histological evidence of residual lymph node or identifiable vascular or neural structures. If a vessel wall is identifiable on H&E, elastic or other stains, it should be classified as venous invasion (V1/2) or lymphatic invasion (L1). Similarly, if neural structures are identifiable, the lesion should be classified as perineural invasion (Pn1). The presence of tumour deposits does not change the primary tumour T category but changes the node status (N) to pN1c if all regional lymph nodes are negative on pathological examination.

M—Distant Metastasis

M0	No distant metastasis
M1	Distant metastases

- M1a: Metastasis confined to one organ (liver, lung, ovary, non-regional lymph node(s)) without peritoneal metastasis
- M1b: Metastasis in more than one organ
- M1c: Metastasis to the peritoneum with or without other organ involvement

References

Williams GT, Quirke P, Shepherd NA. *Dataset for colorectal cancer*, 2nd edn. London: Royal College of Pathologists, 2007.

Courtney ED, West NJ, Kaur C et al. (2009) Extramural vascular invasion is an adverse prognostic indicator of survival in patients with colorectal cancer. *Colorectal Dis* **11**: 150–6.

Crozier JE, Leitch EF, McKee RF, Anderson JH, Horgan PG, McMillan DC (2009) Relationship between emergency presentation, systemic inflammatory response and cancer-specific survival in patients undergoing potentially curative surgery for colon cancer. *Am J Surg* **197**: 544–9.

Waldner M, Schimanski CC, Neurath MF (2006) Colon cancer and the immune system: the role of tumor invading T cells. *World J Gastroenterol* **12**: 7233–8.

Shirouzu K, Isomoto H, Kakegawa T (1993) Prognostic evaluation of perineural invasion in rectal cancer. *Am J Surg* **165**: 233–7.

Distribution of disease

It is important to understand the spreading pattern of CRC to be able to evaluate the extent of disease before deciding on appropriate treatment.

Macroscopic appearance

- Ulcerative: atypical malignant ulcer with rolled edges and a necrotic base. This tends to infiltrate deeply and is more likely to perforate.
- Polypoidal: a proliferative lesion protruding into the lumen of the bowel
- Stenosing or annular lesions: a circumferential lesion of variable size. Short obstructing lesions are typically seen in the sigmoid colon
- Diffuse infiltrative disease: an extensive lesion infiltrating the bowel wall over many centimetres.

Pattern of spread

Direct spread

Intramural

- Significant intramural spread of rectal cancer is associated with poor prognosis but spread >2cm is rare
- 5cm margin recommended in colon cancer and where possible in rectal cancer although no increase in local recurrence is observed with a 2cm margin.

Radial

Radial spread results in invasion of adjacent tissues or organs and is the most important mode of local spread in rectal cancer. Pre-operative evaluation of the CRM is important in rectal cancer to determine neoadjuvant treatment (Fig. 7.9). A positive CRM is associated with a high rate of local recurrence and reduced survival. Colon cancer involving adjacent structures is often only recognized at operation but if radical en bloc resection is feasible, survival comparable with non-advanced tumours can be achieved.

Lymphatic spread

- Resection of the LN-bearing mesentery associated with the primary tumour is vital for the accurate staging of disease and to determine adjuvant treatment
- Lymphatic spread of CRC occurs in a stepwise progression with paracolic nodes initially involved followed by nodes along the main vascular branches to the portal vein and liver. Skip metastases occur in <5%
- LN size is not an accurate predictor of metastasis which makes both pre-operative and intraoperative nodal staging unreliable
- In rectal cancer distal lymphatic spread is rare and associated with advanced disease. Lateral spread to nodes around the internal iliac arteries is more common with lesions below the peritoneal reflection
- Risk of LN metastasis is related to depth of invasion. 10% of T1 and 25% of T2 tumours are node positive. This has implications for the local treatment of rectal cancer
- Lateral lymph node dissection (LLND) in rectal cancer may reduce local recurrence and relapse-free survival in patients with enlarged nodes following CRT
- High vs low ligation of the IMA does not affect survival
- Sentinel LN techniques have been described in CRC although specific benefit has not yet been established.

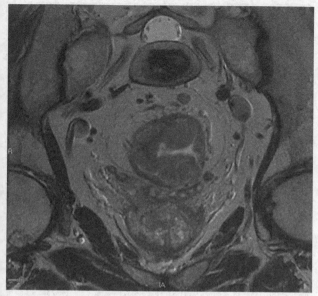

Fig. 7.9 T3 rectal cancer with threatened anterior CRM.

Haematogenous spread

CRC may spread via the bloodstream to various organs, liver being the most common (50%). Lung is the second most common site (20%). Other infrequent sites are adrenal glands, kidneys, bones, and brain.

Venous invasion is a well established risk factor for distant metastasis.

Transcoelomic spread

Spread within the peritoneal cavity initially occurs close to the tumour with small discrete nodules arising from cells shed from the 1° tumour. As disease advances, plaques become more widespread, omentum is involved, and ascites is produced. Peritoneal involvement is a poor prognostic factor (median survival <6 months).

Ovarian metastases (Krukenberg tumours) present in 3–14% (bilateral in 50%) and may arise through this mechanism. Haematogenous spread is also implicated.

Spread by implantation

Spread may occur by implantation in a variety of areas: peritoneum, suture lines, abdominal wall (Fig. 7.10), haemorrhoidectomy scars.

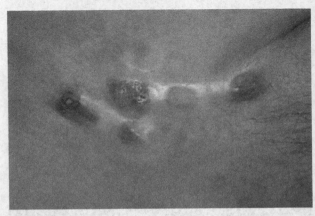

Fig. 7.10 Port site metastasis.

References

Quirke P, Durdey P, Dixon MF, Williams NS (1986) Local recurrence of rectal adenocarcinoma due to inadequate surgical resection: histopathological study of lateral tumour spread and surgical excision. *Lancet* **2**: 996–9.

Wibe A, Rendedall PR, Svensson E et al. (2002) Prognostic significance of the circumferential resection margin following total mesorectal excision for cancer. *Br J Surg* **89**: 327–34.

Alexander RJT, Jaques BC, Mitchell KG (1993) Laparoscopically assisted colectomy and wound recurrence. *Lancet* **341**: 249–50.

Ogura A, Konishi T, Beet GL et al. (2019) Lateral nodal features on restaging Magnetic Resonance Imaging associated with lateral local recurrence in low rectal cancer after neoadjuvant chemoradiotherapy or radiotherapy. *JAMA Surgery* **154**(9): e192172.

Management of colon cancer

Presentation

Despite the introduction of the bowel screening programme, most CRCs are diagnosed in symptomatic patients. As one might expect, asymptomatic patients diagnosed through the screening programme have a better prognosis compared to those who present with symptomatic disease.

Symptomatic patients present either electively or as an emergency with obstruction or perforation. Stage for stage, those who present as an emergency with obstruction or perforation have a poorer prognosis.

Many have non-specific symptoms that can also occur in a variety of other conditions. However, those who present to primary care with rectal bleeding (especially dark red blood and blood mixed in stool), change in bowel habit, or weight loss have the highest likelihood of having a CRC.

It is expected that introduction of the qFIT test for patients with any bowel related symptoms will lead to faster referral and better discrimination of those at increased risk of harbouring a CRC (➔ Colorectal assessment, Chapter 2, p.33).

Elective symptoms include:
- Altered bowel habit–loose stools more concerning than constipation. Affects up to 75% of patients
- Rectal bleeding—more common in left sided and rectal lesions
- Abdominal pain—uncommon as an isolated symptom
- Iron deficiency anaemia—occurs in up to 10% of patients
- Palpable abdominal or rectal mass—noted in 10–25% of patients
- Weight loss.

Evaluation of disease extent

Colonic assessment
- It is important to assess the whole colon pre-operatively where possible to exclude synchronous lesions which present in 3–9%
- Benign polyps will be found in 12–60% of those with one carcinoma and in 55–80% of those with synchronous lesions
- Biopsy confirmation of malignancy should be sought where possible (Fig 7.11)
- Colonoscopic tattooing of the lesion (other than those in the rectum and caecum) should be carried out to aid intraoperative identification
- Where a stenosing lesion does not allow full colonoscopic assessment CT colonography should be considered
- In the emergency setting, intraoperative colon assessment should be attempted although manual palpation is frequently inaccurate.

Distant disease
- In the UK, ~22% of patients will present with stage IV CRC
- All patients require careful clinical examination and then assessment of disease spread to identify those with distant disease
- A contrast-enhanced CT chest/abdomen/pelvis can assess locoregional extent and confirm or exclude liver and lung metastases
- Individual methods of investigation are discussed elsewhere (➔ Radiological investigations: large bowel and rectum, Chapter 2, p.48) (Fig 7.12)
- PET-CT or routine MRI of the liver are not indicated in standard assessment of CRC although may be considered if there is concern regarding the presence of metastatic disease.

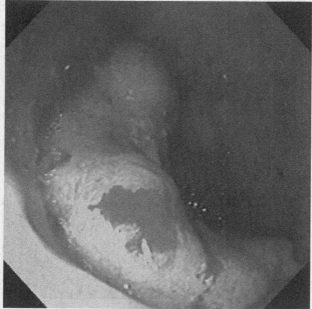

Fig. 7.11 Endoscopic view of colorectal cancer.

Tumour markers
- CEA is not helpful in screening for colorectal cancer but should be performed once a diagnosis of CRC has been made
- ↑ pre-operative CEA (>5ng/ml) is a poor prognostic indicator for patients with an equivalent TNM stage but normal CEA
- Failure of ↑ pre-operative CEA to return to normal after resection raises concern regarding the possibility of metastatic disease.

Indications for surgery
- The primary aim should be complete surgical resection of disease (minimum curative resection rate 80%)
- Patients with involvement of adjacent structures/organs should be considered for extended *en bloc* resection
- Select group of patients with localized metastatic disease, e.g. hepatic, pulmonary, ovarian, adrenal, peritoneal, will be suitable for surgery with curative intent after thorough pre-operative assessment. This may be as a synchronous procedure or following resection of the 1° tumour
- Resection of the 1° tumour may be appropriate for palliation in patients with irresectable metastatic disease, e.g. anaemia, obstruction
- Each case with distant disease should be considered on its merits with careful discussion at an MDT meeting.

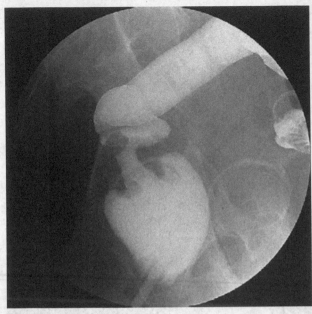

Fig. 7.12 Barium enema showing a malignant stricture.

The multidisciplinary team

All cases of CRC should be discussed at an MDT meeting. The team should consist of:
- Appropriately trained colorectal surgeons carrying out a minimum of 20 resections/yr
- Clinical oncologist with or without a medical oncologist
- Diagnostic radiologist with an interest in GI radiology
- Histopathologist with an interest in GI pathology
- Clinical nurse specialist
- Palliative care specialist
- Meeting coordinator.

A record should be kept of clinicians attending the meeting, patients discussed, and any management decisions made. The team should maintain links with other professionals involved in the management of GI disease including gastroenterologists, hepatobiliary surgeons, dieticians, geneticists, and of course the patient's GP.

Pre-operative preparation

- The patient should be in the best physical state after a thorough assessment of co-morbidities and risk of anaesthesia

- They should have a good understanding of their diagnosis and proposed treatment to allow informed consent to be given
- Their diagnosis and pre-operative imaging should be reviewed by the team carrying out the procedure
- Where appropriate, a stoma therapist should visit before surgery and acceptable stoma sites should be marked
- Bowel preparation in combination with pre-operative oral antibiotics should be considered (➲ Mechanical bowel preparation, Chapter 10, p.482).
- An enhanced recovery regime should be used where possible (➲ Enhanced recovery, Chapter 10, p.498).

General principles of surgery for colon cancer

- A curative procedure requires all tumour to be removed with adequate margins of healthy bowel (5cm) along with its associated vascular pedicle and nodal basin
- As for rectal cancer, it is also critical to ensure clear CRM in colon cancer. An involved colonic CRM is an important predictor of recurrence, risk of death, and reduced survival and is independent of stage
- Around 10% of cases show local invasion to adjacent organs. This should be removed *en bloc*. It is not possible to differentiate inflammatory from malignant adhesions during surgery; therefore, resection should be radical (avoid 'pinching off')
- Oncological principles of resection are the same regardless of approach, i.e. open, laparoscopic, or robotic surgery
  - In experienced hands, laparoscopic colon surgery facilitates a faster, less painful recovery with fewer complications and does not negatively impact recurrence or survival
  - Given the faster recovery, node positive patients who undergo a laparoscopic resection are more likely to be considered for postoperative adjuvant chemotherapy
- Midline incisions (for specimen extraction in laparoscopic surgery or as the primary incision in open surgery) can be easily extended to give wide access and avoid scarring sites which may be subsequently used for stoma formation
- Small transverse incisions can be used, especially in frail elderly patients, although evidence of improved outcome is lacking
- Tumours of the ascending colon and proximal transverse are treated by right hemicolectomy (➲ Right hemicolectomy, Chapter 11, p.526)
- Tumours of the transverse colon and splenic flexure are generally treated by extended right hemicolectomy although extended left hemicolectomy may be considered
- Tumours of the descending and sigmoid colon are treated by either left hemicolectomy or sigmoid colectomy depending on exact position (➲ Left hemicolectomy, Chapter 11, p.534)
- Subtotal colectomy and IRA may be required for synchronous lesions, polyposis syndromes, or in obstructed cases

- Irrespective of the surgical technique, it is important to achieve a complete clearance of the regional nodes along the major vessels supplying the tumour
  - There is a direct correlation between the number of nodes removed and survival
  - At the very least, the specimen should contain 12 or more nodes
  - The presence of <12 nodes in a Stage II/Dukes B cancer is associated with a poorer prognosis, as it may reflect an inadequate resection and partly because this group is likely to also contain patients with node positive disease who would not routinely be offered post-operative adjuvant chemotherapy
- Ureteric stents may be placed at the beginning of the surgical procedure to aid identification in patients with large pelvic tumours or undergoing re-operative surgery (Radical pelvic surgery, Chapter 11, p.566)
- Intestinal continuity is restored by anastomosis which may be sutured or stapled depending on surgeon preference. Sutured anastomosis using an interrupted serosubmucosal technique may be preferable when bowel ends are oedematous
- The 'no touch' technique has not been proven to improve outcome although minimal tumour handling is still recommended. Early isolation of the vascular supply before mobilizing the colon does not confer a survival advantage
- Intraluminal 'cytotoxic' lavage with sterile water or povidone–iodine has no proven benefit in terms of local recurrence or survival
- Palliative procedures may involve limited resection, by-pass, or defunctioning stoma, directed by symptom control and quality of life.

Complete mesocolic excision (CME)
- As for rectal cancer surgery, there is an increasing understanding of the correlation between quality of surgical resection and oncologic outcome in colon cancer surgery
- CME techniques (initially advocated by Hohenberger et al.), use sharp, precise dissection along embryologic fascial planes which envelop the mesentery of the colon.
- A complete *en bloc* excision of draining nodes by performing a central vascular ligation is an important component of the technique
- Hohenberger's seminal paper reported a reduction in local recurrence from 6.5 to 3.6%. Five-year survival increased from 82 to 89% after adopting the technique
- Several centres have incorporated CME into their laparoscopic and robotic surgery practices with similar improvement in results
- Some studies have suggested that the technique may be associated with an increased risk of complications including post-operative ileus
- Good quality data from prospective randomized trials comparing 'conventional' and CME colonic resection for cancer is lacking
- Currently, published evidence does not clearly support the superiority of CME. In time however, it may be that CME can be recommended as the new standard of care for colon cancer resection.

Obstructing or perforated cancers
Management of malignant large bowel obstruction (➜ Large bowel obstruction, Chapter 8, p.422) and colonic perforation (➜ Colonic perforation, Chapter 8, p.428) is covered later in this book.

Synchronous cancers
↑ risk of metachronous adenoma and carcinoma, but survival is equivalent to most advanced-stage tumour. An extended resection may be necessary, e.g. sub-total colectomy ± IRA and avoids the risk of two anastomoses, but segmental colectomies can be considered depending on location.

Polyp cancers
Malignant polyps and their management have been discussed earlier in this chapter (➜ Colonic polyps, p.320).

Ovarian metastasis
More common in young, pre-menopausal women. If metastatic lesions are identified pre-operatively, oophorectomy is appropriate. The role of prophylactic oophorectomy has not been proven.

Pregnancy
CRC during pregnancy is rare (incidence 1/50,000). Management depends on stage, presentation, gestational age, and religious beliefs. Survival is equivalent stage for stage, but presentation is often delayed. <20 weeks' gestation, cancer management should be prioritized. Surgical resection is compatible with a viable intrauterine pregnancy. Need for adjuvant therapy should be considered when deciding whether to continue the pregnancy. In the later stages, surgery should be delayed if possible until after delivery, which may be scheduled early.

Locally advanced primary colon cancer and neoadjuvant therapy
Locally advanced CRC tumours should be carefully assessed for resectability. Invasion into adjacent structures or organs is not a contra-indication and multivisceral resection should be considered where appropriate.
• There is no consensus on who should be considered for neoadjuvant chemotherapy (NAC). It might be appropriate in the following scenarios:
  • The resection margins are close or threatened despite considering an extended resection
  • A curative resection is not possible without tumour shrinkage
  • The tumour has a significant inflammatory component
  • For medical reasons, it is not possible to consider immediate surgery
• The FOxTROT trial randomized patients with resectable T3/4 colon cancer to surgery or to a 6-week course of oxaliplatin-based NAC before surgery. Preliminary results show
  • NAC did not ↑ anastomotic leak rate or other complications
  • NAC was associated with a ↓ in risk of incomplete resection to 5% versus 10% in the straight to surgery group
  • At 2yrs of follow-up, NAC was associated with a non-significant trend towards a lower recurrence rate (14% versus 18%).

Outcomes

- Much of the literature on outcomes after surgical treatment does not differentiate between patients with colon and rectal cancer
- Operative mortality should be <3% for elective procedures and <15% in the emergency setting
- Anastomotic leak rate should be <4%
- Complications following colorectal surgery are discussed in detail later (➔ General complications, Chapter 10, p.502)
- Survival is related to stage at presentation (Box 7.4)
- Crude survival rates ↑ in ♂ and ♀ over past three decades from 22 to 52%
- Patients from an affluent background have a 5–9% improvement in outcome compared with those from more deprived groups.

Table 7.1 5 year net survival colorectal cancer

CRC stage	Percentage of cases (%)	5yr survival (%)
1	18	92
2	26	84
3	30	65
4	26	10

Source: Data from Office for National Statistics Cancer Survival by Stage at Diagnosis in England 2019. Survival data shown for patients diagnosed between 2013–2017. Unknown and unstageable disease data excluded

References

Association of Coloproctology of Great Britain and Ireland (2017) Guidelines for the management of colorectal cancer. *Colorectal Disease* **19**(Supplement).

MacDermid E, MacKay G, Hooton G et al. (2009) The colorectal cancer multi-disciplinary team is associated with improved patient survival. *Colorectal Dis* **11**: 291–5.

Seymour MT, Morton D et al. (2019) FOxTROT: an international randomised controlled trial in 1052 patients evaluating neoadjuvant chemotherapy for colon cancer (abstract). *J Clin Oncol* **37**(15 suppl: abstr 3504).

Amri R, Bordeianou LG, Sylla P, Berger DL (2015) Association of Radial Margin Positivity With Colon Cancer. *JAMA Surg* **150**(9): 890–8.

Hohenberger W, Weber K, Matzel K et al. (2009) Standardized surgery for colonic cancer: complete mesocolic excision and central ligation—technical notes and outcome. *Colorectal Dis* **11**: 354–64.

Management of rectal cancer

- The assessment and management of rectal cancer follows similar oncological principles as colon cancer. The importance of visualization of the entire colon, tumour markers, and general preoperative assessment have been covered in the preceding chapter (➔ Management of colon cancer, p.344)
- Several areas require special consideration regarding rectal cancer and particular attention needs to be placed on the importance of resection technique, which is fundamental to outcome.

Evaluation of disease extent

Local assessment

- Careful assessment of the tumour should be carried out by DRE and sigmoidoscopy. Information available includes fixity (80% accuracy), distance from the dentate line to the distal margin, and the number of quadrants involved
- MRI of the pelvis to assess extent of local invasion should be carried out in all patients. High spatial resolution MRI can accurately predict threatened CRM (sensitivity 88%) helping decision-making about neoadjuvant treatment. MRI may also identify high risk features such as mesorectal LN involvement with a positive predictive value of ~70% and negative predictive value of ~90%. Extramural venous invasion and extra-mesorectal LN involvement may also be detected (Figs 7.13 and 7.14)
- ERUS is more accurate in early, low rectal tumours and can be considered prior to local excision
- Histological confirmation should be achieved in all cases in order to confirm diagnosis and differentiate between adenocarcinoma versus other pathologies such as squamous carcinoma.

Distant disease

- Distant disease should be excluded with a contrast enhanced CT chest/abdomen/pelvis in all patients, unless contraindicated
- MRI liver may be required to clarify nature/number of liver lesions
- PET-CT is not routinely performed unless there is concomitant resectable, metastatic disease and synchronous or staggered resection of the primary and metastatic disease is being considered
- Individual methods of investigation have previously been discussed in more detail (➔ Radiological investigation: large bowel and rectum, Chapter 2, p.48).

Local recurrence

Local recurrence (LR) frequently signifies incurable disease and can be challenging to palliate effectively. Thorough pre-operative local staging, accurate surgical resection and proportionate neoadjuvant therapy are key to reducing rates of LR. The goal is to remove the rectum with clear proximal, distal, and circumferential resection margins in order to minimize the risk of LR.

- Tumour location, stage, and MRI-predicted resection margin, extra-mesorectal LNs are the most important pre-operative factors
- Tumour grade, histological types, neural/vascular invasion, border configuration, tumour budding also play a role

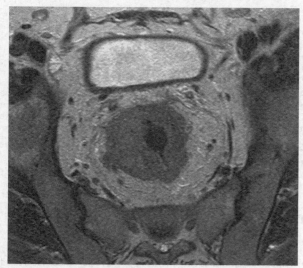

Fig. 7.13 Axial scan showing T3 disease with involvement of anterior mesorectal fascia (1 o'clock position) prior to radiotherapy.

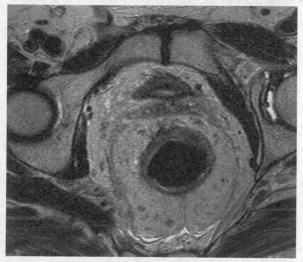

Fig. 7.14 Post-treatment MRI showing the tumour in Fig. 7.13 has retracted from the mesorectal fascia following radiotherapy.

- Total mesorectal excision ↓ rates of local recurrence and improves survival (Fig. 7.15)
- LR ↑ in low rectal cancer and after abdominoperineal resection of the rectum (APER) due to ↑ involved margins
- LR ↑ after local excision probably 2° to unrecognized LN metastases
- Inadvertent tumour perforation ↑ LR
- No difference in LR between open and laparoscopic approach.

APER was the operation of choice for rectal cancer until the middle of the last century. Modern anterior resection was first developed at the Mayo Clinic (Rochester, MN, USA). More recently modern stapling devices have revolutionized sphincter-saving surgery for rectal cancer.

General principles of surgery for rectal cancer

- Rectal resection (anterior or APER) can be performed as an open, laparoscopic or robotic procedure and the best approach is determined by surgeon experience, tumour size, and location. In experienced hands, all techniques appear to have equivalent oncologic outcome with a faster recovery and fewer complications with a minimally invasive approach
- The procedure of choice for upper third rectal cancer is anterior resection (◑ Anterior resection, Chapter 11, p.542). Total mesorectal excision (TME) is not always required although dissection in the mesorectal plane should be adhered to with a 5cm distal margin
- Tumours of the middle and lower third of the rectum should be treated by TME where possible. A distal margin of 1cm is acceptable in order to facilitate sphincter preservation (Fig 7.15)
- A clear circumferential margin of >1 mm is critical to reduce risk of local recurrence
- High ligation of the IMA may be required to give adequate length for a low pelvic anastomosis, but does not confer survival advantage
- Extended lymphadenectomy in unselected patients does not appear to improve outcome and may compromise functional results. If enlarged lateral compartment nodes (e.g. pudendal) respond and disappear after pre-operative CRT, a lateral compartment lymphadenectomy is not required. However, patients who show persistently enlarged lateral compartment nodes (>7mm or malignant appearance) after CRT should undergo LLND
- Autonomic nerves should be preserved where possible to maintain bladder and sexual function
- The rectum can be lavaged prior to anastomosis in left sided resections with povidone–iodine ('cytocidal washout'). There is no evidence to show a benefit in terms of LR or survival
- Colopouch or side-to-end anastomosis may reduce frequency, urgency, and soiling in the first year after low anterior resection
- Anastomotic leak is ↑ in anastomoses <5cm from anal verge. A defunctioning stoma should be considered in these cases to reduce the clinical consequences and permanent stoma rate. Neoadjuvant radiotherapy does not increase the risk of anastomotic leak.
- Leak rate following anterior resection should be <8%
- Recommended rates for APER are <30%
- ↑ LR following APER may be due to 'coning in' at the distal limit of the abdominal part of the dissection (◑ Abdominoperineal excision of the rectum, Chapter 11, p.550) (Fig 7.16)

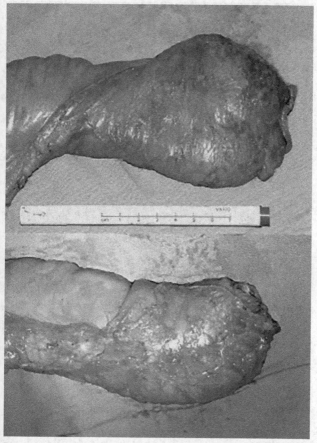

Fig. 7.15 TME resection specimen.

- Locally advanced rectal cancer invading adjacent organs and/or sacrum may require multivisceral resection/pelvic exenteration. This may be best performed within specialist centres.

Transanal total mesorectal excision (TaTME)

Operative excision of low rectal cancers can be technically challenging, especially using a laparoscopic approach in patients with a narrow pelvis (usually males), obesity, and very low tumours where sphincter preservation is being considered. The synchronous laparoscopic assisted TaTME was first performed in 2010.

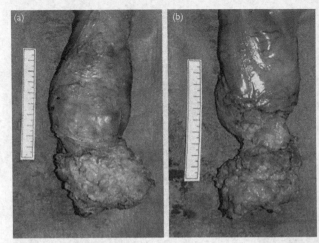

Fig. 7.16 APER specimen. (b) 'Waisting' compared with the desired cylindrical specimen shown in (a).

A standard laparoscopic mobilization of the left colon and upper rectum is performed. Using a transanal minimally invasive platform (e.g. Gelpoint® Applied Medical, CA, USA), a second operator performs a synchronous transanal mobilization of the lower rectum. After joining the dissection of the abdominal operator, a stapled or handsewn anastomosis is fashioned.

- Early results are encouraging with low anastomotic leak rates and good TME specimen quality
- Long-term outcomes and the results of randomized trials are awaited
- There is an increasing recognition of the potential for unique complications with the procedure including the risk of serious pelvic sidewall bleeding, damage to adjacent structures including the prostate, urethra, and vagina
- As with the introduction of laparoscopic and robotic colorectal surgery, it is important that surgeons who wish to undertake this new technique should participate in an appropriate training and mentorship programme.

Local excision

Small, early T1, N0 cancers may be appropriately treated with transanal local excision. However, this represents a very small group and MRI and endorectal US are not always able to accurately identify nodal involvement or differentiate between T1 and T2 disease. Currently, local excision can only be recommended for

- Mobile, T1 lesions in mid and low rectum
- Well or moderately differentiated tumours
- No lymphovascular or perineural invasion
- No evidence of locoregional nodal disease
- Patient willing to comply with close post-operative surveillance.

A variety of transanal approaches have been used. Although newer techniques may facilitate resection of higher lesions, none have shown clear oncologic superiority. Techniques include traditional transanal approach (good for very low lesions), TEM, TAMIS which are covered in more detail in the operative section of this text (➲ Transanal endoscopic microscopic, Chapter 11, p.580).

The risk of nodal involvement is 0–2% in Sm1 lesions (depth of invasion is <1000 micrometres) but around 8% for Sm2 and 23% for Sm3 lesions. If final pathology of a locally excised cancer shows Sm3 invasion, involved resection margins (<1mm), poor differentiation, lymphatic or vascular invasion, tumour budding or a T2 cancer, further treatment should be considered, e.g. formal resection or chemoradiotherapy depending on patient fitness.

Careful follow-up with regular MRI and endoscopic assessment of the scar is recommended after local excision.

Endocavitary radiation

Pioneered by Papillon, radiation therapy is delivered directly to the tumour through a 3cm diameter applicator inserted through a special proctoscope. Used to treat small, early, low grade tumours in patients unfit for surgery, with excellent rates of local control reported (~90%). Morbidity is low, with complications including radiation proctitis, ulceration, and stenosis. Treatment can be given on an outpatient basis.

Rectal cancer and metastatic disease

It is important to determine if all disease is potentially resectable in those who present with a synchronous rectal primary and metastatic disease (e.g. liver or lungs). A PET-CT is helpful in this setting

- Consideration may be given to initial chemotherapy followed by either short-course RT (SCRT) or long-course CRT.
- For patients with symptomatic primary tumours, initial SCRT followed by chemotherapy may be considered
- Long-course CRT followed by chemotherapy may be considered for high risk, locally advanced rectal cancers
- A synchronous resection of the primary and liver metastases may be considered. However, more commonly, a staged resection is performed. Final decision-making depends on patient fitness as well as the planned extent of resection of the primary and metastatic disease.

Local palliative techniques

Palliative resection may be indicated in exceptional circumstances, but a defunctioning stoma is the more common surgical approach to palliation. External beam RT may improve symptoms of bleeding and pelvic pain. Several less invasive approaches are available for palliation.

Fulguration

Debulking of tumours can be achieved using electrocautery. This may need to be repeated to keep growth under control and maintain a lumen. Haemorrhage is the main complication.

Laser

Nd-YAG laser can be used in obstructing tumours to improve the lumen or for palliation of bleeding, urgency, and tenesmus. Initial symptom control can be achieved in 80–90% after 2–5 treatments.

SEMS

Self-expanding metallic stents are described elsewhere (➲ Large bowel obstruction, Chapter 8, p.422).

Cryotherapy

Cryotherapy has been used to induce tumour necrosis. This should be done under anaesthesia and produces rectal discharge. Radiofrequency ablation (RFA) has also been described.

References

Heald RJ, Ryall RDH (1986) Recurrence and survival after total mesorectal excision for rectal cancer. *Lancet* **1**: 1479–82.

Williams NS (1984) The rationale for preservation of the anal sphincter in patients with low rectal cancer. *Br J Surg* **71**: 575–81.

Pollett WG, Nicholls RJ (1983) The relationship between the extent of distal clearance and survival and local recurrence rates after curative anterior resection for carcinoma of the rectum. *Ann Surg* **198**: 159–63.

Wolmark N, Fisher B (1986) An analysis of survival and treatment failure following abdomino-perineal resection and sphincter-saving resection in Dukes' B and C rectal carcinoma. A report of the NSABP clinical trials. *Ann Surg* **204**: 480–9.

Glynne-Jones R, Wyrwicz L, Tiret E, Brown G, Rödel C, Cervantes A, Arnold D (2017) ESMO Guidelines Committee. Rectal cancer: ESMO Clinical Practice Guidelines for diagnosis, treatment and follow-up. *Ann Oncol* **28**(suppl 4): iv22.

Balyasnikova S, Read J, Wotherspoon A et al. (2017) Diagnostic accuracy of high-resolution MRI as a method to predict potentially safe endoscopic and surgical planes in patients with early rectal cancer. *BMJ Open Gastro* **4**: e000151. doi:10.1136/bmjgast-2017

Adjuvant treatment

Adjuvant treatment

Surgery remains the mainstay of management for patients with colorectal adenocarcinoma. Decisions for patients with CRC are commonly made by consensus within a multidisciplinary team setting. Scenarios in which non-surgical treatment may be considered include treatment given before (neoadjuvant) or after (adjuvant) definitive surgery and the treatment of metastatic disease.

Typically, the aim of neoadjuvant therapy is to shrink the tumour, thereby increasing the prospect of resecting the tumour with a clear or uninvolved CRM. Post-operative adjuvant therapy is given to patients who have undergone a curative resection in order to treat any residual occult micrometastases that ultimately would manifest as overt metastatic disease.

Adjuvant chemotherapy

- Adjuvant chemotherapy given after resection of Stage III (equivalent to Dukes C) colon cancer confers a 20–30% survival advantage and a 30% reduction in risk or disease recurrence
- Other groups may also benefit:
  - Although lacking an evidence base, Stage III rectal cancer patients commonly also receive chemotherapy in the UK
  - Carefully selected patients with Stage II CRC with adverse histological features (some of whom may have a prognosis poorer than many Stage III patients' may also derive benefit from adjuvant chemotherapy (Table 7.2)
- Typically, several chemotherapeutic drugs are given over 3–6 months
- Most regimens are based around 5-FU and oxaliplatin
- Older patients gain a similar survival advantage with adjuvant chemotherapy compared to younger patients. However, they may be less tolerant of the side effects, particularly of oxaliplatin. Single agent 5-FU chemotherapy or a non-oxaliplatin containing regimen is often considered in patients aged >70yrs
- Side effects are common and include mucositis, nausea, vomiting, diarrhoea, fatigue, neutropaenia, and hand-foot syndrome. 5-FU has a cardiotoxic effect. Oxaliplatin frequently causes a cold-induced peripheral neuropathy and cumulative dose toxicity can cause persistent and often painful peripheral neuropathy that can be disabling
- The risk of chemotherapy related mortality is 0.5–1%.

Commonly used drugs and drug regimens

FOLFOX
- Comprised of **Fol**inic acid, 5-**F**luorouracil, and **Ox**aliplatin
- Typically, the 5-FU is given as a 48-hr infusion.

CAPOX
- Comprised of **Cap**ecitabine and **Ox**aliplatin.

5-Fluorouracil
- Belongs to family of drugs called anti-metabolites
- Pyrimidine analogue inhibits thymidylate synthase (TS) and incorporates into cell DNA/RNA inducing cell cycle arrest and apoptosis
- 5-FU may be given as an outpatient continuous infusion via a central venous catheter. This reduces side effects and improves efficacy compared to bolus IV infusion regimens such as the MAYO regimen.

Table 7.2 Prognostic factors in Dukes' B disease*

Factor	Score
Vascular invasion	1
pT4 disease (peritoneal involvement)	1
pT4 disease (perforation)	2
Mesocolic margin involvement	1

*Prospective study of 268 Dukes' B colon cancer patients undergoing rigorous histopathological review; patients lacking any of the above adverse features have risk of recurrence comparable with that of Dukes' A patients. Score of 2 confers risk at least equivalent to Dukes' C disease.

Source: Data from Petersen VC, Baxter KJ, Love SB, et al. Identification of objective pathological prognostic determinants and models of prognosis in Dukes' B colon cancer. *Gut* 2002;51:65–69.

Folinic acid
- Enhances effect of 5-FU by inhibiting TS
- The term leucovorin refers to a reduced folinic acid.

Capecitabine
- Oral prodrug selectively converted to 5-FU by enzymes found mostly in tumour cells
- Oral administration is convenient. Compared to IV bolus 5-FU (MAYO regimen), it has a lower risk of neutropenia, stomatitis, and alopecia but increased risk of neurotoxicity, diarrhoea, thrombocytopenia, and severe hand-foot syndrome.

Tegafur–uracil (UFT)
- Tegafur converts to 5-FU in the liver while uracil slows breakdown of 5-FU
- This is another oral pro-drug and alternative to bolus/infusional 5FU.

Oxaliplatin
- Platinum-based agent which cross-links DNA, inhibiting replication and transcription
- Febrile neutropenia, diarrhoea, and cold-induced peripheral neuropathy are more common in those who receive an oxaliplatin-5-FU regimen vs 5-FU alone
- >90% will suffer from a transient cold-induced sensory neuropathy, which is graded as severe in 13%. Peripheral sensory neuropathy of lesser severity may persist for more than 2yrs.

Treatment rationale
- Single-agent 5-FU/folinic acid (FA) regimens improve overall survival by 8–12% in Stage III disease
- Additional advantage (20–30%) is achieved if oxaliplatin is added to 5-FU/FA (FOLFOX), but at the expense of additional toxicity (myelosuppression and persistent sensory peripheral neuropathy)
  - The MOSAIC trial showed higher survival rates in stage III disease when oxaliplatin was added to a 5-FU based regimen (73 vs 69% at 6yrs and 67 vs 59% at 10yrs)
  - Stage II patients did not seem to gain significant benefit from the addition of oxaliplatin to the regimen

- The oral fluoropyrimidines (capecitabine and UFT) are suitable 5-FU substitutes. CAPOX regimens show a similar improvement in survival in stage III disease compared to FOLFOX regimens
- Until recently, adjuvant chemotherapy was typically given for 6 months. Recent studies have shown that a 3-month regimen in 'low' risk stage III patients (i.e. T1-3N1) obtain a similar survival benefit but with fewer side effects compared to a 6-month regimen. In this setting the CAPOX regimen may be chosen for the 3-month regimen rather than 6 months of FOLFOX
- There is a smaller but definite survival advantage in patients with high risk stage II (Dukes B) cancer. High risk factors include:
  - T4 tumours, especially if perforated or obstructed
  - Poorly differentiated
  - Lymphovascular or perineural invasion
  - <12 nodes in specimen
- MSI-H/deficient MMR tumours (Lynch syndrome-related tumours and the 15% of sporadic cancers which are MSI-H) appear to be insensitive to 5-FU therapy. Single agent 5-FU therapy is unlikely to be of benefit and an oxaliplatin-based regimen should be considered in stage III cancer
- Trials in which adjuvant chemotherapy demonstrated survival advantage generally commenced treatment within 8 weeks of resection. Although conflicting results are reported from individual studies, two meta-analyses have reported a significant negative impact if chemotherapy was delayed beyond 8 weeks for one analysis and beyond 12 weeks in the second
- The use of other drugs and biological agents that show activity in CRC (irinotecan, bevacizumab, cetuximab, and panitumumab) have not been shown to offer additional benefit in the adjuvant setting.

Adjuvant therapy with aspirin

- Large scale observational studies have shown that long-term use of aspirin is associated with a significant reduction in the overall risk of a number of cancers including colorectal, gastric, oesophageal, pancreatic, prostate, and ovarian cancer
- It is estimated that aspirin use for five or more years is associated with a 25–35% reduction in the incidence of CRC and a 40% reduction in CRC-related mortality
- Aspirin and NSAIDs downregulate the COX-2 pathway which is upregulated in 80–85% of CRC
- The beneficial effects of aspirin must be counterbalanced by ↑ risk of complications from GI bleeding and haemorrhagic stroke
- Observational studies also suggest that aspirin may also have a beneficial effect in reducing recurrence rates and CRC-related mortality, even if initiated at the time of cancer diagnosis
- At least one large prospective randomized trial is currently assessing the impact of regular aspirin after curative treatment of early CRC (ADD-ASPIRIN trial).

References

Chan G, Chee, CE (2019) Making sense of adjuvant chemotherapy in colorectal cancer. *J Gastrointest Oncol* **10**(6): 1183–92.

Qiao Y, Yang T, Gan Y et al. (2018) Associations between aspirin use and the risk of cancers: a meta-analysis of observational studies. *BMC Cancer* **18**(1): 288.

Neoadjuvant treatment

Rectal cancer

- Non-surgical treatment strategies in patients with localized rectal cancer are best delivered pre-operatively when treatment is better tolerated and more effective
- Historically, local tumour recurrence has been a significant form of relapse; the advent of TME is associated with lower rates of LR
- UK rectal cancer management is based on high quality TME surgery, accurate pre-operative local tumour staging, and histological assessment of CRM—achievement of a clear CRM is of prognostic significance, for both local and systemic disease control
- The likelihood of achieving a clear CRM can be determined pre-operatively using high resolution, thin-slice MRI
- Multidisciplinary team evaluation of rectal cancer patients maximizes the proportion achieving a clear CRM; patients felt at risk of an involved CRM receive pre-operative treatment to produce tumour regression and facilitate a CRM-negative procedure
- Pre-operative treatment for CRM-threatened patients commonly comprises a 5–6-week course of pelvic RT with concomitant chemotherapy (usually 5-FU or capecitabine/UFT-based). Resection is undertaken 12–14 weeks later
- This regimen is also known as long-course CRT. The main indications for CRT are
  - Tumour where pre-operative investigations show invasion of the mesorectal fascia, i.e. predicted positive or close (<2mm) CRM
  - T3 or node positive lower 1/3 tumours (assessed on a case by case basis, i.e. early T3 invasion (<5mm) or node positive patients without extranodal extension may be suitable to proceed to surgery
  - T2N0 lower 1/3 tumours which are likely to require an APER. CRT may enable a sphincter-saving operation or even a complete clinical response (cCR), thus avoiding surgery altogether (this indication is not universally accepted as standard practice)
- Up to 2/3 of patients with a threatened CRM who undergo CRT will subsequently undergo rectal resection with a clear CRM
- It is unclear if post-resection adjuvant chemotherapy following CRT is beneficial although it is usually given based on extrapolation from surgery-only colorectal cancer studies
- Total neoadjuvant therapy is occasionally used in patients with locally advanced and bulky primary rectal cancer. A more intensive induction chemotherapy (e.g. FOLFOX) is followed by CRT
- For patients not felt at risk of involved margins, the risk of LR is small and many patients can proceed to immediate resection
- Additional small but significant improvements in local control (and possibly disease-free survival) can be achieved with short-course pre-operative radiotherapy (SCPRT), given as a 1-week course of treatment immediately before resection
- SCPRT is associated with toxicity, particularly long-term bowel dysfunction. The shorter duration of therapy may be beneficial in less fit patients and those that require additional systemic chemotherapy for metastatic disease

- For rectal cancer patients of appropriate fitness who develop LR, consideration should be given to resection. Results of surgery may be improved if pre-operative CRT is used. If resection is not possible, such treatment has a valuable role in palliation.

Non-operative 'Watch-and-Wait' strategy in rectal cancer

- Pre-operative long-course CRT can result in a pathologic complete response (pCR) in 8–24% of patients
- The likelihood of achieving a pCR depends on the initial tumour stage, bulk, and timing of surgery after completion of CRT
- Patients with a pCR can expect 5-yr survival rates of 85–90% (data collected from studies where the majority of patients had low rectal cancers)
- A cCR in distal rectal cancers based on clinical assessment, MRI, and endoscopy can have similar outcomes to those with a pCR
- Tumour shrinkage continues for up to 12 weeks after completion of radiotherapy, so final assessments on whether a cCR has occurred should be deferred until this time
- Dr Angelita Habr-Gama and others have developed a non-operative 'Watch-and-Wait' approach for distal rectal cancers with a cCR
- Local recurrence rates after cCR in distal rectal cancers vary between 10–30%
- Most local recurrences will occur in the first 12 months
- With careful and frequent monitoring (endoscopy and MRI), most such recurrences can be successfully 'salvaged' with resectional TME or APER surgery (local excision is not recommended)
- 5–10% in a Watch-and-Wait regimen will develop distant metastases, which is equivalent to a comparable group undergoing surgery
- If a patient with a distal rectal cancer is being considered for Watch-and-Wait management, clinicians should follow current local guidelines on frequency of clinical, MRI (usually 4 monthly in first year), and endoscopic assessment (2–3 monthly in first year) to identify recurrences early.

Colon cancer

The use of neoadjuvant chemotherapy in locally advanced colon cancer is currently under evaluation in clinical trials (➔ Locally advanced primary colon cancer and neoadjuvant therapy are discussed earlier in this chapter, under the heading of Management of colon cancer, p.344).

References

Heald RJ, Moran BJ, Ryall RD, Sexton R, MacFarlane JK (1998) Rectal cancer: the Basingstoke experience of total mesorectal excision, 1978–1997. *Arch Surg* **133**: 894–9.

(1997) Swedish Rectal Cancer Trial participants. Improved survival with preoperative radiotherapy in resectable rectal cancer. *N Engl J Med* **336**: 980–7.

Kapiteijn E, Marijnen CA, Nagtegaal ID et al. (2001) Preoperative radiotherapy combined with total mesorectal excision for resectable rectal cancer. *N Engl J Med* **345**: 638–46.

Habr-Gama A, Perez RO, Nadalin W et al. (2004) Operative versus nonoperative treatment for stage 0 distal rectal cancer following chemoradiation therapy: long-term results. *Ann Surg* **240**(4): 711–18.

Treatment of metastatic disease

~25% of patients with CRC present with metastatic disease and at least 1/3 of patients who undergo curative treatment will subsequently develop metastatic disease. Given that most patients with metastatic CRC (mCRC) will not be cured, it is important to remember that treatment is palliative in intent. However, interventions such as chemotherapy may improve quality of life by improving symptoms and can significantly prolong survival. Patients with potentially resectable liver metastases are discussed elsewhere in this chapter (❍ Liver resection, p.376).

The median survival of patients with mCRC receiving best supportive care (6 months) is improved using single-agent fluoropyrimidine treatment (12 months) and is further enhanced using combination chemotherapy. Median survival times approaching three years are not unexpected and 1 in 5 patients may live for five years. Both RT and chemotherapy have significant roles in the palliation of disease-related symptoms. Performance status (PS) is a key factor in determining patients' suitability for specific therapies, with patients of PS 3–4 regarded as unsuitable for chemotherapy (Table 7.3).

Chemotherapy

- To determine appropriate treatment, patients with metastatic disease should undergo thorough radiological staging with CT
- The MDT should consider patients with metastatic disease restricted to the liver or lung for resection. RFA or other therapies may also be considered (❍ Ablation of liver metastases, discussed later in this chapter, p.378)
- Studies of perioperative chemotherapy in patients felt to have potentially resectable disease suggest disease-free survival benefit for those patients undergoing surgery
- If resection is initially precluded, patients should be re-assessed for surgery following chemotherapy as a proportion may become resectable
- Best response rates are achieved with the use of combination chemotherapy, incorporating either oxaliplatin or irinotecan (topoisomerase I inhibitor) with a fluoropyrimidine such as 5-FU or capecitabine. Up to 50% of patients respond with time to progression in clinical trials approximating 8 months
- Single-agent fluoropyrimidine treatment may be appropriate in certain patients depending on their co-morbidity, PS, and extent of disease
- Whether patients of poor performance status (e.g. PS 2) are best served by (less toxic) single-agent treatment or (more active but potentially more toxic) combination therapy is unclear
- Biomarker expression increasingly plays a critical role in determining which drugs should be administered in patients with mCRC
- The roles of monoclonal antibodies to epidermal growth factor receptor (EGFR), e.g. cetuximab/panitumummab and vascular endothelial growth factor (VEGF), e.g. bevacizumab, are evolving. These biological agents enhance response and time to tumour progression in certain situations
- Responses to second-line therapy are less frequent and of shorter duration.

Table 7.3 WHO performance status

0	Asymptomatic: Fully active and able to carry on all pre-disease performance without restriction
1	Restricted in physically strenuous activity but ambulatory and able to carry out work of a light or sedentary nature, e.g. light housework, office work
2	Ambulatory and capable of all self-care but unable to carry out any work activities. Up and about >50% of waking hours
3	Capable of only limited self-care, confined to bed or chair >50% of waking hours
4	Completely disabled. Cannot carry out any self-care. Totally confined to bed or chair

Commonly used drugs and drug regimens

Many of the drugs and drug regimens used in adjuvant therapy are also used as first-line treatment in mCRC (◔ Adjuvant treatment, discussed earlier in this chapter, p.360).

First-line therapy

FOLFOX: **Fol**inic acid, 5-**F**luorouracil and **Ox**aliplatin
CAPOX: **Cape**citabine and **Ox**aliplatin
FOLFIRI: **Fol**inic acid, 5-**F**luorouracil, and **Iri**notecan
FOLFOXIRI: **Fol**inic acid, 5-**F**luorouracil, **Ox**aliplatin, and **Iri**notecan

- FOLFOX and FOLFIRI have similar activity and usually FOLFIRI is used if oxaliplatin has been used previously, e.g. for adjuvant therapy
- FOLFOXIRI has significant toxicity but is sometimes considered in fit patients who might be candidates for resection of metastatic disease if they get a good response with significant tumour shrinkage. This is called conversion chemotherapy and is particularly used to try and convert non-resectable liver metastases to resectable disease (◔ Liver resection, discussed later in this chapter, p.376).

Biologic drugs

Biologic therapy with anti-EGFR drugs (cetuximab/panitumumab) are added in patients without RAS/BRAF mutations. The triple combination has better response and disease-free survival when compared with doublet chemotherapy.

- Patients with RAS or BRAF V600E mutations do not benefit from treatment with EGFR-targeting agents (cetuximab/panitumumab) Bevacizumab (anti-VEGF) may be considered instead.

Cetuximab

- This chimeric (mouse-human) IgG(1) monoclonal antibody (trade name Erbitux®) blocks EGFR activation
- EGFR signals through the mitogen-activated protein kinase (MAPK) pathway. KRAS is part of this pathway (Fig. 7.17).
- If KRAS is mutated, KRAS signalling is increased and uncoupled from EGFR control

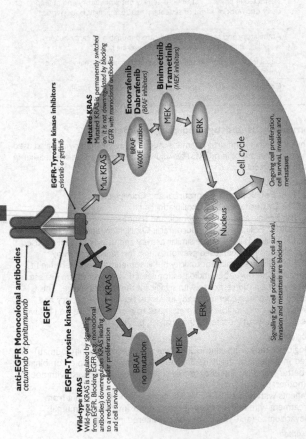

Fig. 7.17 Diagrammatic representation of the targets for anti-EGFR therapy and the relevance to KRAS mutations

- KRAS mutations are seen in at least 40% of CRC and ~75% of patients with mCRC have an EGFR-expressing tumour
- Cetuximab is only indicated in an EGFR-expressing tumour which is also KRAS normal/wild
- Patients with progressive KRAS wild type, BRAF-mutated cancers have been treated with a combination of an anti-EGFR drug plus BRAF inhibitor plus MEK inhibitor, e.g. combination therapy with cetuximab, encorafenib, binimetinib (Fig. 7.17).

Bevacizumab
- Humanized monoclonal antibody that inhibits VEGF-A (trade name Avastin®)
- It is contraindicated if there is a recent history of arterial thromboembolism and if surgery is planned within 8 weeks after cessation of therapy (increased risk of impaired would healing, perforation, and fistulae).

Newer drugs active in metastatic CRC
- Aflibercept is a recombinant fusion protein consisting of portions of human VEGF receptors which are fused to the Fc portion of human Ig1. It is relatively non-immunogenic and is used in the second-line setting in combination with FOLFIRI
- Regorafenib is active against a variety of kinases including those associated with VEGF receptors. It is administered orally
- Many cancers can inactivate T cells (which have important anti-cancer functions). They do this by producing inhibitory molecules including Programmed Cell Death 1 ligand 1 or 2 (PD-L1-2). These molecules bind to PD-1 and PD-2 on the surface of T cells, thereby inactivating T cell function. Immune checkpoint inhibitors such as nivolumab and pembrolizumab block PD-L1 from binding to PD-1. They may have a role in treating relapsed MSI-H or MMR deficient CRC.

Radiotherapy
- RT is useful in palliating pain from bone metastases and for the unpleasant symptoms of uncontrolled pelvic disease.

References
Salvatore L, Aprile G, Arnoldi E et al. (2017) Management of metastatic colorectal cancer patients: guidelines of the Italian Medical Oncology Association (AIOM). *ESMO Open* **2**: e000147.

Recurrent colorectal cancer

Recurrent colorectal cancer is observed in 30–40% of patients following surgical resection with curative intent. Recurrence may be local, distant, or a combination. 70% of recurrences occur within the first 2yrs after operation, while relapse after 5yrs is uncommon. Isolated recurrence amenable to surgical resection is infrequent but 5yr survival of 25–30% can be achieved. Symptomatic recurrence is less likely to be resectable and has a poorer overall survival. For these reasons, to be able to treat recurrent CRC effectively, some form of follow-up is required for detection of asymptomatic disease.

Colorectal cancer follow-up

Rationale

- Should lead to early detection of metastatic disease, local/anastomotic recurrence as well as metachronous and pre-malignant lesions (polyps)
- Allows audit of surgical outcomes
- Meta-analyses suggest intensive follow-up improves overall survival (~10%) and ↑ detection of isolated asymptomatic LR
- Improved survival has to be balanced against earlier detection of incurable disease in the majority of patients who relapse
- ~3–7% develop metachronous lesions and 20% polyps following resection of cancer, suggesting colonoscopic surveillance is indicated although survival benefit has not been proven.

Delivery

CEA

- Carcinoembryonic antigen as a marker of recurrence has sensitivity of 64% and specificity of 90% using cut-off >5ng/ml
- ↑ by smoking, liver disease, active IBD, chronic obstructive pulmonary disease (COPD), pulmonary TB, and other advanced malignancies. Reduced in poorly differentiated tumours
- May be measured 3–6 monthly at outpatient clinical review to guide further radiological/endoscopic investigation.

CT

- Annual abdominal CT in the first 2–3yrs is a common component of an intensive follow-up regime
- Allows assessment of both liver disease and locoregional recurrence.

Colonoscopy

- Colonoscopy to exclude metachronous lesions/polyps and anastomotic recurrence is recommended following similar intervals to polyp surveillance (◑ Colonic polyps, discussed earlier in this chapter, p. 320).

An example follow-up schedule is displayed in Box 7.5 although the optimal intensity/modality for follow-up of CRC has not been proven. Follow-up should be tailored to the age and co-morbidity of the patient. Patients unfit for further intervention clearly will not benefit from intensive follow-up.

Box 7.5 Example follow-up protocol for colorectal cancer

1–3 Months
Post-operative visit for clinical review/examination
CEA baseline measurement

6 Months
Outpatient visit for clinical review/examination
CEA measurement
Colonoscopy if incomplete pre-operative visualization

1 Year
Outpatient visit for clinical review/examination
CEA measurement
CT abdomen

18 Months
Outpatient visit for clinical review/examination
CEA measurement

2 Years
Outpatient visit for clinical review/examination
CEA measurement
CT abdomen

3 Years
Outpatient visit for clinical review/examination
CEA measurement
CT abdomen
Colonoscopy

Surgical management of recurrent colorectal cancer

Rationale

- 7–33% of patients who relapse have isolated locoregional disease
- Without treatment, outcome is universally poor, often with disabling complications, e.g. severe pain, ureteric/GI obstruction
- 5yr survival following resection of isolated recurrence including liver and lung ranges between 20–45%
- Survival is closely correlated with resection margin (R0 > R1 > R2)
- Extensive surgery with potentially significant morbidity should only be considered in patients where negative margins are achievable
- Short disease-free interval may predict poor outcome but is not an absolute contraindication to resection.

Contraindications to radical surgery for recurrent rectal cancer

- Nerve root involvement above S1/2
- Invasion of sacrum above S1/2
- Extensive para-aortic node involvement
- Tumour invasion through the sciatic notch
- Bilateral ureteric obstruction (relative contraindication)
- Circumferential involvement of pelvic wall.

Work-up
- The key to a good outcome in these patients is a thorough pre-operative work-up to exclude other sites of recurrence
- Recurrent disease will most commonly be diagnosed through follow-up surveillance including CEA and CT
- MRI/ERUS may be used to complement CT for pre-operative planning
- PET-CT has an increasingly pivotal role in excluding irresectable disease with higher sensitivity and specificity than CT/MRI (Fig. 2.13). It is especially useful for discriminating between scar tissue and active tumour including investigation of raised CEA
- If a lesion cannot be characterized radiologically, histological proof should be sought first or at least signs of progression on serial imaging before proceeding to radical surgery.

Management
- Pre-operative chemoradiation should be considered depending on previous adjuvant/neoadjuvant treatment
- Intraoperative radiotherapy (IORT) is suggested to improve outcomes although facilities for delivery are limited
- The most common site of resectable local disease is the pelvis after rectal cancer resection. Extent of resection will vary from converting someone who has had an anterior resection to an APER to total pelvic exenteration with sacrectomy ($\ominus$ Radical pelvic surgery, Chapter 11, p.566)
- Often in these patients, reconstruction will involve the use of myocutaneous flaps to close the perineal defect, e.g. rectus abdominus, inferior gluteal artery perforator (IGAP)
- A multidisciplinary surgical approach is required for advanced cases
- Involvement of S1/2 or pelvic sidewall and bilateral ureteric obstruction suggests irresectability
- Other sites that may be cured by radical surgery include recurrence involving tail of pancreas and stomach after resection of a splenic flexure tumour and duodenum and head of pancreas after resection of a hepatic flexure tumour
- Patients with para-aortic LN recurrence will sometimes be salvaged by retroperitoneal LN dissection
- Management of hepatic metastases ($\ominus$ Liver metastases, p.374) and abdominal wall recurrence ($\ominus$ Tumours of the abdominal wall, p.408) are described later in this chapter.

Peritoneal carcinomatosis
On occasion, colorectal cancers may present with peritoneal carcinomatosis. It can also be a feature of recurrent CRC. In 25% of cases, there is no evidence of other sites of metastatic disease. The best management in this scenario is not clear, although traditionally all patients with carcinomatosis were treated with palliative intent.

There is an increasing trend towards aggressive cytoreductive surgery (CRS) to remove as much macroscopic disease as is possible, followed by heated intra-peritoneal chemotherapy (HIPEC) as long-term cure can be achieved in a minority of patients. A similar approach has found more widespread acceptance in the management of pseudomyxoma peritonei ($\ominus$ Pseudomyxoma peritonei, discussed later in this chapter, p.400). There are a number of areas of uncertainty in the management of such patients.

- Long-term survivors after CRS and HIPEC may have a biologically less aggressive cancer
- It is unclear if the HIPEC component adds an additional survival advantage over high quality CRS
  - Early results from the PRODIGE-7 trial suggest that the addition of HIPEC did not increase survival
- It is unclear if combination chemotherapy with oxaliplatin /irinotecan-based chemotherapy ± biologic therapy can have a similar impact on disease eradication or prolonged survival
- The best results for CRS and HIPEC come from very specialized centres and these skills (with associated low morbidity) are not easily transferred to non-specialist colorectal surgery units.

It is likely that CRS ± HIPEC does have a positive effect on median survival for some and can result in long-term survival for a small percentage of patients. However, it is not clear how to select out such patients and some who undergo CRS ± HIPEC are likely to have derived a similar benefit from combination chemotherapy with less morbidity and mortality.

References

Colorectal cancer. NICE guideline [NG151] Published 29 January 2020. https://www.nice.org.uk/guidance/ng151

Renehan AG, Egger M, Saunders MP et al. (2002) Impact on survival of intensive follow up after curative resection for colorectal cancer, systematic review and meta analysis of randomised trials. *BMJ* **324**: 813–15.

Liver metastases

Approximately 50% of CRC patients will be diagnosed with liver metastases, either at the time of presentation or as a result of disease recurrence. Of those who develop liver metastases half will have disease confined to the liver but only ~10% will have operable disease. 90% of cancer deaths are the result of metastasis.

Pathophysiology of metastasis

- Metastasis is the dissemination of malignant cells from the primary tumour to a distant organ. It is a complex multistage process
- The first step in the pathway involves clonal expansion of cells with an invasive phenotype and the ability to break away from the primary tumour site
- Reduced adhesion by downregulation of E-cadherin is thought to be vital to this process, with upregulation after arrival at distant sites
- Intravasation is an extension of invasion, with cells penetrating the endothelium of immature vessels formed by tumour neovascularization
- In the bloodstream, cells form clumps or emboli which must survive physical damage, filtration, and immune recognition before arresting at the metastatic site by either adhesion to the endothelium or lodging in capillaries due to their size
- Extravasation is followed by apoptosis due to either hostile tissue microenvironment, dormancy, or proliferation
- The exact molecular signals involved in each stage of the process are not fully understood.

Investigation

- Investigation of liver metastases involves local staging and exclusion of extrahepatic disease
- Safety and efficacy of hepatic resection is greatly facilitated by contrast-enhanced spiral CT ± MRI allowing for tumour characterization, staging, and accurate identification of position in relation to major vasculature (Fig. 7.18)
- PET-CT can further improve patient selection and optimize long-term surgical outcomes
- PET-CT identifies disease not recognized on CT in up to 20%
- The risk of local tumour dissemination with biopsy of a liver metastasis is thought to be low (and much higher in primary hepatocellular carcinoma). However, biopsy is not usually considered if CT/MRI are consistent with a diagnosis of metastatic disease and prior histology has confirmed the diagnosis of CRC
- Laparoscopic inspection ± US can be performed as part of the diagnostic work-up to exclude irresectable disease and avoid non-therapeutic laparotomy.

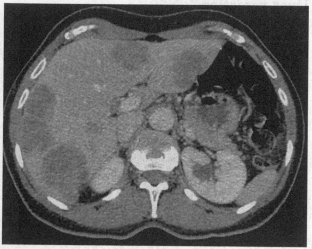

Fig. 7.18 Liver metastases.

Management

The majority of patients with liver metastases will have inoperable disease and should be selected for either chemotherapy (median survival 18 months, ➲ Treatment of metastatic disease, discussed earlier in this chapter, p.366) or supportive care (median survival 6 months, ➲ Palliative care, discussed later in this chapter, p.380). Liver resection is the only therapy shown to be potentially curative for liver metastases (median survival 40 months, ➲ Liver resection, discussed in the next section, p.376). A combination of resection and ablative techniques may be required for complete eradication of disease (➲ Ablation of liver metastases, discussed later in this chapter, p.378). Approximately 10–20% of patients who have isolated non-resectable liver disease can ultimately be converted to undergo resection after neoadjuvant chemotherapy. Patients should therefore be classified as having either potentially convertible or unconvertible metastatic liver disease.

Liver resection

Liver resection is the treatment of choice for resectable colorectal liver metastases (CRLM).

Selection

- Assessment of co-morbidity and fitness for surgery is clearly important, particularly a history of liver disease and its likely influence on hepatic reserve
- Contraindications to liver resection include irresectable extrahepatic disease and insufficient future liver remnant
- MDT review is important in all patients with CRLM.

Poor prognostic factors

- ↑ number of lesions, size >5cm and bi-lobar disease
- Short disease-free interval (DFI)
- LN +ve primary tumour
- Serosal disease (T4) in primary tumour
- CEA >200ng/ml
- Previously, it was thought that lesions larger than a fixed size or more than a fixed number of deposits should be viewed as a contra-indication to surgery. It is now felt that there should be no fixed contraindications and patients should be considered for surgery if it is technically possible to resect/ablate all with a view to cure (and maintain sufficient remaining liver volume).

Perioperative management

- Insufficient liver remnant can be addressed by pre-operative portal vein embolization ± 2-stage hepatectomy
- Sudden haemorrhage is the most important intraoperative consideration. Suitable monitoring, vascular access, and cross-matched blood to permit rapid transfusion should be in place
- Low central venous pressure (CVP) anaesthesia may reduce blood loss
- Pringle manoeuvre may help temporarily to control bleeding from intrahepatic arterial branches
- Both anatomical (mono-, bi-, tri-segmentectomy, hemi-, extended hemi-hepatectomy) and non-anatomical (metastasectomy) resections are commonly used
- Parenchymal transection is performed with a combination of ultrasonic dissection, crush-clamp dissection, ligation, suturing, and diathermy
- Negative histological margin alone is important as width of resection margin has no impact on survival, recurrence risk, or site of recurrence
- Many centres now undertake liver resection laparoscopically with low blood loss, less post-operative pain, and more rapid recovery
- Repeated liver resection is possible with outcomes in those deemed suitable (5–10%) similar to that for initial resection.
- A staged resection can be considered for extensive bilobar disease that cannot be resected in a single operation. As many lesions as can be safely removed in a first operation is followed either by portal vein embolization to promote hypertrophy of the remaining remnant or chemotherapy to stabilize the remaining disease. Once the remaining liver has hypertrophied to an adequate size, a second resection is considered

- Synchronous liver and colonic resection is feasible and may reduce total hospital stay. A synchronous approach may also reduce morbidity with no effect on long-term survival. However, a staged resection may be considered best if either the liver or CRC resection is viewed as being a 'higher risk' procedure. If a staged resection is felt best, traditionally the CRC resection is performed first. However, an individualized approach is appropriate
- Consideration may also need to be given to pre-operative CRT for rectal cancers or neoadjuvant chemotherapy.

Conversion chemotherapy and adjuvant chemotherapy

- Pre-operative chemotherapy (termed conversion chemotherapy) has the ability to render 15–30% of patients with initially unresectable CRLM suitable for resection with comparable outcomes
- Pre-operative neoadjuvant chemotherapy has also been considered in patients who present with resectable CRLM and a primary still *in situ* as this offers a chance to see if further metastatic disease develops over the initial few months after presentation
- The role and optimal regimen for neoadjuvant chemotherapy is still a matter of ongoing research although doublet therapy with FOLFOX and FOLFIRI is commonly given. However, it is increasingly recognized that these patients may have liver damage that increases the technical difficulty of surgery and increases the risk of complications
- Neoadjuvant chemotherapy is often reserved for patients with higher risk CRLM or when there is concern regarding the resectability of the liver disease
- Although there is a clear role for post-operative adjuvant chemotherapy after resection of Stage III and some Stage II primary CRC, there is no definite role for adjuvant chemotherapy after curative resection of CRLM. It is often considered in patients who are viewed as higher risk for recurrent disease and those who are chemotherapy naïve.

Outcomes

- Surgical mortality <3%
- Morbidity ~20% and increased with more extended resections
- Complications include bleeding, abscess, bile leak, and liver failure
- 5yr survival 25–60%, 10yr survival 17–33%.

References

Chow FC, Chok KS (2019) Colorectal liver metastases: An update on multidisciplinary approach. *World J Hepatol.* **11**(2): 150–72. doi:10.4254/wjh.v11.i2.150

Ablation of liver metastases

Hepatectomy is currently the treatment of choice for patients with CRC liver metastases. Unfortunately, curative surgery is only possible for ~10% of patients. The majority are unsuitable because of advanced stage, distribution of disease, or co-morbidities precluding major surgery. However, advances in neoadjuvant chemotherapy mean that 10–20% of patients who initially were felt to have unresectable disease may be considered for hepatic resection.

Radiofrequency ablation

RFA is an attractive alternative for patients for whom resection is not an option or in combination with hepatectomy for the ablation of multiple metastases (Fig. 7.19). It may be suitable for patients who have had surgery and now require further non-surgical treatment or for patients with a low volume disease who prefer a less invasive treatment. RFA can also be used to treat tumours located close to major hepatic or portal veins.

Ideally, it is best used for smaller lesions (<3cm) and with a limited number of lesions (<5), although suitable lesions up to 5cm may be considered (e.g. if away from major vessels which act as a heat sink).

Technique
- Thermoablative technique that destroys tissue by heating to temperatures often exceeding 100°C resulting in coagulative necrosis
- High frequency alternating current passes between passive, large surface area skin electrodes and an active electrode placed in the tumour
- The needle electrode can be placed by percutaneous, laparoscopic, or open route under transcutaneous or intraoperative US guidance
- For larger tumours multiple placements of the electrode may be required, aiming to include a 1cm 'margin' of normal liver parenchyma
- Flow of blood in large vessels leads to a 'heat sink' effect with poorer tissue heating and destruction.

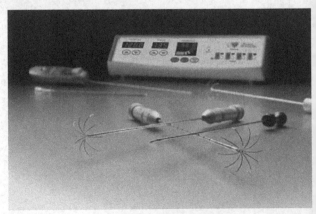

Fig. 7.19 Radiofrequency ablation equipment.
Reproduced courtesy of Boston Scientific, Natich, MA, USA.

Outcome
- Local recurrence rates 5–60%
- 5yr survival rates of 17–51% have been reported, although comparison is difficult as patients often have poorer prognosis disease
- Data on long-term outcome is lacking as is randomized comparison of RFA and surgery. NICE (National Institute of Health and Clinical Excellence) recommends that RFA should be used with special arrangements for informed consent and in the setting of audit or research
- Complications rates of 0–33% are reported, including liver abscess, bile duct stricture, needle track seeding, liver infarction, and bowel perforation. Mortality 0.1–0.3%.

Alternative techniques

- Other thermoablative techniques include laser-induced thermotherapy and microwave ablation (MWA)
  - MWA is less susceptible to heat sink and charring of tissues which limit the effectiveness of RFA
- Percutaneous ethanol injection causes cell death by dehydration. Success has been limited in colorectal liver metastases
- Cryotherapy employs liquid nitrogen or argon to freeze lesions with cycles of freezing and thawing leading to irreversible cell damage. Complications include liver cracking and cryoshock
- Stereotactic body radiation therapy (SBRT) involves hypofractionated, high precision radiation therapy. Local control rates of 65–80% are reported, but follow-up is short.
- Transarterial chemoembolization (TACE) combines embolization of the affected segment of liver with delivery of chemotherapy via sustained release particles. This therapy may be combined with ablative techniques to improve efficacy.
- Selective internal radiation therapy (SIRT), uses transarterial infusion of radiolabelled microspheres (Yttrium-90), infused into the arterial system
- Hepatic arterial chemotherapy infusion (HAI) has also been used to administer high dose chemotherapy but it is unclear if it offers any real benefit over standard chemotherapy.

Reference

Chow FC, Chok KS (2019) Colorectal liver metastases: An update on multidisciplinary approach. *World J Hepatol* **11**(2): 150–72. doi:10.4254/wjh.v11.i2.150

Palliative care

Palliative care is the active, holistic care of patients with advanced, progressive illness. Central to this is the management of symptoms as well as psychological, social, and spiritual support. Focus is on achieving best possible quality of life. Many aspects can be applied in conjunction with other more aggressive forms of treatment.

Management of pain in patients with cancer

~2/3 of patients will require strong opioids to alleviate pain. Of these, ~88% can have their pain adequately controlled if the basic principles outlined in the WHO and SIGN guidelines are followed (Table 7.4).

Evaluation
- Accurate assessment of pain to determine the cause, type, and severity as well as its effect on the patient
- The patient should be the prime assessor of the pain.

Tips for successful pain control
- Prescribe analgesia regularly along with 'rescue' or 'breakthrough' analgesia (this should be 1/6 of the total opioid dose)
- Anticipate likely side effects and warn patient, e.g. prescribe laxative
- Prescribe an anti-emetic for first 5–7 days of starting an opioid
- Patients on NSAIDs who are at high risk of GI complications should be prescribed gastric protection (e.g. a PPI)
- Don't combine weak and strong opioids or two weak opioids.

Route of administration
- Morphine should be given orally if possible
- SC infusion may be appropriate if the oral route is unavailable
- To convert from oral morphine to SC diamorphine divide the total dose of oral morphine by 3
- Sometimes topical morphine may be used, e.g. in pressure sores. A mixture of morphine in instillagel or intrasite can be given 10mg/10ml and applied to the painful area as needed.

Table 7.4 WHO analgesic ladder

Step 1: mild pain(pain score <3/10)	Step 2: mild to moderate(pain score 3 to 6/10)	Step 3:moderate to severe(pain score >6/10)
Paracetamol ± NSAID ± adjuvants	Opioid for mild to moderate pain e.g. codeine + step 1 non-opioids ± adjuvants	Opioid for moderate to severe pain, e.g. morphine + step 1 non-opioids ± adjuvants
Pain increasing or persisting →	Pain increasing or persisting →	Freedom from cancer pain

Adapted from WHO Guidelines for the pharmacological and radiotherapeutic management of cancer pain in adults and adolescents. Copyright © World Health Organization, 2018

Adjuvant analgesics

A group of drugs that can be used in addition to opioids and non-opioids to relieve pain in specific circumstances.

- Corticosteroids, e.g. dexamethasone 6–12mg daily
  - Useful in liver capsule pain, neuropathic pain, and bony pain
- Anti-depressants, e.g. amitriptyline 10–100mg nocte (titrated slowly)
  - Useful for neuropathic pain
  - Can be combined with gabapentin in severe neuropathic pain
- Anti-epileptics, e.g. gabapentin
  - Start at 100–300mg daily and titrate slowly (max dose 900mg tid)
  - Useful for neuropathic pain
- NMDA receptor channel blockers, e.g. ketamine
  - Used in specialist palliative care only
- Anti-spasmodics, e.g. hyoscine butylbromide
  - Useful for colic and other spasm-like pain.

Non-drug treatments for pain

- RT or chemotherapy may be of benefit in some patients
- In a small minority pain can be difficult to control with conventional analgesia, e.g. neuropathic pain syndromes in patients with locally advanced colorectal malignancy. Consideration of anaesthetic techniques including nerve blocks and intrathecal analgesia may be appropriate
- TENS (transcutaneous electrical nerve stimulation)
- Acupuncture.

Nausea and vomiting

Nausea and vomiting (N+V) are common symptoms in patients with advanced cancer (frequency 40–70%) who rate them almost as distressing as pain. Symptoms should be carefully evaluated to devise a management plan aimed at the likely cause and tailored to individual patient response.

Evaluation and assessment

- Enquire about nausea and vomiting separately
- Time of day, duration, triggers, effect of vomiting, pattern of vomiting, and content of vomitus are all important clinical features
- Further evaluation will include examination of oropharynx, abdomen, DRE, fundi, bloods, and consider AXR
- Address reversible causes, e.g. medication (opioids), hypercalcaemia, constipation, uraemia, gastric irritation, infection, cough.

Management

- Although mechanisms of nausea/vomiting are complex and often multifactorial, the choice of anti-emetic depends on the most likely cause
- It is often necessary to use drugs in combination (Table 7.5)
- It is often better to give SC drugs (e.g. continuous SC infusion (CSCI)), as oral absorption may be unreliable
- Best practice is to prescribe anti-emetics regularly, rather than PRN.

Table 7.5 Commonly used anti-emetics

Drug	Action	Indications
1. Metoclopramide	D2 receptor antagonist	Gastric stasis and irritation
	Prokinetic	Toxin-related N+V
2. Cyclizine	Anti-cholinergic	Movement-induced N+V
	Anti-histamine	Cerebral tumours, GI tract infiltration/irritation
3. Haloperidol	D2 receptor antagonist	Toxin-related N+V, e.g. drugs, hypercalcaemia, renal failure. Often in combination with 1 or 2
4. Levomepromazine	Long-acting phenothiazine	Broad spectrum
	Effective at multiple receptors	Useful as second-line or in combination
5. Ondansetron	5-HT3 antagonist	Chemo + RT-induced N+V

NB: do not combine 1 + 2 as they interact

Medical management of bowel obstruction

Medical management in patients with inoperable bowel obstruction can be effective in relieving symptoms while avoiding the 'drip and suck' technique, which can be distressing to patients and families. Most patients will require a syringe driver as oral absorption is unreliable due to gut oedema and vomiting.

Corticosteroids
- Consider dexamethasone 8–16mg SC daily
- Prescribe before midday due to insomnia and agitation if given later
- Thought to reduce peritumoral inflammatory oedema and improve intestinal transit which may improve symptoms and relieve obstruction. Evidence for this is equivocal but a 3–4 day trial may be appropriate.

Patients without colic
- Review medication, discontinuing drugs which reduce peristalsis
- Use a prokinetic agent, e.g. metoclopramide 30–120mg/24h in CSCI
- Review regularly and stop if worsening colic.

Patients with colic
- Stop prokinetic agents, e.g. metoclopramide.
- Use cyclizine 150mg/24h in CSCI if nausea/vomiting problematic
- Can be combined in CSCI with hyoscine butylbromide 80–120mg/24h to relieve colic.

Persistent nausea or vomiting
- Persistent nausea or vomiting in either scenario (i.e. with/without colic) would warrant either
  - Adding haloperidol 2.5–5mg (sometimes higher doses required) or
  - Switching anti-emetic to levomepromazine 6.25–25mg
- Avoid 5-HT3 antagonists as these can be constipating.

Anti-secretory agents

- Indicated if despite a trial of corticosteroids and first- or second-line anti-emetic, the patient remains symptomatically obstructed
- If large volume vomiting is present, it may be necessary to consider anti-secretory agents earlier
- Hyoscine butylbromide 80–120mg/24h via CSCI. Anti-secretory and anti-spasmodic but possibly less effective than octreotide
- Octreotide 300–900mcg/24h via CSCI
- It may be necessary to combine both drugs if colic is a particular problem as only hyoscine butylbromide is anti-spasmodic.

General measures

Mouth care

- Dry mouth is extremely common and a significant source of morbidity.

Laxatives

- Review laxative regime—bulking agents are contraindicated
- Avoid stimulant laxatives if colic present
- If complete obstruction, then all laxatives are contraindicated
- Movicol 1–3 times daily (up to 9 sachets/24h) altered to response
- Some patients may need rectal intervention.

Fluids

- IV fluids may be appropriate depending on the individual situation
- In general fluids can be given SC (rather than IV) being careful about the volume of fluid. >1–1.5litres in 24h may lead to worsening of symptoms as they increase volume of bowel secretions.

Management of tenesmus

Tenesmus is the painful sensation of fullness in the rectum, often due to local tumour. Pathophysiology of tenesmoid pain may be neuropathic from lumbosacral nerve infiltration or associated smooth muscle spasm.

- Prevent and treat associated constipation which may add to symptoms
- Trial of opioid analgesia, although efficacy in this type of pain is low
- NSAIDs, e.g. diclofenac
- Adjuvant analgesics for neuropathic pain, e.g. gabapentin
- Nifedipine modified release 10–20mg bd
- Consider local anti-tumour treatment, e.g. RT, laser treatment
- May require anaesthetic input for consideration of nerve block.

References

Mercedante S, Cassucio A, Mangione S (2007) Medical treatment for inoperable malignant bowel obstruction: a qualitative systematic review. *J Pain Symptom Manage* **33**: 217–23.

Scottish Intercollegiate Guidelines Network. *Control of pain in adults with cancer: a national clinical guideline.* Edinburgh: SIGN, 2008.

Zech DF, Gond S, Lynch J, Hertel D, Lehmann KA (1995) Validation of World Health Organization guidelines for cancer pain relief: a 10 year prospective study. *Pain* **63**: 65–76. http://www.palliativecareguidelines.scot.nhs.uk

Anal cancer

Anal cancer is rare, comprising ~2.5% of GI malignancies. It has an incidence of <1 in 100,000. It is potentially curable and one of the few malignancies where treatment paradigms have shifted from surgical to non-surgical. Chemoradiation is now central to management. Surgery retains an important role in salvage of locoregional failure.

Background/aetiology

- More common in ♀; overall incidence ↑ and greatest in >75yr olds
- Risk factors for the disease include:
  - Lifetime number of sexual partners
  - Genital warts
  - Receptive anal intercourse especially among men
  - Men who have sex with men (MSM)
  - Smoking
- Epidemiological and molecular studies strongly suggest association with the human papilloma virus, which is present in more than 90% of cases (particularly serotype 16) (➲ Sexually transmitted infections, Chapter 12, p.626)
- Immune suppression (transplant patients/HIV population) is important in disease promotion.

Clinical features

- Anal tumours arise within either the anal canal or anal margin Fig. 7.20. These tumours predominantly involve the canal but may extend on to the perianal skin within 5cm of the anal margin.
  - 85% are squamous cell cancers (SCCs) arising within anal canal
  - Tumours arising from transitional epithelium above dentate line were previously called basaloid/cloacogenic/junctional cancers. These are now referred to as nonkeratinizing SCCs
  - Anal adenocarcinomas arising from anal glands are rare. They are staged as for anal SCC but treated as rectal adenocarcinoma
  - Tumours arising at or distal to squamous mucocutaneous junction, within 5cm of anal verge and can be seen in their entirety on gentle traction of perianal skin, are termed perianal cancers. These are also treated as anal canal SCC
  - Primary rectal SCCs are very rare and treated as anal cancer
- Most will present with local anal symptoms including pain and bleeding. Not infrequently they are misdiagnosed as haemorrhoids
- Large tumours of the canal may disrupt the function of the sphincter and lead to incontinence
- Occasionally anal malignancy may be found incidentally within tissue excised as treatment for haemorrhoids
- A biopsy should be obtained in all cases to confirm the diagnosis.

Staging

- Tumour staging is clinical; all patients require biopsy/assessment of the primary tumour which may be done under general anaesthetic. Consider screening ♀ for cervical cancer (Table 7.6)
- Consider screening 'at risk' groups for HIV
- <20% are node positive at presentation. Perform fine needle aspiration (FNA) on any suspicious/enlarged nodes. Clinical examination and CT scan are not sensitive and 50% of enlarged nodes are reactive on FNA
- Above the dentate line, drainage is to inferior mesenteric/internal iliac nodes while below dentate is predominantly inguinal nodes
- CT, MRI, and PET-CT are performed to exclude metastatic disease.

Table 7.6 TNM staging of SCC of anal canal

T—Primary Tumour	
Tx	Primary tumour cannot be assessed
T0	No evidence of primary tumour
Tis	Carcinoma *in situ*: Bowen disease, high-grade squamous intraepithelial lesion (HSIL), anal intraepithelial neoplasia II-III (AIN II-III)
T1	Tumour 2cm or less in greatest dimension
T2	Tumour more than 2cm but not more than 5cm in greatest dimension
T3	Tumour more than 5cm in greatest dimension
T4	Tumour of any size invading adjacent organ(s), e.g. vagina, urethra, bladder*
Note	* Direct invasion of the rectal wall, perianal skin, subcutaneous tissue, or the sphincter muscle(s) alone is not classified as T4.
N–Regional Lymph Nodes	
Nx	Regional lymph nodes cannot be assessed
N0	No regional lymph node metastasis
N1	Metastasis in regional lymph node(s)
• N1a:	Metastasis in inguinal, mesorectal, and/or internal
• N1b:	iliac nodes
• N1c:	Metastasis in external iliac node
	Metastases in external iliac and in inguinal, mesorectal and/or internal iliac nodes
M—Distant Metastasis	
M0	No distant metastasis
M1	Distant metastasis

Anal intraepithelial neoplasia (AIN)

- AIN is an important premalignant lesion (similar to cervical intraepithelial neoplasia), which can progress to SCC of the anal canal
- Improved understanding of the oncogenic pathway of anal and genital cancers and the importance of HPV infection has led to a unified pathological classification for anogenital intraepithelial neoplasia
- Low-grade AIN (LGAIN)
  - Condyloma or AIN grade I with mild dysplasia
  - Not thought to be premalignant but can progress to HSIL
- High-grade AIN (HGAIN)
  - AIN grade II with moderate dysplasia or AIN grade III with severe dysplasia
  - Considered a premalignant condition
- Risk ↑ in HIV infection, MSM, multiple sexual partners, receptive anal intercourse, smoking, and immunosuppression
- Lesions may be visible as flat/raised, white, pigmented/non-pigmented areas in anal canal and perianal skin
- Many are asymptomatic or give rise to non-specific symptoms, e.g. pruritus, burning, bleeding
- High resolution anoscopy and acetic acid facilities assessment and mapping of nature and extent of changes
- The natural history is not clear. LGAIN lesions may regress but HGAIN may progress to SCC
  - ~10–20% HGAIN progresses to SCC over 40–50 months
  - ~12–25% LGAIN progresses to HGAIN over 18–36 months
  - Concomitant HIV infection may increase the risk of progression
- Screening may be indicated in high risk groups, e.g. HIV +
- HPV vaccination reduces incidence of LGAIN and HGAIN and may also prevent further HGAIN developing after treatment
- HPV vaccination is currently offered in UK to girls and boys aged 12–13yrs
- LGAIN may be followed for 12 months to ensure no progression
- HGAIN should undergo high resolution anoscopy and a treatment plan initiated. Specialist referral may be appropriate
- If well localized, excision/ablation (photodynamic therapy, RFA, laser, cautery, liquid nitrogen)
- Topical treatment with imiquimod, 5-FU, and trichloroacetic acid is used when there is more extensive involvement
- Recurrence rates are high, especially for HGAIN. Active surveillance after treatment of HGAIN may be effective in reducing risk of SCC.

Treatment of anal cancer

Non-surgical

- Treatment is predominantly non-surgical and chemoradiation (rather than RT alone) is the modality of choice; commonly infusional 5-FU and mitomycin C chemotherapy are given synchronously with radical pelvic RT over 5–6 weeks
- Mitomycin C (MMC) is an important component of treatment. Its substitution by cisplatin confers no additional advantage. Capecitabine can be used in place of 5-FU
- Neoadjuvant chemotherapy prior to chemoradiation is not recommended

- It is likely that total dose of external beam RT is a significant prognostic factor for both local control and survival
- Three dimensional conformal RT (3D-CRT) and intensity-modulated RT (IMRT) are designed to minimize toxicity and maximize local control and show promising results in anal cancer
- Gaps during treatment are best avoided; the use of a brachytherapy boost after initial external beam radiation treatment is no longer used
- Prophylactic bilateral low-dose irradiation of clinically uninvolved groin nodes is commonly used to eradicate possible subclinical microscopic disease. For patients with involved nodes the affected groin will, however, be treated to full dose
- Acute skin morbidity is reversible but may be severe for 10–14 days after treatment
- Other acute toxicities include diarrhoea, tenesmus, cystitis, stomatitis, and myelosuppression
- Patients who have undergone resection of all macroscopic disease (e.g. after haemorrhoidectomy) but in whom there is concern over residual microscopic tumour (commonly when surgical margins uncertain or involved) may be adequately served by reduced radiation doses
- No changes to treatment are necessary for HIV positive patients. Those with a low CD4 count may have increased side-effects
- Those with a past history of HIV/AIDS related complications (e.g. opportunistic infections or other malignancies) are more likely to develop side effects with treatment and may require a dose reduction or omission of MMC, but outcomes are similar to non-HIV patients
- Late morbidity needs to be viewed in the context of the surgical alternative (APER) but includes anal ulceration, stenosis, necrosis, incontinence, enteritis, vaginal stenosis, late bladder effects, and (rarely) pelvic insufficiency fractures. Patients of child-bearing potential will be rendered infertile by pelvic radiotherapy
- Late toxicity may necessitate a colostomy in 6–12% of patients who are otherwise disease-free.

Surgical
- Females with T4 disease breaching the vaginal mucosa or incontinent patients may benefit from a defunctioning stoma prior to treatment
- Small (T1N0) tumours not encroaching upon the sphincter and <1cm in size may be adequately treated by wide local excision. Long-term survival is comparable to CRT.

Outcome
- Patients should be initially assessed 4–6 weeks after treatment and further assessed at 12 weeks if they have an incomplete response
- Induration is not uncommon and may persist for several months, but a biopsy should be taken if there is concern of persistent tumour
- Locoregional control and survival decrease with increasing T and N stage. The American SEER database reports an overall 5yr relative survival of 68%, comprising
  - 82% with local disease only
  - 65% with locoregional disease
  - 32% with distant disease

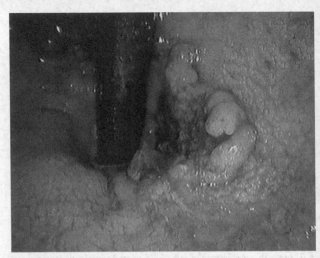

Fig. 7.20 Anal cancer on retroflexion at colonoscopy.

- Relapse beyond 3yrs is highly unusual
- Patients who relapse should be carefully re-staged with CT and PET-CT before considering surgical options
- Block groin dissection may be considered in the event of isolated inguinal relapse although, if previously unirradiated, further chemoradiation may remain an option
- Patients with central pelvic relapse or persistent disease following treatment may require an extensive procedure ranging from APER to pelvic exenteration (➔ Radical pelvic surgery, Chapter 11, p.566)
- Multidisciplinary support with urology, gynaecology, and plastic surgery is often desirable
- Complications following non-surgical management including fistula and incontinence may also require surgical intervention
- A colostomy may be required in ~15–35% of patients due to recurrent disease or CRT-related late complications. Typically, 70–80% of colostomies are required for recurrent disease
- Risk factors for colostomy are tumour >5cm (↑ risk of recurrent disease) and history of prior excision (CRT-related complication).

References

Ajani JA, Winter KA, Gunderson LL et al. (2008) Fluorouracil, mitomycin and radiotherapy vs. fluorouracil, cisplatin and radiotherapy for carcinoma of the anal canal. *JAMA* **299**: 1914–21.

Eng C, Messick, C, Glynne-Jones R (2019) The management and prevention of anal squamous cell carcinoma. *Am Soc Clin Onc Educat Book* **39**: 216–25.

Rare anal tumours

Adenocarcinoma

- Accounts for 5–15% of anal cancers
- May arise from anal glands or in a chronic fistula
- More aggressive than SCC with significantly poorer prognosis
- Treatment involves APER and combined modality therapy.

Neuroendocrine carcinoma (small cell carcinoma)

- 1% of malignant anal canal tumours
- High grade poorly differentiated carcinoma with high mitotic rate
- Usually metastatic at presentation (60–80%)
- 1yr survival ~15%. May be improved by cisplatin-based chemotherapy.

Melanoma

- Often confused with benign pathology, e.g. thrombosed haemorrhoid
- May present as pigmented or amelanotic lesion
- Frequently presents at advanced stage with metastatic disease
- Local excision or APER should be considered although prognosis is usually poor despite treatment (5yr survival <20%)
- Adjuvant therapy has no proven efficacy.

Basal cell carcinoma (BCC)

- 0.1% of anal cancers
- More common in ♂ after 5th decade
- Usually presents as a nodule which ulcerates as it grows
- Local excision as for BCC at other sites.

Paget's disease

- Extramammary Paget's can affect perianal region, axilla, groin, scrotum, penis, and buttock (Fig. 7.21)
- Intraepithelial adenocarcinoma that may eventually develop into invasive disease arising from apocrine glands
- Usually eczematous-type lesion presenting with itch
- Associated with Paget's at other sites and synchronous malignancy, e.g. GI, skin, prostate
- Lesions should be mapped taking multiple biopsies followed by local excision for non-invasive disease. Skin grafting or rotational flaps may be required for closure
- Radical surgery ± inguinal lymphadenectomy may be required for invasive disease
- Radiotherapy treatment may also be considered.

Buschke–Lowenstein tumour (verrucous carcinoma)

- Giant condyloma accuminatum is a rare variant of genital warts affecting anywhere in the perineum
- May be locally invasive (50%) but does not metastasize
- Associated with HPV and more common in ♂
- Malignant transformation to invasive SCC may occur
- Treatment is by radical local excision, but recurrence rates are high
- Grafts/flaps frequently required following excision.

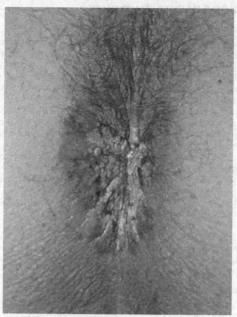

Fig. 7.21 Perianal Paget's disease.

Neuroendocrine tumours

Introduction

- Previously, described as carcinoid tumours, the current preferred terminology refers to a blanket term of neuroendocrine neoplasms (NEN) which is comprised of well differentiated neuroendocrine tumours (NETs) and poorly differentiated neuroendocrine carcinomas (NECs). The term carcinoid should only be used in relation to the carcinoid syndrome
- These are rare tumours with an annual incidence of 2–5 per 100,000
- The has been at least a 5-fold increase in incidence over the last 40 years. This may be related in part to increased detection with high resolution CT scans
- Indolent NETS may remain undiagnosed during life (post-mortem incidence ~8%)
- 60% are GI in origin. Within the GI tract, the ileum is the most common site (~45%) followed by the rectum (~20%), appendix (~15%), colon (~10%), and stomach (~5–10%). The incidence of small rectal NETs has increased with the introduction of bowel screening
- Other sites include pancreas and lung
- Up to 30% of GI NETs are functional, producing serotonin as well as other vasoactive substances, e.g. histamine, corticotrophin, dopamine, prostaglandins, substance P, which may lead to carcinoid syndrome (see later, under the heading Metastatic NETs).

Pathology

- Arise from the cells of the diffuse endocrine system most commonly enterochromaffin cells, located in neuroendocrine tissue
- Stain positive to markers of neuroendocrine tissue including chromogranin A, synaptophysin, neuron-specific enolase, and serotonin
- Size may be a predictor of outcome, but it is increasingly recognized that differentiation and grade (assessed by measuring the Ki67 proliferation index and mitotic index) are perhaps the most important determinants of prognosis.

Classification

A recent WHO change in classification has stressed the premise that all NENs, including NETs, have a malignant potential and should not therefore be referred to as benign or malignant.

- Well differentiated NET
  - May be subclassified into low, intermediate, or high grade (G1, 2, 3) based on mitotic rate and Ki67 proliferation index
  - G1 and G2 tumours tend to behave in a benign/indolent fashion
  - Well differentiated high grade (G3) NETs may behave in a more aggressive fashion, although they still have a better prognosis than poorly differentiated neuroendocrine carcinomas
- Poorly differentiated neuroendocrine carcinoma (High grade G3 tumours that are similar to small or large cell NECs occurring in the lung). Tend to behave very aggressively.

Investigation and staging

- Carcinoid of the colon, rectum, or ileum may be diagnosed incidentally on colonoscopy
- Small bowel imaging, e.g. capsule endoscopy, MR enteroclysis may be useful in locating a small bowel primary
- Patients are often diagnosed on CT when presenting with liver metastases
- CT/MRI are widely used for staging particularly for colorectal lesions (Figs 7.22 and 7.23)
- Somatostatin receptor scintigraphy (SRS: Indium-111 pentetreotide imaging (OctreoScan)) is useful in functioning tumours for staging extent of disease
- PET-CT is also valuable in assessing metastatic NET with an unknown primary
- Echocardiography should be carried out in carcinoid syndrome to exclude carcinoid heart disease which is a significant cause of mortality
- PET has shown improved sensitivity to SRS for localization
- 5-HIAA, a metabolite of serotonin, can be measured in the urine and is useful in the diagnosis of functional carcinoids particularly foregut and midgut tumours. It is also used to monitor treatment
- Chromogranin A assay may also be useful.

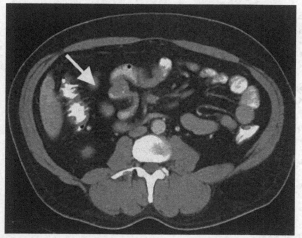

Fig. 7.22 Carcinoid tumour of jejunum with mesenteric lymph node mass (arrow).

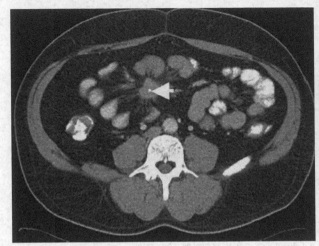

Fig. 7.23 Desmoplastic reaction has tethered adjacent bowel loops (arrowhead).

Small bowel NETs

Background
- Median age of presentation 60–70yrs
- Usually present late with obstruction or abdominal pain
- Small bowel NETs have a strong predilection to metastasize which is independent of tumour size
- 25% are multicentric while 2/3 have distant spread at presentation
- Most occur within 60cm of the ileocaecal valve
- Carcinoid syndrome is more common in small bowel NETs (20%).

Management
- For localized disease small bowel resection combined with wide mesenteric resection is recommended
- Vascular control and resection of regional draining LNs may be complicated by extensive mesenteric fibrosis
- Debulking surgery may be indicated in the presence of metastases for symptom control
- 5yr survival is 75% for localized disease, 40% with distant disease, and worse still in patients with carcinoid syndrome (20%).

Appendix

⮕ Tumours of the appendix, discussed later in this chapter, p.396.

Colon and rectum

Background
- Median age of presentation is between 5th and 7th decade
- Presentation is similar to adenocarcinoma with diarrhoea, rectal bleeding, abdominal pain, weight loss, and anorexia

- Most are diagnosed on colonoscopy to exclude adenocarcinoma
- NETs of the colon usually occur in the caecum and 2/3 of patients have either nodal or distant metastases at presentation
- Rectal NETs are usually localized at presentation and are usually asymptomatic
- Carcinoid syndrome is rare as hindgut NETS tend to be non-secretory.

Management

- Colonic NETs are treated in a similar fashion to adenocarcinoma
- NETs of the rectum are usually <1cm and can be treated by local resection
- Tumours >2cm have usually local or distant spread and anterior resection is recommended for local disease
- The management of tumours measuring 1–2cm is controversial and some have suggested that those with ulceration or invasion of the muscle wall should have a radical resection
- 5yr survival for localized disease is 70–80% compared with 20% with metastases.

Metastatic NETs

- 'Carcinoid syndrome' refers to a group of symptoms that may occur with metastatic NETs through release of a variety of vasoactive peptides including serotonin, histamine, and tachykinins
- Symptoms include diarrhoea, wheezing, episodic flushing, and right-sided valvular heart disease
- It has been reported to occur in 8–35% of patients with NETs
- The risk of developing metastatic disease correlates with tumour size, differentiation, tumour grade, and location of NET
- Somatostatin analogues have a central role in the diagnosis and treatment of metastatic NETs
- Radiolabelled octreotide can localize previously undetected primary or metastatic disease
- Octreotide is also highly effective in relieving symptoms of patients with carcinoid syndrome (symptomatic improvement in 80%, tumour stabilization in 50%)
- Liver resection is indicated in patients with resectable disease (5yr survival 60–80%)
- Combination therapy with liver resection/ablation/chemoembolization ± debulking/ resection of the primary may be indicated for palliation
- Very well selected patients may be candidates for liver transplantation, although long-term cure is unlikely
- IFN α can be given with octreotide, but side effects limit use
- Cytotoxic chemotherapy (cisplatin + etoposide) may be used in a select group with poorly differentiated neuroendocrine carcinoma
- Radionuclide-labelled somatostatin analogues have been used in SRS-positive tumours refractory to medical treatment.

Reference

Ramage JK, Goretzki PE, Manfredi R et al. (2008) Consensus guidelines for the management of patients with digestive neuroendocrine tumours. *Neuroendocrinology* **87**: 31–9.

Tumours of the appendix

Appendiceal tumours comprise a diverse group of rare tumours which account for ~1% of intestinal neoplasms. A neoplasm is found in approximately 1% of appendicectomy specimens. They can broadly be categorized into three main groups: epithelial tumours, NETs, and a diverse range of other tumours including metastatic disease (Table 7.7).

Table 7.7 Classification of appendiceal tumours

Epithelial tumours	Notes
Adenoma	May manifest as abdominal pain. Adenoma tissue confined to mucosa with intact muscularis mucosa
Low grade appendiceal mucinous neoplasms (LAMNs)	Previously called appendix cystadenoma. Pushing invasion through muscularis mucosa, but no infiltrative invasion. Low grade cellular atypia
High grade appendiceal mucinous neoplasms (HAMNs)	Pushing invasion through muscularis mucosa, but no infiltrative invasion. High grade cellular atypia
Colonic type invasive adenocarcinomas • Mucinous type • Intestinal type • Signet ring	Mucinous tumours are graded according to differentiation. Well differentiated mucinous adenocarcinomas more likely to produce peritoneal spread and pseudomyxoma Intestinal type behave in a similar fashion to colorectal adenocarcinoma Signet ring type are poorly differentiated and behave in an aggressive fashion
Goblet cell adenocarcinomas (GCAs)	Previously called goblet cell carcinoids and adenocarcinoids. Occurs exclusively in the appendix
Neuroendocrine tumours	Divided into well differentiated (grades 1, 2, and 3), poorly differentiated neuroendocrine carcinoma (large cell and small cell types) and mixed neuroendocrine and non-endocrine neoplasms (MiNENs).
Other tumours	
Lymphoma, GIST, desmoids, sarcomas, metastatic disease, and non-carcinoid NETs	

Presentation
• Acute appendicitis is the most common presentation for both benign and malignant appendiceal tumours
• Malignant tumours may also present with an abdominal mass, pain, perforation, or malignant ascites
• Pseudomyxoma peritonei (PMP) typically present with ascites.

Appendiceal adenocarcinoma

- Appendiceal colonic-type adenocarcinomas are the most common malignant neoplasm of the appendix
  - Mucinous type accounts for 37% of cases
  - Non-mucinous colonic type accounts for 27% cases
- Average age at presentation is 60 years
- Nodal involvement and metastatic disease may be present
- Although treated as for CRC, these tumours appear to have a poorer prognosis and higher risk of recurrence compared to CRC
- There may be a role for CRS and HIPEC with advanced peritoneal carcinomatosis.

Goblet cell adenocarcinoma (GCA)

- Very rare tumours with features of both adenocarcinomas and NETs but behave like appendiceal adenocarcinomas
- Account for ~20% of cases of appendiceal cancer
- Patients typically in their 50s at presentation
- Up to 40% have metastatic disease at presentation
- Prognosis for GCA is worse than for NETs but better than appendiceal adenocarcinoma.
- Appendicectomy may be adequate with early, localized disease
- Right hemicolectomy should be considered for the following:
  - T3 tumours
  - Involvement of the base of the appendix/caecum
  - Poorly differentiated tumours
  - Tumours >2cm in size
- If proceeding to right hemicolectomy, consideration should be given to BSO in women and possibly localized stripping of the peritoneum in the RIF, given the poorer prognosis
- There is no definite role for post-operative adjuvant chemotherapy.

Neuroendocrine tumours

- Benign NETs are the most common tumour of the appendix
- They are discovered as an incidental finding in every 150–300 appendicectomies
- 75% of tumours occur at the tip of the appendix
- Typically found in younger patients in their 20s
- Majority are asymptomatic
- Tumour size is the best predictor of outcome. Metastases from tumours <2cm are rare while 1/3 of patients with tumours >2cm develop either nodal or liver metastases
- 30% develop other malignancies including GI and breast
- Well differentiated NETs are divided into low, intermediate, and high grade according to their proliferative rate
- On rare occasions and usually in the presence of metastatic disease, they can give rise to carcinoid syndrome
- Simple appendicectomy is appropriate treatment in well differentiated tumours <1 cm in size
- Tumours between 1–2cm with good prognostic features (clear margins, no mesoappendiceal invasion, low proliferative rate) are also adequately treated with simple appendicectomy

- Consideration should be given to right hemicolectomy for tumours >2cm or those with poor prognostic features
- Tumours >2cm require follow-up with CT and SRS
- Screening for synchronous/metachronous malignancies should be carried out
- 5yr survival for localized disease is 94% compared with 83% for regional disease and 31% for distant disease
- Poorly differentiated neuroendocrine carcinomas are similar to large cell and small cell lung tumours and behave in an equally aggressive fashion.

Appendiceal mucinous lesions

A distended, mucus-filled appendix is called a mucocoele. The term describes the macroscopic appearance of the appendix and does not offer an insight into the underlying pathology. Mucinous lesions of the appendix may be categorized as follows:

- Non-neoplastic mucinous lesion of the appendix
  - These are simple retention mucocoeles and do not contain neoplastic epithelium that develop after obstruction of the lumen of the appendix
- Neoplastic appendiceal mucinous lesions
  - Serrated lesions of the appendix
  - Mucinous appendiceal neoplasms. Low grade appendiceal mucinous neoplasm (LAMN) and high grade appendiceal mucinous neoplasm (HAMN)
  - Mucinous adenocarcinoma of the appendix
- Appendiceal mucinous neoplasms are rare and patients typically present in the 50s and 60s
- They may present with pain, RIF mass, pressure effects on retroperitoneum, or progressive abdominal distention due to rupture and the development of PMP
- Appendicectomy ± caecectomy should be considered for all appendiceal mucinous lesions, both for diagnosis and treatment
- A right hemicolectomy may be considered for ruptured lesions
- Additional treatment may need to be considered for more advanced or recurrent disease which may present as PMP. It may be appropriate to seek advice or refer to a specialized centre (➔ Pseudomyxoma peritonei, discussed in next section, p.400).

Pseudomyxoma peritonei

PMP describes a rare syndrome (incidence of 1 per million) where diffuse collections of gelatinous material and mucinous implants are found affecting the abdominal peritoneum and omentum 'jelly belly'. Traditional thinking was that PMP developed after rupture of an LAMN, HAMN, or mucinous adenocarcinoma of the appendix, resulting in diffuse involvement of the peritoneum. Most tumours are non-invasive and slow-growing with a prolonged asymptomatic phase. Presentation is usually at an advanced stage.

More recently, the term has been used to include patients with progressive abdominal distention due to peritoneal mucinous carcinomatosis from a wide variety of GI and extra-GI mucin-producing tumours. These two groups can thus be defined

- Acellular and low grade PMP (due to rupture of a LAMN or even benign mucocoele)
- High grade and high grade with signet ring PMP.

Presentation

- The most common presentation is with abdominal distension
- ♀ may present with an ovarian mass
- Alternative presentations include appendicitis, mucinous tumour found in a hernial sac, or as an unexpected finding at laparotomy
- Metastasis to solid organs is rare (<2% LN or liver metastases).

Histology

- A broad spectrum of histology has been reported making diagnosis difficult. There is no universally accepted classification system
- PMP arises from the appendix unless proven otherwise by a normal appendix or conclusive evidence for an alternate primary site
- The spectrum of peritoneal disease ranges from the more low grade diffuse peritoneal adenomucinosis (DPAM) to peritoneal mucinous carcinomatosis (PMCA).

Investigation

- Diagnosis is often at laparotomy
- CT is the gold standard, showing mucinous ascites and septated soft tissue densities, possibly with surrounding calcification (Fig. 7.24)
  - A mass may be seen in the region of the appendix or ovaries
  - Accumulation near the diaphragm and liver gives rise to a scalloped appearance
  - CT-based scoring systems can be used to assess extent of disease and resectability.

Management

- Evidence supporting specific treatment modalities is lacking due to the rarity of the disease and poor understanding of the natural history and the diverse group of patients who are not categorized as having PMP
- For asymptomatic patients with low grade PMP, some advocate a conservative approach
- CRS/HIPEC is increasingly advocated for all fit patients as it offers the potential for long-term cure. This treatment should be carried out in a national centre specializing in the management of PMP

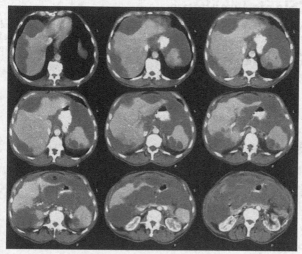

Fig. 7.24 CT showing pseudomyxoma peritonei.

- Surgery may involve anterior parietal, right/left subphrenic and pelvic peritonectomy, omentectomy + splenectomy, cholecystectomy, and visceral resections (right colon, rectosigmoid, total colon, small bowel, TAH)
- Chemotherapeutic agents include 5-FU, mitomycin C, and cisplatin.

Outcome

- Surgery is usually prolonged with median blood loss >2l
- Morbidity (30–50%) and mortality (5%) following surgery are high
- Prognosis is related in part to disease extent and distribution, ability to perform a surgical clearance, and most importantly, to the underlying pathology. Low grade PMP carries the best prognosis
- Sugarbaker's group reported 5 and 10yr survival of 81 and 70% in 1419 patients with low grade/acellular mucin PMP, 59 and 49% respectively in 700 patients with mucinous carcinomatosis and 78 and 63% in those with intermediate histology undergoing CRS/HIPEC
- Repeated CRS/HIPEC is feasible.

References

Sugarbaker PH (2006) New standard of care for appendiceal epithelial neoplasms and pseudomyxoma peritonei syndrome? *Lancet Oncol* **7**: 69–76.

Yan TD, Black D, Savady R, Sugarbaker PH (2007) A systematic review on the efficacy of cytoreductive surgery and perioperative intraperitoneal chemotherapy for pseudomyxoma peritonei. *Ann Surg Oncol* **14**: 484–92.

Chua TC, Moran BJ, Sugarbaker PH et al. (2012) Early- and long-term outcome data of patients with pseudomyxoma peritonei from appendiceal origin treated by a strategy of cytoreductive surgery and hyperthermic intraperitoneal chemotherapy. *J Clin Oncol* **30**(20): 2449.

Colonic lymphoma

Primary lymphoma of the large bowel is rare, accounting for 0.2–0.4% of all malignant tumours of the large bowel. Isolated colonic lymphoma makes up 10–20% of all GI lymphomas, with stomach and small bowel the more commonly affected sites.

Background

- Peak incidence in 50–70yr age group, with male predominance
- Caecum most commonly affected site (60–70%) followed by rectum
- Thought to arise from mucosa-associated lymphoid tissue (MALT) or acquired lymphoid tissue 2° to inflammation or autoimmune disease.

Pathology

- Non-Hodgkin's lymphoma is most common, in particular diffuse large B-cell type (DLBCL)
- Other types include MALT, mantle cell, and Burkitt's (rarely isolated)
- Patients with coeliac disease and IBD are at ↑ risk (enteropathy-associated T-cell lymphoma)
- Immunosuppression and HIV also risk factors
- Hodgkin's lymphoma affecting the colon is rare.

Presentation

- Patients with large bowel lymphoma present in a similar fashion to those with adenocarcinoma although diagnosis is often at a late stage
- Abdominal pain and weight loss are the most common symptoms
- Altered bowel habit, rectal bleeding, or a palpable mass may be present.

Investigation

- May be diagnosed on biopsy following colonoscopy or CT
- Diagnosis at emergency laparotomy for complications not uncommon
- Multiple lymphomatous polyposis is a rare phenotype which may mimic FAP
- Once the diagnosis is established the patient should be staged by CT chest/abdomen/pelvis and bone marrow biopsy to exclude generalized disease
- Histopathology in this area should be reviewed by a pathologist with a special interest in lymphomas as histology is complex, varying from low grade tumours where no treatment may be required, to very aggressive lesions with a poor prognosis irrespective of treatment.

Management

- Localized disease should be treated by surgical resection followed by chemotherapy depending on tumour histology and whether there is LN involvement
- Advanced disease is treated with chemotherapy and/or RT. In these patients surgery may sometimes be necessary for residual disease or a complication of treatment such as perforation or stricture formation
- 5yr survival ranges from 30 to 55%.

Gastrointestinal stromal tumours

GISTs represent 1% of all primary GI tumours with an estimated incidence of 10–15 per million. The median age at diagnosis is 60yrs. The stomach and small bowel are the most commonly affected sites, with 5–15% presenting in the colon and rectum.

Pathology

- Arise from the interstitial cells of Cajal (gut pacemaker cells)
- Differentiated from leiomyosarcomas of bowel by staining positively for CD117 antigen (C-KIT)
- Prognosis is related to the size of the tumour and the number of mitoses per high power field on histology.

Presentation

- Those arising in the large bowel usually present with abdominal pain, obstruction, or rectal bleeding
- Usually sited in the wall of the rectum or caecum
- Often, they will not have ulcerated through the mucosa and histological diagnosis may only be confirmed after resection. Tumour predominantly extraluminal displacing surrounding structures.

Management

Localized disease

- Unlike adenocarcinomas, GISTs rarely metastasize to LNs and the goal of surgery is to achieve macroscopic clearance of tumour
- Neoadjuvant treatment of rectal GISTs may downstage the tumour making a less radical procedure feasible
- Adjuvant therapy with imatinib (tyrosine kinase inhibitor) may delay relapse in certain high risk groups, although effect on overall survival will not be known until completion of ongoing adjuvant trials
- Long-term follow-up is required as these tumours can recur many years after resection
- Recurrence is usually either local or with liver metastases and radiological screening at least annually is recommended for high risk tumours
- 5yr survival after surgical resection of the primary tumour is ~50%.

Recurrent/metastatic disease

- For inoperable lesions radiological-guided biopsy is mandatory as the response to medical therapy is ~90% with a median survival for responders of 5yrs (previously 12 months pre-imatinib)
- In addition, some patients will become operable and can be cured of their disease
- Second-line tyrosine kinase inhibitors are available for patients who become resistant and progress on imatinib.

Rare pelvic tumours

The pelvis can be the site of a group of congenital and neoplastic lesions. This includes tumours of the presacral or retrorectal space which often present late, having reached a considerable size. Diagnosis and management have progressed in recent years, with advances in radiological imaging, adjuvant therapy, and a more aggressive surgical approach. The treatment of these complex lesions often requires several specialties and can be optimized by an experienced MDT.

Presentation

- Pelvic tumours produce few symptoms and the incidental diagnosis of a large asymptomatic tumour is often the norm
- A minority of patients present with vague, long-standing low back pain or perineal pain, and occasionally there may be perineal discharge which leads to confusion with anal fistula or pilonidal disease
- Larger tumours may present with constipation, faecal or urinary incontinence, and sexual dysfunction due to sacral nerve root involvement
- Most presacral tumours can be palpated on DRE. Typically, an extrarectal mass is felt displacing the rectum with a smooth, intact overlying mucosa. The proximal limit, degree, and extent of fixation and relationship to other pelvic organs can be assessed
- Rigid or flexible sigmoidoscopy can be used to examine the overlying mucosa and rule out transmural penetration of the tumour
- A careful neurological examination is mandatory for presacral lesions.

Radiological imaging

- Radiological evaluation includes plain radiographs, CT, MRI, and ERUS
- Plain radiographs of the sacrum identify bony expansion, destruction, and/or calcification of soft tissue masses
- CT and MRI are the most important modalities for diagnosis and surgical decision-making, as well as in the assessment of response to neoadjuvant treatment
- CT can determine whether a lesion is solid or cystic and the involvement of adjacent structures such as bone, bladder, ureters, and rectum
- The multiplanar images and improved soft tissue resolution from MRI allow planning of the surgical approach, assessment of the extent of spinal cord involvement, and level of sacrectomy, if required
- MR angiogram/venogram can add information regarding anatomy
- ERUS may help characterize retrorectal tumours and their relationship to the muscular layers of the rectum.

Biopsy

- Pre-operative biopsy of resectable presacral tumours remains controversial
- As a general principle, biopsies are useful if they are representative of the lesion and will help define management, e.g. use of pre-operative neoadjuvant therapy or surgical approach, and/or extent of resection
- Biopsies are indicated for most solid and heterogeneously cystic presacral tumours

- A route that will allow resection of the biopsy tract during subsequent resection is employed, e.g. transperineal or parasacral
- Transperitoneal, transvaginal, and transrectal biopsy should be avoided.

Surgery

- Individual cases are discussed at an MDT meeting pre-operatively and the surgical approach, resection, and reconstruction are planned
- Insertion of a temporary vena caval filter may be required, as post-operative anti-coagulation may be contraindicated
- Bilateral ureteric stents are required for large tumours
- Resections are performed using anterior (abdominal), posterior (perineal), or a combined abdominoperineal approach
- Low pelvic or presacral tumours can be resected using a posterior approach in the prone jack-knife position. The anococcygeal ligament, coccyx, and the lower sacrum may be resected with the lesion
- Larger tumours extending above the S3 level often require a combined anterior and posterior approach
- The magnitude of the operation depends on the extent and nature of the tumour, but can involve mobilization of the rectum, formation of an end colostomy, harvesting of a rectus abdominus flap, and bilateral ligation of the internal iliac arteries followed by repositioning in the prone jack-knife position for composite sacrectomy and myocutaneous flap reconstruction. Some units perform the abdominal and perineal operations as two distinct procedures, allowing for a period of resuscitation in the intensive care unit.

Developmental cysts

- Retrorectal lesions are more common in women (incidence ~1 in 40,000 hospital admissions). The majority are benign, although even in benign lesions malignant transformation can rarely occur.

Epidermoid cyst

- Congenital lesion developing in ectopic remnant of ectodermal tissue
- Thin-walled and lined by stratified squamous epithelium
- Contains a mix of desquamated debris, cholesterol, keratin, and water.

Dermoid cyst

- Ectodermal origin but unlike epidermal cysts, contain skin appendages
- Lesion containing 'fat balls' on MR suggests the diagnosis and represents sebum in the cyst
- May cause post-anal skin dimpling and become infected. Can be confused with perianal/pilonidal abscess.

Teratoma

- Arises from pluripotent cells in the primitive streak—containing tissue from all three embryologic layers: endoderm, mesoderm, and ectoderm
- Most common neonatal neoplasm (1 in 30,000 live births)
- Suggested on imaging by well defined lesion with mixed cystic and solid components possibly with calcifications (Fig. 7.25)
- Recurrence occurs in 10–20% and can be malignant.

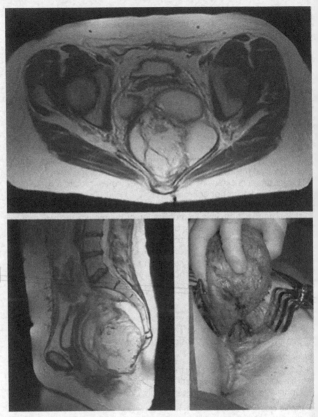

Fig. 7.25 Presacral teratoma.

Enteric cysts

Tailgut cyst
- Cystic hamartomas or mucus-secreting cyst
- Formed by persistent remnant of the primitive hindgut (the post-cloacal extension or tailgut which normally involutes)
- Multiloculated cyst lined by squamous, cuboidal, or transitional epithelium.

Rectal duplication cyst
- From sequestration of developing hindgut
- Multiloculated cyst often with smaller satellite cysts surrounding and lined by intestinal epithelium.

Chordoma

- Most common retrorectal malignancy
- Locally aggressive bone tumour arising from remnants of the foetal notochord
- Predominantly involve the axial skeleton, with 50% affecting sacrococcygeal region
- Metastasize in 20–40% with 40% 10yr survival.

Anterior sacral myelomeningocele

- Occurs when the meningeal sac herniates anteriorly through a defect in the sacrum.
- Should be excluded by MRI prior to resection of presacral tumour

The pelvis can be the site of a range of soft tissue, cartilaginous, and bone sarcomas including liposarcoma, leiomyosarcoma, desmoid, Ewing's sarcoma, chondrosarcoma, and osteogenic sarcoma. It may also be the site of neurogenic tumours including neurilemomas. GISTs covered separately (⊙ Gastrointestinal stromal tumours, discussed earlier in this chapter, p.403).

References

Jao SW, Beart RW Jr, Spencer RJ et al. (1985) Retrorectal tumors. Mayo Clinic experience, 1960–1979. *Dis Colon Rectum* **28**: 644–52.

Cody HS 3rd, Marcove RC, Quan SH (1981) Malignant retrorectal tumors: 28 years' experience at Memorial Sloan-Kettering Cancer Center. *Dis Colon Rectum* **24**: 501–6.

Tumours of the abdominal wall

Lipoma

- Lipomas of the abdominal wall are common
- Usually superficial and rarely (<1%) undergo malignant transformation
- Suspicious features include rapid recent growth, lesions >5cm, and lesions deep to fascia. In these cases, MRI is indicated and, if suspicious, core biopsy should be performed
- If core biopsy confirms sarcomatous change, a staging CT of chest/abdomen/pelvis should be performed and the patient referred to a specialist soft tissue sarcoma service
- Outlook for patients with sarcomas of the abdominal wall depends on size and grade but ~60–70% will be cured by adequate surgery (Fig. 7.26).

Metastatic tumours

- Most malignant tumours of the abdominal wall are metastatic from a primary GI malignancy
- Occurs in ~1% of patients following curative resection of CRC
- Usually accompanied by diffuse intra-abdominal disease
- Occasionally it will be the sole source of recurrence and in properly staged patients with CT ± PET, wide surgical excision is indicated.

Desmoid tumours

- Abdominal wall desmoid tumours (fibromatosis) are benign fibrous neoplasms originating from musculoaponeurotic structures
- Although benign may be infiltrative and locally aggressive
- Trauma and oestrogens suggested to be involved in aetiology
- Usually observed in females
- Can occur at any age (mean 40yrs)
- Present with a hard, painful mass in the abdominal wall muscle
- Diagnosis is confirmed by core biopsy and examination by a pathologist with an interest in soft tissue tumours
- Generally managed by wide excision (>1cm) margin and abdominal wall reconstruction with either a synthetic or biological implant
- Biological implants should be considered in pre-menopausal females
- Desmoid tumours associated with pregnancy often grow rapidly and reduce significantly after delivery. Treatment is best delayed until after pregnancy
- Desmoid tumours associated with FAP (Gardner's syndrome) often recur locally and patients may have accompanying mesenteric fibromatosis (◆ Genetic disorders and polyposis syndromes, discussed earlier in this chapter, p.328)
- LR after adequately excised abdominal wall fibromatosis is otherwise observed in 10–20% of patients
- Sulindac and tamoxifen may have efficacy. Use is predominantly for irresectable lesions.

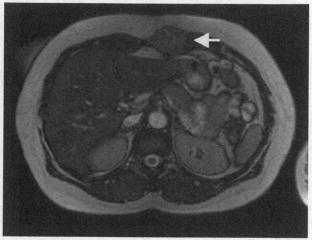

Fig. 7.26 MRI (T2 weighted) showing an abdominal wall sarcoma (arrow) arising from the left rectus muscle.

Emergency presentations

Appendicitis

The first appendicectomy for appendicitis was performed by Morton in 1887 and since then it has become the most common abdominal condition requiring emergency surgery. Although the prevalence of appendicitis is decreasing, it still affects ~7% of the population of Western countries.

Aetiology

The exact aetiology is not clear, but appendicitis seems to arise 2° to luminal obstruction. Luminal distension leads to compromise of the vascular and lymphatic channels, with ischaemia, bacterial overgrowth and translocation. Inflammation can result in perforation with localized/generalized peritonitis depending on the host response.

Luminal obstruction may be due to lymphoid hyperplasia 2° to infection, faecoliths, parasites, neoplasia and foreign bodies (FBs). Domestic hygiene and dietary factors have been implicated although fibre does not seem to play an important role. A familial tendency has been noted but may be partly environmental rather than genetic.

Presentation

- The classical presentation is of vague central abdominal pain migrating to the RIF with associated nausea/vomiting and anorexia
- Localized peritoneal irritation may cause pain on walking, coughing or movement
- Patients have a dry tongue with foetor and a low-grade pyrexia
- Tenderness/percussion rebound is maximal at McBurney's point and Rovsing's sign may be positive (pressure in LIF gives pain in RIF)
- Typical presentation may only occur in ~50% patients and depends on the position of the appendix (Fig. 8.1)
- Urinalysis may be positive for blood and protein if in close contact with ureter. Psoas irritation may give 'psoas stretch sign'. Diarrhoea is reported to be a feature with pelvic appendix. Retrocaecal appendix may give vague symptoms and with a long appendix pain may be in RUQ
- Presentation is more non-specific at the extremes of age, with increased morbidity/mortality
- 2–6% of patients present with a palpable appendix mass.

Diagnosis

- Differential diagnosis includes mesenteric adenitis, gastroenteritis, terminal ileitis, MD, caecal carcinoma, renal stone disease, pyelonephritis and cholecystitis
- In female patients mittelschmerz pain, ovarian cysts, ruptured ectopic pregnancy and PID should also be considered (→ Pelvic inflammatory disease p.610)
- The value of history and examination ± active observation should not be underestimated
- Normal WCC and CRP have a good negative predictive value after 12h of onset of symptoms
- Clinical scoring systems help improve diagnostic accuracy, but sensitivity is still increased by use of US scan/CT

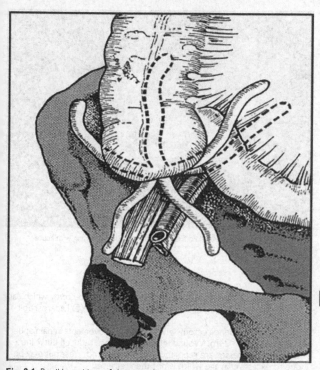

Fig. 8.1 Possible positions of the appendix.

Reproduced with permission from Silen, W (Eds.) (2010). *Cope's Early Diagnosis of the Acute Abdomen*, 16th Edition. Oxford, UK: Oxford University Press.

- Graded-compression US scan reduces rates of negative appendicectomy particularly in females, with diagnostic accuracy of up to 90%. It is quick and non-invasive but highly operator dependent. Appendix 'not visualized' may be a useful negative predictor
- CT is the most sensitive/specific (~95%) radiological investigation for acute appendicitis. Appendicular diameter (>8mm) is probably the most useful feature. It is particularly useful in older patients where the differential diagnosis is wider (Fig. 8.2)
- Laparoscopy should be carried out early in patients where there is diagnostic uncertainty, but symptoms fail to settle
- Diagnosis in pregnancy becomes progressively more difficult, with perforation rates increasing up to the 3rd trimester. Leucocytosis is not helpful in pregnancy. US is the first-line investigation. Low dose CT or MRI can be used in cases where US scan is equivocal.

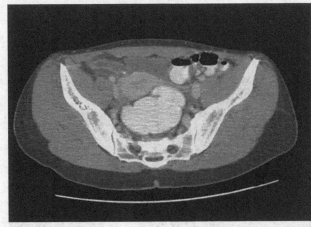

Fig. 8.2 CT showing tubular fluid filled structure in RIF in keeping with acute appendicitis.

Treatment

Appendicitis
- The recognized treatment for appendicitis is appendicectomy which can be carried out by an open or laparoscopic approach (⊕ Laparoscopic appendicectomy p.524)
- Laparoscopic appendicectomy gives minor improvements in pain and hospital stay (↓ <24h). Wound infection rates are reduced but ↑ intra-abdominal abscesses are reported. The reason is not clear but may be due to excessive lavage which is not then retrieved
- Appendicectomy should be carried out at laparoscopy if no other firm diagnosis is reached as macroscopic assessment of the appendix is inaccurate (negative predictive value 60–70%). Appendicectomy is routinely carried out at open surgery if the appendix looks normal
- Complications include wound infection, intra-abdominal abscess, bleeding, ileus, SBO, faecal fistula, retained appendix and stump appendicitis
- Prophylactic single dose antibiotics reduce post-operative infective complications, with multiple dosing advised if established peritonitis
- Rate of negative appendicectomy is 10–15%.

Antibiotic therapy for acute appendicitis
- Several recent studies have reported good outcomes with antibiotic therapy for acute uncomplicated appendicitis
- It is important to confirm the diagnosis and exclude other pathology with a CT scan before considering antibiotic treatment
- Studies suggest:
  - 20-30% of patients ultimately undergo surgery in first year (either during index admission or subsequently)

- After 5 years of follow up surgery is avoided in around 60% of patients)
- Overall complications may be lower in the antibiotic group than those undergoing surgery

Currently, most guidelines recommend an operative approach to acute appendicitis. If a conservative approach with antibiotic therapy is to be used, it is important that CT confirms a diagnosis of uncomplicated appendicitis and patients are followed up appropriately.

Appendix mass

- Appendix mass/abscess can be safely treated conservatively with IV antibiotics ± percutaneous drainage
- Success of conservative treatment >90%
- Operative management may increase post-operative complications, hospital stay and likelihood of colonic resection
- Recurrence of symptoms is <10% and is most common within the first 6 months
- Interval appendicectomy is not necessary unless recurrent symptoms.

Table 8.1 Alvarado scoring system

	Mnemonic (MANTRELS)	Value
Symptoms	Migration	1
	Anorexia/foetor	1
	Nausea/vomiting	1
Signs	Tenderness RIF	2
	Rebound	1
	Elevated temp >37.3°C	1
Laboratory	Leucocytosis	2
	Shift to the left	1
Total score		

Adapted with permission from Alvarado, A., A practical score for the early diagnosis of acute appendicitis. *Annals of Emergency Medicine;* 15(5):557–64. Copyright © 1986 Published by Mosby, Inc., Elsevier. DOI:https://doi.org/10.1016/S0196-0644(86)80993-310

Reference

Salminen P, Tuominen R, Paajanen H et al. Five-year follow-up of antibiotic therapy for uncomplicated acute appendicitis in the APPAC randomized clinical trial. *JAMA* 2018;**320**(12): 1259–65

Meckel's diverticulum

Introduction

Meckel's diverticulum is named after German anatomist Johann Meckel the Younger (1809). It is one of a group of abnormalities due to failed involution of the ophalomesenteric duct connecting the yolk sac to the fetal intestine until the 8th week of gestation. Other anomalies include meso/omphalodiverticular bands, enterocysts and omphalomesenteric fistulae. MD is the most common congenital abnormality of the small bowel.

As a true diverticulum it contains all layers of the intestinal wall and is usually found within 100cm of the ileocaecal valve arising from the antimesenteric border of the ileum. 50% contain heterotopic mucosa which may be gastric (most common), pancreatic, duodenal or even colonic. Length varies from 1 to 10cm, with 100cm the longest recorded.

Clinical features

- Incidence thought to be 1–4% with a 2:1 male to female ratio
- Lifetime risk of complications ~5%
- Complications include bleeding, intussusception, obstruction, perforation, volvulus, diverticulitis, Littre's hernia and neoplasia
- Complications more common in paediatric patients, with bleeding the leading cause. Bleeding is caused by ileal ulceration due to acid secretion from HGM. *Helicobacter* is not thought to play an important role
- Obstruction is the most common complication in adults.

Diagnosis

- Diagnosis is problematic and commonly made either incidentally or at laparotomy for acute abdomen
- Diagnosis for unexplained abdominal symptoms or occult bleeding requires a high index of suspicion
- Plain x-rays are non-specific and accuracy of barium studies is ~50%
- Technetium-99m pertechnetate scan ('Meckel's scan') has accuracy for bleeding of 90% in children and ~60% in adults. Cimetidine (inhibits luminal secretion) and glucagon (reduces radionuclide washout) may be used to increase accuracy to ~90%
- Wireless capsule endoscopy has shown sensitivity and specificity >90%.

Management

- Symptomatic MD should be resected
- Simple diverticulectomy or limited small bowel resection should be carried out. Enterotomies should be closed transversely to avoid narrowing the lumen (Fig. 8.3).
- Small bowel resection is preferred for bleeding, perforated base, palpable mass or neoplasia and short diverticulae when HGM in the base is more likely
- Management of incidentally detected MD is still a matter of debate
  - Some argue increased morbidity after resection outweighs the small risk of subsequent complications
  - HGM is less common in incidental MD (10% compared with 50%)
  - No studies are available showing long-term complications in incidental MD left *in situ*

- Selective resection has been proposed if features seen more frequently in symptomatic patients are identified: age <50yrs, male sex, MD >2cm or abnormal features in the diverticulum
- Others claim recent results show minimal post-operative morbidity, favouring resection in all patients.

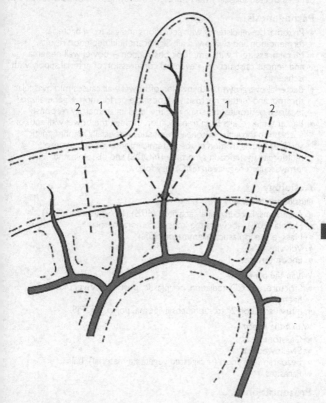

Fig. 8.3 Meckel's diverticulum resection.

Small bowel obstruction

SBO accounts for 5% of acute surgical admissions and carries a mortality of ~2%. The majority of patients presenting with SBO will settle with conservative management. 20–40% of patients will require surgery. ~10% of patients treated surgically will re-present with symptoms of SBO within 1 yr.

Pathogenesis

- Proximal bowel distends with secretions and gas from bacterial fermentation and swallowed air. Significant fluid depletion results.
- Mural pressure ↑ with lymphatic obstruction → bowel wall oedema and venous obstruction → eventual compression of arterial supply with ischaemia
- Bacterial overgrowth with invasion of bowel wall causes microvascular thrombi and further necrosis with possible perforation + generalized/localized peritonitis depending on the local inflammatory response
- Bacteraemia results from translocation through the bowel wall and/or absorption through peritoneal lymphatics (especially diaphragmatic surface) with activation of the systemic inflammatory response. multiorgan dysfunction syndrome (MODS) and disseminated intravascular coagulation (DIC) may follow.

Aetiology

Outside the bowel wall
- Adhesions, i.e. congenital/acquired (60%) (⊃ Adhesions p.512)
- Hernia (20%)—beware the 'missed' femoral hernia
- Mass, e.g. neoplastic, inflammatory (5%)
- Volvulus (5%)
- Endometriosis.

Within the bowel wall
- Stricture, e.g. CD, radiation, neoplastic, post-operative, mural haematoma
- Intussusception 2° to submucosal lipoma, polyp, e.g. PJS.

Within the lumen
- Gallstone ileus
- Swallowed FBs
- Bezoarsm, e.g. food (undigested vegetable material), hair
- Parasites.

Presentation

- Colicky central abdominal pain
- N+V (early onset suggests more proximal obstruction)
- Constipation (a later feature in SBO)
- Abdominal distension (depends on level of obstruction)—Fig. 8.4
- Diffuse abdominal tenderness due to bowel wall stretch
- Dehydration
- High pitched bowel sounds (becomes silent after chronic obstruction or with ischaemia)
- Fever, tachycardia, hypotension and peritonism indicate possible strangulation/ischaemia/perforation
- Differential diagnosis includes paralytic ileus, ischaemic bowel, pseudo-obstruction and pneumonia.

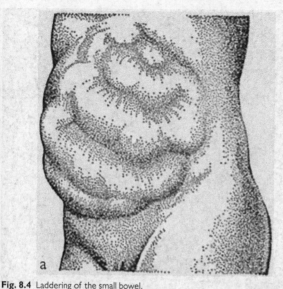

Fig. 8.4 Laddering of the small bowel.
Reproduced with permission from Silen,W (Eds.) (2010). *Cope's Early Diagnosis of the Acute Abdomen*, 16th Edition. Oxford, UK: Oxford University Press.

Investigations

- *Bloods* including arterial gases. ↑ WCC indicates possible strangulation. Electrolyte abnormalities are common. Lactic acidosis may be 2° to dehydration/sepsis
- *Plain AXR.* Sensitivity reduced in partial obstruction or where bowel loops are fluid filled. Other findings include thumb-printing, calculus, absence of large bowel air, pneumatosis intestinalis
- *Water-soluble contrast study.* Contrast seen in colon <24 h after ingestion suggests partial obstruction. There is a high likelihood of resolution with conservative management (sensitivity/specificity 96%). May also be therapeutic by reducing bowel wall oedema and increasing smooth muscle contractility.
- *CT.* Sensitivity and specificity >90%. May indicate level of obstruction as well as the cause, e.g. malignancy, hernia, volvulus. Features of portal venous gas, mesenteric venous congestion, pneumatosis, bowel wall oedema and absent/abnormal wall enhancement suggest ischaemia/strangulation (Fig. 8.5).

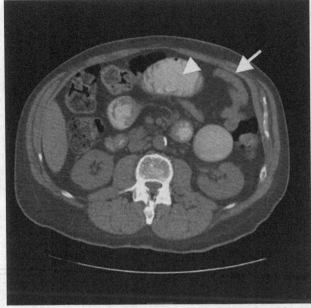

Fig. 8.5 Adhesive mid small bowel obstruction. Distended jejunal loops (arrowhead) with collapsed ileal loops (arrow) and an abrupt transition point with no cause identified.

Management

- Nasogastric decompression ('drip and suck')
- Correct electrolyte abnormalities and treat sources of sepsis
- Early water-soluble contrast (100ml gastrograffin) should be given either orally or NG to differentiate partial from complete SBO
  - In partial obstruction a trial of conservative management is indicated. Patients should not be allowed to undergo prolonged periods (>48h) of conservative management as outcomes are worse
  - Operative management is required for complete obstruction on water-soluble contrast.

Non-operative

Indications

- Partial obstruction (as defined by water-soluble contrast)
- Previous abdominal surgery
- Advanced malignancy.

Operative

Indications

- Complete obstruction on water-soluble contrast
- Generalized/localized peritonitis
- Visceral perforation
- Irreducible hernia
- Failed non-operative management.

Relative indications

- Virgin abdomen
- Palpable mass.

Procedure

- Full pre-operative resuscitation should be carried out where possible
- Midline laparotomy is the standard approach. Extend any previous midline wound to enter the abdomen in virgin territory
- Identify cut-off between collapsed and dilated bowel and identify cause
- Decompression may be required to improve handling of the bowel. This can be by milking proximally to an NG tube on suction or through an enterotomy
- Decision regarding resection and anastomosis or diverting stoma will depend on the cause of obstruction, viability of the bowel and the general condition of the patient. There is no substitute for good clinical judgement
- Extent of adhesiolysis is also a clinical judgement. Not all adhesions require division as further adhesion formation is inevitable
- Removal of FB should be through an enterotomy made proximal to the obstruction in more normal small bowel
- Anastomosis should be used with caution in radiation enteritis, connective tissue disease, chronic peritonitis, mesenteric ischaemia
- Laparoscopy has been described but should only be considered by experienced laparoscopic surgeons.

Reference

Abbas S, Bissett IP, Parry BR. Oral water soluble contrast for the management of adhesive small bowel obstruction. *Cochrane Database Syst Rev* 2007;(**3**):CD004651.

Large bowel obstruction

LBO can be divided into mechanical and non-mechanical obstruction (➔ Acute colonic pseudo-obstruction p.426). Mechanical obstruction of the large bowel causes proximal bowel distension with collapse of bowel distal to the level of obstruction. If the ileocaecal valve is competent small bowel distension will not be evident and a closed loop obstruction will develop.

Causes of mechanical obstruction

- Colonic tumours (>60%)
  - 20% of colonic malignancies present with obstruction
- Diverticular disease (10%) (➔ Diverticular disease: background p.214)
- Volvulus (5%) (➔ Colonic volvulus p.238)
- Other causes include:
  - Inflammatory strictures (UC/Crohn's)
  - Endometriosis (➔ Endometriosis, p.606)
  - FB
  - Extrinsic compression (intra-abdominal malignancy)
  - Hernia
  - Adhesions
  - Intussusception. More common in children. In adults may be ileocolic or colocolic, with 90% due to pathology (70% tumours).

Presentation

- Abdominal distension (Fig. 8.6)
- N+V (late with more distal obstruction)
- Colicky central abdominal pain in right-sided obstruction. Vague lower abdominal pain for more distal obstruction
- Altered bowel habit, weight loss or bleeding PR may be reported in malignant obstruction
- Signs of peritonism may suggest ischaemia or perforation
- Previous history of diverticulitis, volvulus, abdominal surgery, etc. may be relevant

Investigation

- Plain AXR. Absence of small bowel dilatation suggests a competent ileocaecal valve. Intramural gas indicates evidence of ischemia. (Fig. 8.7)
- Erect CXR looking for evidence of perforation or metastatic disease
- Water-soluble contrast enema. Useful to exclude pseudo-obstruction but may miss non-obstructing lesions and does not assess extent of local/distant disease.
- CT with IV and oral/rectal contrast has largely replaced other modalities. Sensitive, accurate and has a good negative predictive value. Can distinguish between benign or malignant causes with staging of associated pathology
- Colonoscopy. May be useful to exclude synchronous lesions, obtain pre-operative biopsies or for placement of SEMS.

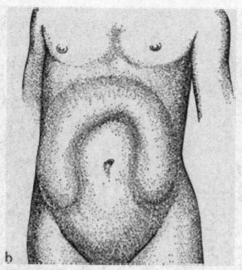

Fig. 8.6 Large bowel distension.

Reproduced with permission from Silen, W (Eds.) (2010). *Cope's Early Diagnosis of the Acute Abdomen*, 16th Edition. Oxford, UK: Oxford University Press.

Management

Supportive

- Fluid resuscitation and correction of electrolyte imbalance
- NG tube decompression if vomiting or small bowel distension is a feature
- IV antibiotics may be indicated if signs of sepsis.

Non-operative

- SEMS placed under radiological/endoscopic guidance may avoid the ↑ morbidity and mortality of emergency surgery and the need for a colostomy (Fig. 8.8)
- Technical success in ~95% of cases of malignant obstruction, depending on location (clinical success in 85–90%)
- Not suitable in low rectal lesions due to anal discomfort, tenesmus, incontinence and migration
- May act as bridge to elective resection or allow a window for neoadjuvant therapy
- Good palliation for left-sided lesions in patients not suitable for surgery
- Higher incidence of migration/clinical failure when used for benign disease
- Complications include migration (10%), re-obstruction (more common in palliative rather than 'bridge' patients) and perforation (4%).

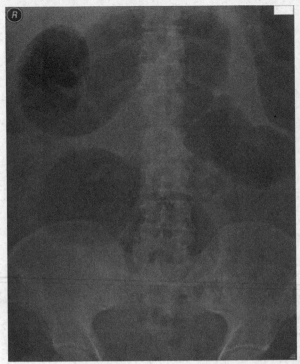

Fig. 8.7 Large bowel obstruction.

Surgery

Operative technique will depend on the condition of the patient, the bowel and the underlying cause of obstruction.

Malignant large bowel obstruction

- Midline laparotomy is performed with the patient in Lloyd–Davies position to allow access to the rectum (flat for right-sided obstruction)
- Needle decompression through a taenia or introducing a suction catheter through base of appendix improves handling of the colon
- On-table lavage is often performed if anastomosis is considered. An antegrade or retrograde technique can be employed.
- Emerging evidence suggests on-table lavage may be avoided with no increase in anastomotic leak rate
- A one-stage procedure should be the aim, with segmental or subtotal colectomy depending on the viability of the proximal bowel
- Primary anastomosis can be performed with reduced morbidity, mortality (<10%), hospital stay (10 days) and low anastomotic leak rate (<5%) compared with a staged procedure

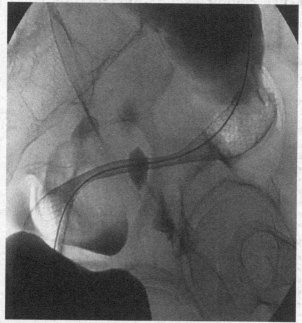

Fig. 8.8 Colonic stenting. Definitive procedure for an 'apple core' lesion in the sigmoid colon of a patient with liver and cerebral metastatic disease with large bowel obstruction.

- Primary anastomosis avoids a potentially challenging procedure to re-establish intestinal continuity following a 2-stage approach
- 40–60% of patients undergoing a Hartmann's procedure never have reversal of their stoma
- If bowel ends are oedematous, sutured anastomosis may be preferable
- In unstable patients or in the presence of peritonitis, exteriorization of bowel ends is recommended
- ~10% of patients have irresectable disease at surgery. Palliation using SEMS or a bypass procedure is preferable to stoma formation.
- Defunctioning stoma can be performed through a trephine wound with loop ileostomy possible under LA (caecostomy should be avoided).

Intussusception
- Involves resection of non-viable bowel and the lead point of the intussusception.

References

Finan PJ, Campbell S, Verma R et al. The management of malignant large bowel obstruction: ACPGBI position statement. *Colorectal Dis* 2007;**9**(Suppl 4):1–17.
Dekovich A. Endoscopic treatment of colonic obstruction. *Curr Opin Gatroenterol* 2009;**25**:50–54.

Acute colonic pseudo-obstruction

Sir William Ogilvie, a British surgeon, first described acute colonic pseudo-obstruction (ACPO) in 1948 when he reported 2 patients with clinical features of LBO without a mechanical cause.

Pathophysiology

- Alteration in autonomic regulation of the bowel is thought to be a major contributory factor, but this has not been proven
- Sympathetic stimulation or reduced parasympathetic supply may be influenced by medication, metabolic disturbance, infections, trauma, etc.

Predisposing conditions

- Trauma (retroperitoneal orthopaedic, burns, post-operative)
- Sepsis, e.g. pneumonia
- Cardiorespiratory disease
- Neurological, e.g. MS, Parkinson's, Alzheimer's
- Hypothyroidism
- Renal failure
- Metabolic imbalance (hypokalaemia, hypocalcaemia, hypomagnesaemia)
- Drugs (opiates, anti-depressants, anti-Parkinsonian).

Presentation

- Abdominal distension that may be acute or chronic
- N+V
- Abdominal discomfort
- Constipation (up to 40% pass flatus ± stool)
- Tympanitic abdomen ± bowel sounds
- Typically, elderly or hospitalised/institutionalised patients
- May present with complications including ischaemic bowel or perforation (3–15%). Mortality in this setting approaches 50%.

Investigations

- Serum electrolytes should be checked as well as stool cultures for *C. difficile*
- Plain AXR shows colonic dilatation predominantly affecting proximal colon. Caecal diameter >12cm ↑ risk of perforation Pneumoperitoneum and pneumatosis should be excluded. Rectal gas makes mechanical obstruction unlikely
- CT/water-soluble contrast enema is essential to exclude a mechanical cause of obstruction as well as non-obstructing colonic pathology.

Management

Intervention depends on patient co-morbidity, clinical status, caecal diameter, duration of distention and presence of complications.

Supportive

- Recommended in all cases of pseudo-obstruction without evidence of ischaemia or perforation
- IV fluid resuscitation with correction of any biochemical imbalance
- Treat sepsis if present
- Avoid or discontinue drugs that delay gut motility (anti-cholinergics, opiates)

- Flatus tube may aid decompression
- Mobilize if possible or regular position changes
- Serial AXR may be helpful, but regular re-evaluation of clinical status will dictate need for further intervention.

Medical

- If no improvement within 48h, duration >4 days or caecal distension >12cm, pharmacological therapy is indicated.

Neostigmine

- A reversible acetylcholinesterase inhibitor which stimulates parasympathetic receptors
- Side effects include hypotension, bradycardia, bronchospasm and abdominal cramps
- IV dose 2mg in normal saline over 3–5min. May be repeated. Cardiac monitoring is recommended
- Contraindications include active bronchospasm, renal insufficiency, mechanical obstruction not excluded, untreated cardiac arrhythmia
- RCTs show improvement in 80–90% of patients with low recurrence (<10%) and no major side effects.

Other medications

- No consistent evidence that erythromycin (motilin receptor agonist) or cisapride (partial 5-HT$_4$ receptor agonist, now withdrawn) resolve symptoms.

Colonoscopic decompression

- Success rates of 70–90% reported but little RCT evidence
- Recurrence of 30–40% may require repeated decompression
- Right-sided intestinal tube can be placed for decompression
- Allows mucosal assessment and excludes mechanical obstruction
- 2% risk of perforation.

Surgery

- Indicated in patients at risk of/presenting with perforation or ischaemia or in patients not responding to conservative, pharmacological or endoscopic treatment
- Defunctioning colostomy/caecostomy for high risk patients in the absence of perforation/ischaemia. Endoscopic caecostomy formation is described
- Subtotal colectomy/right hemicolectomy with exteriorization of ends is recommended for patients with evidence of ischaemia/perforation
- Morbidity and mortality is significant (30-60%).

Reference

Saunders MD. Acute colonic pseudo-obstruction. *Best Pract Res Clin Gastroenterol* 2007;**21**:671–687.

Colonic perforation

Colonic perforation may be the end point of a variety of conditions affecting the bowel and mentioned elsewhere in this text. Management depends on the underlying cause, condition of the patient and the extent of the peritoneal contamination.

Presentation

- Localized or generalized peritonitis
  - worse on movement, coughing or abdominal percussion
- Bowel sounds are usually absent
- Signs of sepsis including tachycardia, hypotension and pyrexia vary with degree and duration of contamination, patient immune response, etc.
- Presentation will be influenced by the underlying aetiology.

Investigations

- Bloods
  - Electrolyte imbalance/dehydration should be urgently corrected
  - Coagulopathy due to sepsis and DIC should be excluded
  - Emergency laparotomy for acute pancreatitis mimicking colonic perforation should be avoided. Amylase may be mildly elevated in perforation
- Erect CXR
  - 80% have air under the diaphragm
- Plain AXR
  - Limited value in perforation, but may show evidence of underlying aetiology, e.g. obstruction, toxic megacolon
- CT
  - The most sensitive imaging modality in perforation. Helps to localize site of perforation (e.g. duodenal, appendicular, colonic, retroperitoneal) and define the most appropriate surgical approach (Fig. 8.9)
  - Localized abscess formation may be amenable to percutaneous drainage
- Laparoscopy
  - Playing an increasing role in the management of perforation
  - Allows localization of perforation site, choice of appropriate access and definitive treatment in certain cases, e.g. perforated duodenal ulcer, laparoscopy and washout for diverticular perforation.

Causes

Diverticular disease (Ↄ Diverticular disease: background p.214)
- Incidence of perforated diverticular disease is 2.66/100,000
- Sequelae range from localized perforation and pericolic abscess to free perforation with generalized peritonitis (Table 5.1)
- NSAIDs, opiates and steroids associated with ↑ risk
- Mortality 10–35%.

Colon cancer (Ↄ Management of colon cancer p.344)
- Up to 10% of colon cancer patients present with perforation
- Perforated colon cancers have worse 30-day mortality (up to 25%) but disease free-survival is not significantly affected. Prognosis is poor, with 5yr survival ~30% related more to advanced stage at presentation (T4).

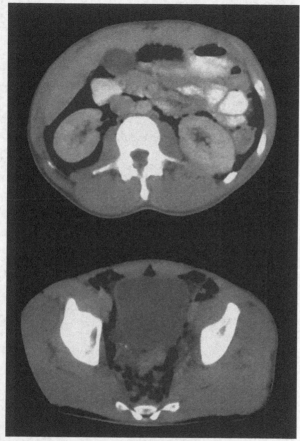

Fig. 8.9 Perforation into the retroperitoneum.

Colitis (⊙ Severe acute colitis and toxic megacolon p.186)
- Includes UC/Crohn's (incidence of perforation 2%) and *C. difficile*
- Perforation is usually in association with toxic megacolon.

Iatrogenic
- Risk of perforation at colonoscopy is 0.08–0.2%, with sigmoid colon (80%) the most common location
- Due to mechanical manipulation (50%), polypectomy (25%) or thermal injury (20%)
- CT colonography is thought to be safer than colonoscopy, with a perforation rate ~0.02% usually related to predisposing colonic pathology
- SEMS associated with 4% perforation rate

Trauma (➔ Colonic trauma p.436)

Vasculitides/connective tissue disorders (➔ Colitis—other p.236)
- Includes mesenteric ischaemia, SLE, Behcet's, polyarteritis nodosa (PAN)
- Wall ischaemia leading to perforation is the final common pathway.

Mechanical obstruction (➔ Large bowel obstruction p.422)
- Perforation may complicate mechanical obstruction of any cause.

Pseudo-obstruction (➔ Acute colonic pseudo-obstruction p.426)
- Risk of perforation ↑ if caecal diameter >12cm
- Overall risk of perforation ~3%
- Mortality with perforation approaches 50%.

Stercoral perforation
- Accounts for ~3% of colonic perforations
- Caused by pressure necrosis from colonic faecal impaction mainly affecting the left colon
- Pre-operative diagnosis is rare
- Segmental resection and exteriorization of bowel ends recommended
- Mortality is high as patients are often frail with significant co-morbidity.

Drugs
- Regular NSAID use is associated with ↑ incidence of colonic complications including perforation. Mechanism of action is through inhibition of prostaglandin synthesis. Can also cause an exacerbation of underlying chronic inflammatory bowel condition
- Anti-angiogenic agents, e.g. bevacizumab, are known to increase risk of colonic perforation in healthy or diseased bowel. Overall colonic perforation rate is 1.5%.

Management
- Fluid resuscitation, analgesia and broad-spectrum antibiotics
- Non-operative management is possible in highly selected cases, e.g. colonoscopic perforation dependent on mechanism and absence of peritoneal signs
- Endoscopic clipping of colonoscopic perforation is described
- Operative procedure will usually be either resection + 1° anastomosis ± defunctioning stoma or resection with exteriorization of bowel ends, depending on extent of contamination and patient fitness
- In colitis a subtotal colectomy is preferred to segmental resection
- Laparoscopic/open washout and drainage for the management of perforated diverticulitis (Hinchey grades II/III) is safe, with morbidity and mortality <5%.

Acute colonic bleeding

Acute colonic bleeding

Rectal bleeding covers a spectrum of presentations from occult to life-threatening haemorrhage. Here we will deal primarily with acute/massive lower GI haemorrhage including the most common causes and suggestions for management.

The overall incidence of acute lower GI haemorrhage is thought to be ~20–30 cases/100,000 population and increases with age. In the majority, bleeding resolves without intervention, but in ~15% it is ongoing, leading to haemodynamic instability. Overall mortality is reported to be ~20% in decompensated patients.

Definition
- No absolute definition for massive lower GI haemorrhage has been agreed but criteria in common use include:
  - Haemorrhage requiring 3–6 units (U) of packed red cells (PRCs)/24h for resuscitation
  - A drop in Hb <10g/dl or haematocrit (Hct) <30%.

Aetiology
Diverticular disease
- Diverticular disease is the most common cause of acute colonic bleeding, accounting for ~50% of cases
- Bleeding affects ~1/5 of sufferers but spontaneously resolves in 80%
- Thought to be due to rupture of vasa recta in apex of diverticulum. The initiating stimulus is unclear but faecolith trauma is suggested. Inflammation does not usually co-exist.
- If patient requires >4U PRCs/24h then >50% will go on to require surgical intervention
- 50% risk of re-bleeding after ≥2 previous episodes.

Angiodysplasia
- Most commonly acquired rather than congenital
- Present in ~50% of >50yrs but usually incidental
- Accounts for up to 40% of cases
- Initially venous occlusion in the submucosa leads to back pressure, incompetence of the pre-capillary sphincter and a direct arteriovenous communication
- Small cherry red area of dilated capillaries can be seen at colonoscopy
- More commonly present with recurrent bleeding and anaemia
- Bleeding is most common from the right colon as is the case with diverticular bleeding
- May be associated with end-stage renal failure, von Willebrand's disease, scleroderma and Osler–Weber–Rendu.

Neoplasia
- Most important in the elective setting but rarely a cause of massive lower GI haemorrhage.

Colitis
- Ischaemic, infectious and inflammatory colitis are rarer causes of acute haemorrhage
- Massive bleeding presents in 1–5% of IBD patients and is the main reason for 5–10% of emergency colectomies.

Anorectal pathology
- Haemorrhoids should not be discounted as a cause of major haemorrhage. Proctoscopy is advised in all patients as suture ligation may be all that is required
- Blood can reflux proximal to the splenic flexure on colonoscopy from a haemorrhoidal source
- Radiation proctitis causes troublesome bleeding but rarely haemodynamic compromise.

Post-procedural
- Rates of post-polypectomy bleeding are 2%, may be delayed or immediate and are increased by use of anti-coagulants
- Anastomotic haemorrhage after bowel resection affects up to 5% but rarely requires intervention.

NSAID related
- NSAIDs may cause ulceration, NSAID-related colitis, ↑ risk of complicated diverticular disease and exacerbation of IBD, all of which could cause bleeding.

Initial management
- Aggressive resuscitation should be commenced depending on signs and symptoms of shock (tachycardia, peripheral vasoconstriction, narrowed pulse pressure, ↓ blood pressure (BP), ↓ urine output, tachypnoea, depressed consciousness). Coagulopathy should be reversed early
- Colour of blood may be helpful, but in massive upper GI haemorrhage fresh rectal bleeding alone is seen in 10–15%
- Patient age and co-morbidity are important in assessing the physiological response to haemorrhage and resuscitation.

Localization
Endoscopic localization
- Upper GI endoscopy and proctoscopy should be first-line investigations
- Colonoscopy is clearly the investigation of choice for colonic bleeding which has spontaneously resolved, but its role in massive ongoing haemorrhage is controversial
- Some groups report localization of source in >90% of cases, but a high level of skill is required and results are not reproduced in other centres
- Blood in the colon reduces visibility and attempts at rapid purging for preparation can lead to fluid overload
- Colonoscopy does allow intervention using bipolar diathermy, heater probe, laser, APC or endoscopic clipping.

Radiological localization

Technetium-99m scintigraphy/labelled red cell scan
- Blood samples are taken, labelled and re-injected
- Scanning at multiple time intervals up to 24h is possible, making the examination useful for slow (0.1–0.5ml/min) or intermittent bleeding
- Intervention and characterization of the bleeding lesion is not possible
- Reported accuracy varies widely from 25 to 90%, with results depending on local expertise and experience.

Selective mesenteric angiography
- Angiography is currently the first-line investigation for massive ongoing lower GI haemorrhage (Fig. 8.10)
- Requires bleeding of 0.5–1ml/min and may be able to suggest the pathology (Fig. 8.11)
- Intervention is possible ,with accuracy up to 90% and successful haemostasis rates of 50–90%
- Selective infusion of vasopressin causes arterial and muscular constriction but has now been largely superseded
- Superselective embolization with polyvinyl alcohol, gel foam or more commonly microcoil embolization is possible at the level of the marginal artery and vasa recta
- Complication rates are low and include ischaemic injury, inadvertent embolization, re-bleeding, puncture site haematoma/pseudoaneurysm, contrast reaction (<1%) and mortality (1 in 40,000).

CT angiography (CTA)
- Sensitivity and specificity of 85 and 95%, respectively, for CTA has been reported
- Less invasive, less interference from movement artefact and may detect bleeding rates <0.5ml/min
- May be more accessible depending on local access to angiography
- In some centres CTA is used first-line before deciding on therapeutic options.

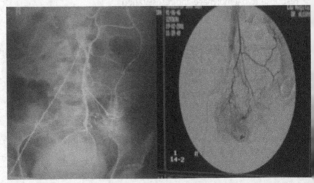

Fig. 8.10 Selective inferior mesenteric artery angiogram showing contrast blush and extravasation from a diverticulum in a patient with torrential rectal bleeding following unsuccessful colonoscopy. Patient treated with embolization without complication.

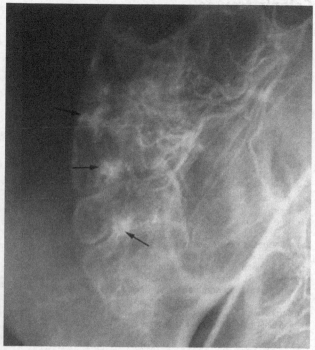

Fig. 8.11 Angiodysplasia in the caecum (arrows).

Surgical intervention

- Despite recent advances localization is still not possible in ~10%
- Where localization has not been possible or haemostasis has failed emergency, laparotomy is required
- If a bleeding site cannot be identified, consider on-table colonoscopy after colonic lavage +/- enteroscopy. Enteroscopy can be either via an enterotomy or orally with manipulation of the bowel over the scope
- If the bleeding site is adequately determined segmental resection can be performed
- If a colonic bleeding site is not identified subtotal colectomy reduces re-bleeding rates compared with segmental resection of the right colon (5 vs 20%). Anastomosis should be avoided
- Exact operative strategy will depend on the need for expediency.

References

Allison D, Hemmingway A, Cunningham D. Angiography in gastrointestinal bleeding. *Lancet* 1982;**2**:30–33.

Anthony S, Milburn S, Uberoi R. Multi-detector CT: a review of its use in acute GI haemorrhage. *Clin Radiol* 2007;**62**:938–949.

Colonic trauma

Abdominal trauma

It should be remembered that colonic trauma may be associated with a variety of other injuries and initial management should be guided by ATLS (advanced trauma life support) principles.

- Resuscitation should follow the ABCDEs of basic trauma care
- Abdominal assessment forms part of the primary survey
- Patients with blunt or penetrating abdominal trauma associated with resistant hypotension require urgent laparotomy
- Patients with penetrating abdominal trauma and peritonitis, evisceration or gunshot wounds require laparotomy
- Stable patients with blunt or penetrating trauma may be managed with serial physical examination ± CT/contrast studies to delineate further the extent of injury.

Colonic trauma

Background

The morbidity and mortality of colorectal trauma has reduced significantly over the last century primarily due to lessons learned from combat situations. Despite the reduction in mortality to ~5%, colonic trauma still carries the high rates of infective complications (20–30%).

- Colonic trauma can be divided into penetrating (96%) and blunt (4%)
- Most common form of penetrating trauma is stabbing (UK) or gunshot wounds (US), with small bowel involved in 30% and colon in 15%
- Blunt trauma most commonly road traffic accidents (RTAs) with deceleration and seatbelt restraints causing tears at points of colonic fixation, burst injuries or devascularization/haemorrhage
- High velocity gunshot wounds cause extensive tissue destruction by producing a temporary cavity 20–25× the diameter of the bullet.

Surgical management

- Successful treatment requires an individualized approach
- Prophylactic antibiotics with combination therapy to cover both aerobic and anaerobic organisms is recommended
- There is strong evidence supporting primary repair for all 'non-destructive' injuries where <50% of the bowel wall is involved
- For injuries involving >50% of the bowel wall, resection with primary anastomosis appears to have similar outcomes to a diversion procedure
- Diversion should be considered if vascularity is dubious or significant oedema of the colon is present
- Shock, gross faecal contamination, surgical delay and multiple associated injuries increase septic complications but are not absolute contraindications to primary repair
- Injuries to the right/left colon or to the mesenteric/anti-mesenteric border can be treated in the same fashion.

Rectal trauma

Rectal trauma

Rectal trauma is thankfully uncommon due to the anatomical protection from the surrounding bony pelvis. It is most commonly due to penetrating trauma from gunshot wounds, stabbing or impalement. Other causes include iatrogenic trauma following endoscopic, urological or obstetric procedures, rectal FBs associated with sexual misadventure or compressed air usually related to a practical joke (Fig. 8.12). Pelvic fracture is the most common cause of rectal injury following blunt trauma.

Assessment

- A high index of suspicion is required as rectal injury may occur from entry wounds in a variety of locations
- DRE should be carried out and, if blood is present a rectal injury must be actively sought. Bony injury following pelvic fracture may be palpable through the rectal wall
- Proctoscopy/sigmoidoscopy to visualize the rectal mucosa directly is the most sensitive investigation
- Contrast studies may help to confirm the diagnosis
- Associated injuries should be excluded, particularly to the genitourinary tract, which may occur in up to 50%
- It should be remembered that anteriorly the peritoneal cavity is only ~5cm from the anal verge, making intraperitoneal injury possible.

Surgical management

- Surgical management of rectal injuries is controversial, with a lack of clear evidence
- Prophylactic combination antibiotics to cover aerobic and anaerobic organisms should be given for at least 24h
- Limited low rectal injuries may be repaired by the transanal route without diversion
- Similarly, intraperitoneal rectal injuries may also be repaired primarily
- Traditional management includes diversion of the faecal stream, rectal repair after debridement, presacral drainage and rectal washout.

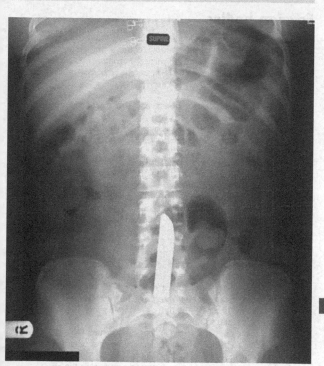

Fig. 8.12 Rectal foreign body.

Foreign bodies

Colorectal FBs are predominantly introduced via the rectum although they can include swallowed FBs which lodge either in the rectum or proximal to co-existing pathology (cancer, diverticular stricture). It is worth remembering that management of rectal FBs can require considerable ingenuity.

Presentation

- Presentation is often delayed due to embarrassment and repeated attempts at self-retrieval
- Reasons include anal eroticism, assault, concealment, therapeutic and diagnostic procedures, attempts to resolve constipation and attention-seeking behaviour
- Often seen in psychiatric patients, prisoners and homosexuals
- The variety of FBs encountered is matched by the different techniques described for their removal
- Accurate history and examination should be taken, including the duration of injury, which may influence management
- Plain radiology will often confirm the position of the object (Fig. 8.12).

Management

Transanal extraction

- Method of extraction will be influenced by the size, shape and position of the FB above or below the rectosigmoid junction
- Transanal extraction should be carried out by an experienced practitioner with care taken not to cause further trauma or migration
- Often requires conscious sedation or regional/general anaesthesia to overcome anorectal spasm
- Rigid or flexible endoscopic techniques can aid removal
- It may be safe to break up some objects allowing spontaneous passage
- Specialist techniques described include
  - Endoscopic snares or a balloon inflated proximal to the FB
  - Obstetric forceps or suction devices
  - Hollow objects can be filled with plaster of Paris with a central wick like a lollipop stick allowing traction to be applied
  - Metal FBs have been retrieved with electromagnets
- After extraction it is vital to examine the rectum by sigmoidoscopy to exclude a rectal tear
- Consideration should be given to a period of observation.

Surgical intervention

- Patients presenting with peritonitis require urgent laparotomy
- Surgical intervention is more likely for FB above rectosigmoid junction
- Laparotomy/laparoscopy with milking of FB via transanal route
- A colotomy ± diverting colostomy may be required if the transanal route is unsuccessful.
- Psychological assessment and support should be offered to all patients.

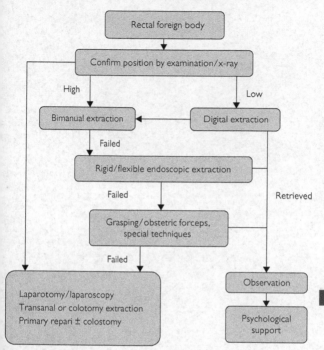

Fig. 8.13 Rectal foreign body management algorithm.

References

Lake JP, Essani R, Petrone P, Kaiser AM, Asensio J, Beart RW Jr. Management of retained colorectal foreign bodies. *Dis Colon Rectum* 2004;**47**:1694–1698.

Clarke DL, Buccimazza I, anderson FA, Thomson SR. Colorectal foreign bodies. *Colorectal Dis* 2005;**7**:98–103.

Fig. 8.12 Flowchart for sketching nonlinear integration algorithm.

References

[1] ...
[2] ...

Stomas

Classification and indications

The 18th century saw several reports of spontaneous and surgically produced colostomies, e.g. faecal fistula after necrosis of incarcerated colon in
hernia. However, colostomies were not routinely fashioned until the start
of the 20th century.

In the 19th century, a number of surgeons performed ileostomies for
obstructing colon cancers. Unfortunately, their patients usually died at subsequent attempts to resect the primary cancer. Maydl may have been the
first to fashion an ileostomy and subsequently successfully resect the primary cancer. However, problems with the construction and management
of ileostomies persisted until the 1960s. Although Brooke's classic 1952
paper on full-thickness eversion of ileostomies gained universal acceptance,
the introduction of karaya gum and the development of stoma therapy as a
specialist field also played an important role in the management of stomas.

Colostomy

End colostomy
- Normally sited in the left lower quadrant
- May be formed as a permanent stoma for patients with
  - Abdominoperineal resection for low rectal cancer
  - Hartmann's procedure (➔ Hartmann's procedure p.538)
  - FI. May be combined with proctectomy
  - Severe anorectal CD although there is a risk of loose stools
  - High anorectal agenesis with a poor functional outcome after
    reconstruction
  - Severe anorectal sepsis or severe anorectal trauma
- A temporary end colostomy may be formed in the following
  circumstances
  - Hartmann's resection (40–60% will never be reversed)
  - Penetrating rectal trauma and compound pelvic fractures involving
    anorectal injury
  - As a staged procedure in management of Hirschsprung's disease.

Loop colostomy
- May be fashioned anywhere along the transverse colon or at the apex
  of a sigmoid loop, so the site depends on the colon used
- Loop colostomies (particularly transverse loop colostomies) are bulky,
  unsightly and difficult to manage because of a high volume of semi-
  formed stool
- They may be inefficient at diverting the faecal stream
- As a consequence, transverse colostomy is no longer viewed as an ideal
  operation, especially if the option of loop ileostomy is available
- There is a theoretical risk of devascularisation if the marginal artery is
  damaged during either formation or reversal which may compromise a
  distal rectal anastomosis
- Mainly used in the following circumstances
  - Defunction an inoperable distal tumour
  - Palliate an obstructing distal tumour
  - Defunction a rectal cancer prior to neoadjuvant chemoradiotherapy
  - Defunction a distal anastomosis or complex anal sphincter repair
  - Defunction the anus following extensive surgery for Fournier's
    gangrene.

Double-barrel colostomy
- Usually fashioned in the left lower quadrant
- Both proximal and distal bowel is brought out through the same ostomy site. This brings both ends into close proximity for ease of reversal
- The resulting stoma can be problematic, particularly if the distal segment becomes ischaemic or retracts.

Ileostomy

End ileostomy
- May be formed as a permanent stoma for patients with
  - UC (most patients undergo RPC)
  - FAP (again, most undergo RPC)
  - After a failed ileal pouch
  - Multiple large bowel cancers, especially in an elderly patient
  - Slow transit constipation
  - Ischaemic colitis
  - Crohn's proctocolitis
- An end ileostomy in isolation (and less commonly as part of a split ileostomy) may be formed as a temporary stoma to ensure complete faecal diversion to protect a downstream colorectal, ileorectal or pouch anal anastomosis. It may also be used to ensure faecal diversion above a Crohn's colitis, perianal CD or an area of colonic or small bowel trauma that has been repaired
- Usually sited in the right lower quadrant of the abdomen, but alternative sites may be chosen depending on the presence of scars, tattoos, etc. (Fig. 9.1).

Loop ileostomy
First described by Turnbull in the Cleveland clinic in the 1960s as an end-loop ileostomy to achieve a more satisfactory, better perfused spout in obese patients with a short or thickened ileal mesentery or in those where there is a high likelihood that the stoma will be permanent (Fig. 9.2). The concept was subsequently adopted as a loop in continuity with the distal bowel in order to defunction downstream anastomoses.
  Loop ileostomies are commonly used in the following situations
- IPAA
- Low anterior resection or colorectal anastomoses
- Ileorectal anastomoses when the rectum is diseased
- Complex anorectal procedures
- Management of slow transit constipation where the extent of dysmotility is uncertain
- Definitive therapy in megacolon.

Deciding to defunction
- Radioisotope marker studies show the exclusion efficiency of everted loop ileostomies to be as high as 99%
- This falls to 85% for patients with a retracted stoma who also pass material per rectum
- There is a clear benefit in defunctioning low rectal anastomoses. The odds ratio for clinically relevant anastomotic leakage is 0.32 and re-operation for leak-related complications is 0.27.

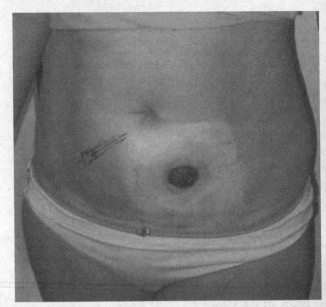

Fig. 9.1 Ileostomies are normally sited in the right lower quadrant of the abdomen, but alternative sites may be chosen depending on the presence of scars, tattoos, etc.

- Functional outcomes after IPAA are similar for those with and without a diverting ileostomy. Non-diversion is associated with an increased risk of anastomotic leak.
- ~5–10% of patients will develop an ileostomy-related complication prior to closure and at least the same percentage will develop a complication related to closure, e.g. infection, obstruction or incisional hernia.

Loop ileostomy vs loop colostomy

Loop ileostomy is favoured by many as the best way to defunction a colonic/rectal anastomosis. Potential advantages of loop ileostomy include:
- ↓ skin irritation, ↓ size and bulk of the stoma, ↓ complications such as peristomal sepsis, parastomal herniation and stomal prolapse
- Loop ileostomies produce less odour, require fewer appliance changes and only 18% of patients complain of problems managing their stoma vs 58% of those with a loop colostomy
- Loop ileostomies are easier to close and closure is associated with fewer complications.

A Cochrane review of randomised trials suggested that except for stomal prolapse, there was no statistically or clinically significant difference between the two; however, a recent meta-analysis of all relevant studies concluded that ileostomy may be preferable to colostomy when used to defunction a distal colorectal anastomosis. Loop ileostomy was associated with a reduction in stoma-related problems and a reduced incidence of wound infection and incisional hernia following closure.

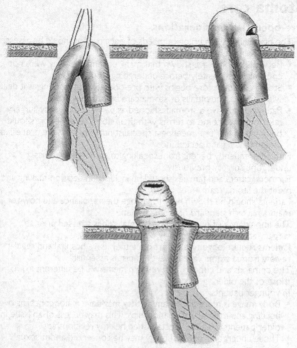

Fig. 9.2 End-loop ileostomy used for patients with a short or thickened mesentery.

Urostomy

- Fashioned in the right lower abdomen, following surgery for bladder cancer, the management of severe urinary incontinence or following pelvic trauma
- The outward appearance is similar to a Brooke ileostomy.

Uncommon stomas

- The Koch continent ileostomy is rarely performed. It involves the formation of an internal reservoir in association with a flat ileostomy.

References

Brooke BM. The management of an ileostomy including its complications. *Lancet* 1952;**ii**:102–104.

Franks K. Colectomy or resection of the large intestine for malignant disease. *Med Chir Trans* 1889;**72**:211–232.

Hüser N, Michalski CW, Erkan M *et al*. Systematic review and meta-analysis of the role of defunctioning stoma in low rectal cancer surgery. *Ann Surg* 2008;**248**:52–60.

Weston-Petrides GK, Lovegrove RE, Tilney HS *et al*. Comparison of outcomes after restorative proctocolectomy with or without defunctioning ileostomy. *Arch Surg* 2008;**143**:406–412.

Güenaga KF, Lustosa SAS, Saad SS *et al*. Ileostomy or colostomy for temporary decompression of colorectal anastomosis. *Cochrane Database Syst Rev* 2009;Issue 3.

Tilney HS, Sains PS, Lovegrove RE *et al*. Comparison of outcomes following ileostomy versus colostomy for defunctioning colorectal anastomoses. *World J Surg* 2007;**31**:1142–1151.

Stoma care

Pre-operative considerations

- The physical and psychological needs of each patient should be assessed by a specialist nurse prior to surgery
  - Repeated audits have shown that many patients feel they were not counselled adequately before undergoing stoma surgery
  - Stoma care therefore begins with pre-operative counselling as it deals with many of the pitfalls of stoma care before they arise
  - Patients who have a stoma fashioned as part of emergency surgery take longer to come to terms with their stoma: every effort should be made to facilitate meeting a specialist nurse to start the process of understanding and acceptance
- Patients frequently benefit from speaking to someone who has undergone surgery previously
- Partners, carers and families should be included in decision-making and meet the stoma team
- Patients should be shown how to change their appliance and how to maintain a high standard of stoma hygiene
- The importance of protecting peristomal skin is stressed prior to surgery and reinforced regularly post-operatively
- Patients require ongoing support once they leave hospital and regular review from a stoma care nurse therapist is essential
- The demands and concerns of young patients will be different from those of the older age group
- In younger patients
  - Body image is more important as they may have major concerns over building and maintaining relationships. This may be less of an issue in older patients who are in established healthy relationships
  - Those undergoing pelvic surgery may be concerned about sexual dysfunction secondary to nerve injury
  - This dysfunction may be compounded by psychological issues relating to the acceptance of their new stoma
  - Conversely, the freedom from illness results in new-found confidence for some and an improvement in sexual relationships.

Appliances

- Patients should be familiarised with the various types of appliance used at different stages in their care
- Immediately after surgery, a clear and drainable appliance is preferred to facilitate daily inspection of the stoma and the contents of the appliance without having to disturb the stoma (Fig. 9.3)
- Closed appliances are self-contained and discarded with a single use. Typically, these are used for colostomies
- Single-use drainable bags may be used for a few days before being replaced
- Two-piece appliances have a base plate and a detachable pouch that is clipped into place. Typically used for ileostomies, the base plate is changed every 2–4 days

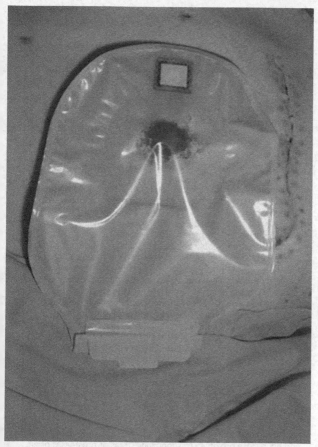

Fig. 9.3 In the early post-operative period, a clear appliance is used to enable inspection of the stoma and contents of the appliance.

- Creation of a neat symmetrical stoma allows the ordering of pre-cut appliances directly from the stoma company. This saves the patient considerable time and helps maintain a healthy stoma
- A range of products have been developed to help manage the problematic stoma, such as convexity base plates for retracted stomas, barrier cream, filler and tape.

Marking a stoma site

- Elective patients should be referred to a stoma nurse specialist well in advance of surgery
- Even in emergency situations patients should be seen by a nurse with expertise in stoma care
- Stoma nurses can do much to improve a poorly constructed stoma, but they can do little to improve the morbidity caused by a poorly sited stoma.

Principles of marking a stoma

- The stoma or the base plate should not encroach on bony landmarks (e.g. iliac crest), the umbilicus, the incision or natural skin creases
- The base plate should lie on an area of flat skin that is easily accessible to the patient
- The skin should be free of skin disorders such as psoriasis and have no moles or papillomas
- The stoma should not lie immediately under the belt or waist band
- The stoma should be easily visible to the patient, especially the inferior aspect
- The stoma should probably be brought through the rectus. If not, there may be a higher risk of prolapse and herniation
- The proposed site should be tested by applying a stoma appliance, ideally when the patient is fully clothed and in the supine position, sitting and standing positions
- Emergency patients can usually flex sufficiently to identify potential skin folds and creases
- In the patient who has not been sited pre-operatively the midpoint between anterior superior iliac crest and umbilicus should be considered
- Beware overweight patients in whom the stoma should be sited higher, as the abdominal wall sags when the patient sits or stands (Fig. 9.4)
- In many situations, consideration should be given to marking both right and left sides to maximise intraoperative surgical options
- The proposed stoma site/sites should be marked with an indelible pen, perhaps covered by an occlusive dressing to stop it being washed off (Fig. 9.4). The alternative is to tattoo the site with India ink.

Additional points

- Special consideration should be given to unusual situations such as high leg amputation and complex pelvic trauma. Stoma sites potentially may end up in close proximity to supporting straps of prostheses or an external fixator
- In Fournier's gangrene the stoma must be placed well away from the site or potential site of sepsis
- Abdominal drains should not be brought out on the same side as a stoma
- The midline wound should pass to the opposite side of the umbilicus to the stoma
- Mucous fistulae should be fashioned well away from the stoma to allow the base plate to be well secured
- With appropriate training a surgeon can site a stoma just as well as a stoma care specialist
- It is important to remember that a poorly chosen site for a permanent stoma may commit a patient to a lifetime of grief.

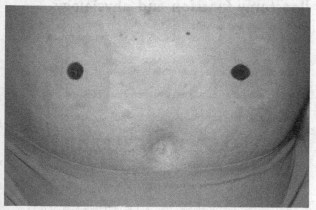

Fig. 9.4 Marking both sides of the abdomen with the mark protected by a clear occlusive dressing. In obese patients a higher than usual site may be considered.

Ileostomy function and physiology

The physiology and function of an ileostomy can be deranged in the initial post-operative period. Function usually then settles into a reasonably predictable pattern of behaviour.

- The normal output is semi-fluid and is ~750ml/day
- Consistency is governed very much by diet, but this does not have to be adjusted unnecessarily
- Patients should be encouraged to eat a balanced diet and chew food well
- If some foodstuffs increase the ileostomy output, these can be excluded/reduced if the result is distressing
- Daytime emptying is frequently governed by social convenience. Many ostomists will empty their appliance when passing urine, even if it is not full
- Night time emptying is a more reliable indicator of function
- 70–80% will be up at least once a night, 40% will be up twice and 15% up ≥3 times
- Patients who have had the ileocolic sphincter retained during the formation of their stoma are disturbed much less often at night
- Ileostomy patients lose excess salt in their stomas. Increased renal absorption will partially compensate for this
- Patients should be encouraged to add salt to their food to increase daily salt intake
- Potassium is usually excreted in the colon. Ileostomy and associated colon resection may therefore lead to potassium retention and borderline hyperkalaemia. The kidneys respond by reducing K^+ re-absorption
- Excessive resection of the terminal ileum leads to reduced absorption of B12, folate and bile salts
- Patients may become B12 and folate deficient. However, this may be related at least in part to a dietary deficiency
- Patients should be encouraged to increase their fluid intake in hot climates and after exercise.

High output ileostomy

- High output ileostomies usually arise following resection of excessive lengths of ileum, usually at the time of initial surgery
- Resection of proximal jejunum can also increase ileostomy output. However, length for length, the ileum is less forgiving
- Small bowel conditions such as CD or coeliac disease should be considered in patients who present with late-onset high output ileostomy
- The water content of a high output ileostomy (1.5–2litres) exceeds normal (750ml). Excessive amounts of sodium, potassium and calcium are lost daily, leading to salt depletion, hypokalaemia and hypocalcaemia
- In mild/moderate cases increased renal re-absorption of sodium compensates for the sodium loss
- Oral salt may be required to prevent total body sodium loss
- Depending on the cause of the high output, carbohydrate and fat along with the fat-soluble vitamins A, D, E and K may be lost. Excess fat in the ileal content may be malodorous

- Loss of amino acids and proteins may lead to hypoproteinaemia
- Rapid transit and excessive resection of the terminal ileum may also result in deficiencies of B12, folate, bile salts and essential minerals
- Management includes the following
  - Fluid restriction (1.5litres/day)
  - Codeine phosphate or loperamide
  - H$_2$ blockers/PPIs to reduce gastric secretions
  - In severe cases, octreotide may be effective at reducing small bowel excretion
  - Vitamin, mineral, salt and dietary supplementation may be necessary.

Stoma formation

Principles when constructing a stoma

- Ideally, all stomas should pass through the rectus muscle
- All stomas should be raised or everted. This ensures a good seal
- All stomas should be matured at the time of the initial surgery
- All stomas should be marked pre-operatively.

End colostomy

- Most colostomies are formed using sigmoid or descending colon
- Problems may arise because of the relatively large sigmoid mesocolon, compared with the sigmoid lumen
- The skin at the site of the stoma is excised as a circle. A near perfect circle ensures that the patients can use pre-cut appliances. The diameter should be 2/3 the width of the flattened colon. Small incisions can always be made bigger
- The skin circle and underlying fat is excised down to the anterior rectus sheath. Excessive fat should not be removed as this can cause a dip close to the stoma and affect placement of the appliance
- A vertical or cruciate incision is made in the anterior rectus sheath. The fibres of the rectus muscle are bluntly dissected, allowing separation of the vertical fibres
- A further incision is then made in the posterior rectus sheath
- The route through the layers of the abdominal wall should be aligned so that the bowel passes through directly rather than obliquely
- The stoma should be fashioned with healthy well-vascularised bowel under no tension
- The defect must be large enough to allow the sigmoid mesocolon and colon itself through the rectus to reach the skin without tension
- To avoid tension, it may be necessary to divide the left colic branch of the inferior mesenteric artery. If there is still tension, the splenic flexure should be mobilised to reduce the risk of retraction
- All colostomies should be deliberately everted at formation, as almost all will retract to some degree within the first 7–10 days
- The bowel is sutured to skin with an absorbable suture
- The sutures should incorporate the full thickness of bowel wall to the subcuticular plane of the skin. Placement of full-thickness skin sutures should be avoided
- Ideally, the surgeon should avoid handling the bowel wall directly with forceps in order to reduce post-operative oedema
- Suturing over areas of protruding fat is unnecessary. Tissue swelling and stoma retraction will cause these small gaps to disappear
- Stoma dehiscence may occur because too many sutures have been placed and tied too tightly, rather than the reverse
- At the end of the operation the stoma appliance should be cut and carefully placed to reduce faecal contamination of the peristomal skin to an absolute minimum
- Some surgeons recommend anchoring the stoma to either the posterior or anterior rectus sheath. Evidence to support this is sparse and the technique runs the risk of local abscess or fistula formation.

Loop colostomy

- This can be performed as an open, laparoscopic or trephine procedure
- Review of the pre-operative CT scan can often identify a degree of sigmoid redundancy
- The patient should be placed on the table in lithotomy position. This allows rectal insufflation to identify proximal and distal limbs of the stoma
- If the sigmoid colon is not sufficiently mobile, it should be mobilised to allow it to be brought through the abdominal wall without tension
- A window is created on the mesenteric border using blunt forceps and a nylon tape or catheter is used to facilitate passage through the stoma aperture
- Once the loop is lying satisfactorily in place, the nylon tape is exchanged with a stoma rod. The bowel should not be stretched against the rod under tension as the sutures will cut out, causing local dehiscence, skin excoriation and leakage from the appliance
- Attention should be paid to fixing the stoma appliance correctly after surgery. This will help to prevent problems in the first few days post-operatively.

End ileostomy

- The stoma trephine is fashioned in the same way as for a colostomy, but with reduced dimensions for the skin and sheath incisions
- An opening that accommodates the tips of the index and middle finger is usually all that is necessary
- In cases where CD can be excluded, the terminal ileum should be divided as close to the ileocolic junction as possible, in order to preserve as much ileal function as possible. Inclusion of the ileocolic sphincter into the stoma may improve stoma function
- Care must be taken to avoid injury to the vascular supply
- The ileum is drawn through so that the mesentery is cephalad (superior) as this will maximise the length of the inferior (anti-mesenteric) lip of the stoma, making it pout into the pouch (Fig. 9.5)
- The stoma is usually matured after closure of all other wounds to minimise contamination
- The ileum is opened and four inverting sutures are placed to produce a 2.5–3cm spout. These should be all placed before tying
- The blunt end of a set of forceps can be used to aid inversion. This is considerably less traumatic than drawing the bowel out from within using a set of Babcock forceps
- The application of GTN paste to the serosal surface may aid eversion by relaxing ileal smooth muscle
- Sutures should not be overly tight. They should be seromuscular at the bowel edge and subcuticular at the skin edge. This reduces the risk of fistula formation and the sutures interfere less with the attachment of the stoma appliance
- Full-thickness skin sutures frequently result in islands of ileal mucosa implanting in the skin at the site of the suture. Mucus production from these implantation sites leads to poor appliance adhesion (Fig. 9.6).

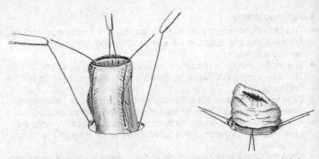

Fig. 9.5 Construction of an ileostomy. The mesentery is placed on the cephalad side in order to ensure that the caudal side of the everted stoma is highest and fits over the edge of the appliance.

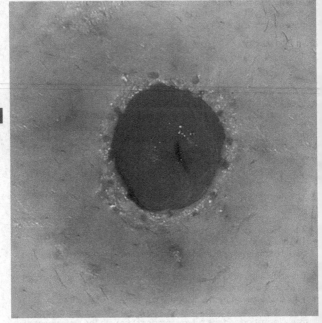

Fig. 9.6 Islands of ileal mucosa implanted in the skin secondary to full-thickness skin sutures used during maturation of the stoma.

Loop ileostomy

- A suitable loop of terminal ileum several centimetres from the ileocaecal valve or start of the ileal pouch should be chosen. This should reach to the proposed stoma site without difficulty
- The loop ileostomy should be fashioned sufficiently far away from the ileocolic junction as to leave plenty of room for ileal–ileal anastomosis if resection of the stoma and adjacent ileum becomes necessary at the time of stoma reversal. Equally a stoma placed in too proximal a position may predispose to a high output ostomy
- Prior to fashioning the stoma, the proximal and distal limb should be clearly identified by placing 2 different coloured sutures alongside each other at the proposed stoma site, e.g. polydioxanone (PDS) and Vicryl. The PDS suture marks the down or distal limb. This ensures that no inadvertent rotation of the limbs occurs (Fig. 9.7)
- The skin incision is made at the pre-marked site, taking into account the requirement for two loops of bowel to be pulled through
- The stoma is matured after all other incisions are closed and dressed to minimise the risk of contamination
- Most surgeons incise the distal (caudal) ileal loop at skin level. The distal limb is then sutured to skin, using only 1/3 of the circumference of the stoma opening
- An alternative method is to incise the bowel 1cm from the distal skin level in order to fashion a modest eversion of the distal limb. This may prevent retraction of the distal limb
- The proximal limb is everted by placing 3 sutures between the ileum (serosubmucosal) and the dermal layer of the skin. These incorporate 2/3 of the diameter of the stoma aperture. These are not initially tied.
- Some surgeons also incorporate a subserosal bite of the ileum at the level of the fascia. However, this may predispose to parastomal fistulation, particularly in patients with CD
- The proximal (cephalad) limb is everted by using the blunt end of a dissection forceps to evert the ileum. At the same time, the assistant places the sutures on the proximal limb under tension to facilitate the eversion. If possible, Babcock forceps and other manipulation of the ileum should be avoided in order to reduce post-operative oedema
- Care must be taken not to introduce a partial twist in the stoma as this can lead to obstruction. The previously inserted marker sutures should ensure that the proximal limb is marked at all times and is the everted limb

Trephine loop ileostomy

- This can usually be performed under direct vision if the patient is placed right side elevated, with head-down tilt
- The ileum can usually be identified by the ileal fat pad which is an anatomical constant
- If adhesions prevent this identification, then laparoscopy or mini laparotomy may be indicated
- Blind formation of a loop ileostomy may result in too proximal a segment of small bowel being used to fashion the stoma.

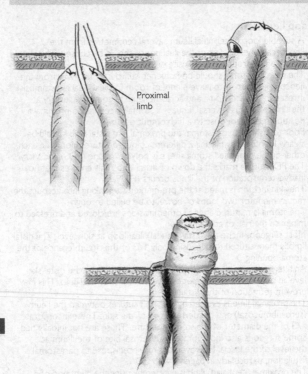

Fig. 9.7 Construction of a loop ileostomy. Sutures mark the proximal and distal limbs, thereby ensuring that the proximal limb is everted. The distal limb encompasses only 1/3 of the diameter of the stoma opening.

Koch continent ileostomy

- This combines a traditional Brooke ileostomy spout with the formation of a terminal ileal reservoir. The formation of an internal nipple valve helps create a continence mechanism
- The advent of pouch-anal surgery has made this operation much less common
- Patients require to self-catheterise to drain the internal pouch
- Problems arise secondary to stricture of the valve mechanism following repeated self-catheterisation and failure of the valve mechanism
- Revisional surgery is problematic and not always successful
- As with ileoanal pouch, conversion of a Koch reservoir to a Brooke ileostomy sacrifices a significant amount of terminal ileum.

Stoma reversal

Procedure

- The principles of reversal of both a loop ileostomy and loop colostomy are the same
- The timing of closure is an important consideration. The risk of complications is higher when stomas are reversed soon after their formation. Parks and Hastings and others have noted that complications (including mortality) related to colostomy closure decreased after 90 days and many continue to use 12 weeks as their standard time when planning routine closure of loop stomas
- It is important to ensure that there is no distal stricture as may be seen following a pouch anal anastomosis
- The use of saline ± adrenaline is helpful to define the anatomy
- Dissection should be close to/on the bowel wall and mesentery. This is a man-made plain and in theory should be bloodless
- The skin is incised close to the stoma to keep the subsequent defect to a minimum
- It should be possible to define anterior rectus sheath, rectus muscle and posterior sheath
- The stoma should be fully mobilised so that it is completely free from the edges of the fascia and abdominal wall
- Extreme care should be taken to avoid serosal injury
- Unrecognised serosal injury is one of the more common reasons for post-operative sepsis. Serosal injuries may be identified by distending both limbs of the stoma with povidone–iodine solution instilled with a catheter-tipped syringe. All serosal injuries should be oversewn
- It may be necessary to extend the fascial and skin openings to mobilise additional bowel so that a tension-free anastomosis can be fashioned
- The anastomosis may be sutured or stapled (functional end–end). A stapled anastomosis may be marginally quicker to perform and is associated with a slightly faster recovery
- When performing a sutured closure, the bowel edges should be freshened and an interrupted serosubmucosal anastomosis performed
- It is not usually necessary to resect the stoma routinely, although this may be the case if the stoma is very indurated or distorted
- Disparity in the size of bowel segments can be corrected using a Cheadle slit.

Complications of stoma reversal

- Transient bowel obstruction is not uncommon following ileostomy closure (12–15%)
- Obstruction may be due to either narrowing of the small bowel lumen at the anastomosis (tissue swelling) or adherence of the anastomotic line to the abdominal wall. This produces acute angulation. Most cases resolve with IV fluids and NG suction
- Although most cases of bowel obstruction settle with conservative management, if surgical intervention is required it should be carried out through a formal laparotomy and not attempted through the trephine.

Reference

Parks SE, Hastings PR. Complications of colostomy closure. Am J Surg 1985;**149**:672–675.

Surgery-related complications

Surgery-related complications

The lifetime cumulative complication rate for stoma surgery is >70%, with many requiring surgical revision.

Risk factors

- Factors that predispose to stoma complications include
  - High BMI
  - IBD
  - Use of steroids and immunosuppressive therapy
  - Diabetes
  - Old age
- Patients with CD are more likely to have problems with stomas (especially stoma retraction). The surgical revision rate is 75% after 8yrs vs 44% for patients with UC
- Patients who receive pre-operative counselling and siting of the stoma are less likely to have an adverse outcome.

Bowel obstruction

- May be secondary to extrinsic compression from adhesions or intraluminal obstruction from a food bolus impacting, usually at the point where the stoma passes through the fascia
- High-grade partial obstruction may result in a high-volume watery stoma effluent
- Initial management is conservative although surgery must be considered in the presence of increasing pain, distension, leucocytosis or rising inflammatory markers.

Stoma ischaemia/necrosis

- Usually presents within 24h of surgery
- More common after end colostomy compared with end ileostomy
- Emergency surgery, obesity and ischaemia as an indication for surgery are associated with a higher incidence of stoma necrosis
- If a stoma becomes black/ischaemic, an attempt should be made to assess the depth and proximal extent of the ischaemia
- Inserting a glass test tube into the stoma may enable visualisation down to the depth of the fascia. Ischaemia deep to this requires re-operation.
- Distal ischaemia or mucosal ischaemia (confirmed by obtaining arterial blood from the muscle following a pinprick) may be managed conservatively although long-term stenosis may follow.

Mucocutaneous separation

- May occur as a result of distal ischaemia, excessive tension on the stoma or creating a skin opening that is too large
- Parastomal infection may also give rise to separation
- Minor degrees of separation are not uncommon
- Significant separation with a gaping defect requires skilled stoma therapy intervention to keep the area clean and pack the area with a paste to prevent extension and abscess formation
- Stoma stenosis may follow.

Parastomal hernia

- Parastomal hernia is a common problem and affects up to 30% of ileostomies and 60% of colostomies. The incidence is likely to increase with time and rates vary according to whether a parastomal hernia is diagnosed on clinical examination, CT scan or in those who have symptoms or come to surgery to repair a hernia
- Predisposing factors include
  - Raised intra-abdominal pressure secondary to obesity, chronic obstructive pulmonary disease, malnutrition and IBD
  - Use of steroids and immunosuppressive drugs
  - Emergency surgery
  - Poor surgical technique. Closure of the lateral space, trephine size, fascial fixation and performing an extraperitoneal stoma have not been clearly shown to affect the incidence of parastomal hernia. Several studies report a 4 to 7-fold increase in the parastomal hernia rate when colostomies were placed through the oblique muscles rather than through the rectus. However, others have not seen any relationship between the stoma site and the risk of parastomal hernia
- Obesity is the only factor that has been consistently shown to contribute to parastomal hernia formation
- Most hernias do not interfere with stoma function and can be managed conservatively
- Larger hernias may become problematic for the patient in terms of stoma care, pain at the stoma and intermittent obstructive symptoms
- Some advocate preventative measures such as abdominal exercises, wearing a stoma support and avoiding excessive weight gain, although there is no firm evidence to support this advice
- Although there have been many proposed classifications of parastomal hernias, none has gained universal acceptance.
- Diagnosis is usually made clinically but a CT scan can help in assessment, especially in obese patients.

Prophylactic mesh reinforcement at primary stoma formation

A recent meta-analysis of 8 randomised trials has confirmed that perioperative placement of a prophylactic mesh when fashioning a primary stoma is a safe and effective means of preventing parastomal herniation. Parastomal hernia rates ranged from 0-59% in the mesh group, compared to 20-94% for controls. There was no significant difference in complication rates

- Most studies have used a pre-peritoneal sublay position behind the rectus sheath and in front of the peritoneum/posterior rectus sheath (Fig. 9.8)
- A square or circle of mesh (6–10cm in length/diameter) with a pre-cut hole is placed at open operation. No fixation is necessary
- The stoma is brought through the opening in the mesh
- There is no apparent increase in the incidence of wound infections
- Reported recurrence rates of 0–22% are approximately half that of controls although longer term follow-up is awaited
- European Hernia Society guidelines strongly recommend use of synthetic mesh when fashioning a primary stoma.
- Prophylactic mesh may also be inserted during laparoscopic stoma formation, but very little high-quality data has been published on outcomes with the technique

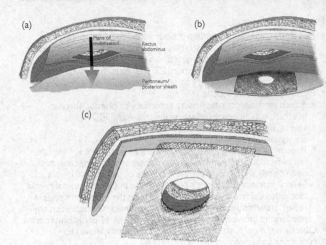

Fig. 9.8 Prophylactic placement of a mesh at the time of the primary operation.

Repair of parastomal hernia
- Repair should only be considered for problematic hernias, i.e. incarceration, obstruction, appliance problems. Although surgeons vary considerably in their threshold for surgical intervention, ~15–30% of patients with a parastomal hernia will ultimately undergo surgical repair
- Minimally symptomatic patients can be managed with the help of a stoma therapist who will advise on appliance modification with or without a support belt
- Patients who are clinically obese should lose weight to decrease the likelihood of further recurrence. Complications are also significantly increased in smokers or patients with poor diabetic control.
- Remember that the 5yr survival for patients undergoing a colostomy for cancer is 50% and the long-term survival following emergency colostomy formation for perforated diverticular disease is also reduced
- Technical factors that should be considered before repair include the size of the abdominal wall defect, the presence of a concomitant incisional hernia, if there have been previous attempts at repair and whether a mesh was used.
- Repair can be fashioned by the following routes
  - Local repair, with or without mesh
  - Transposition with or without mesh
  - Transperitoneal repair (usually with mesh and usually using a laparoscopic approach
- Unfortunately, there are very few good sized RCTs with long-term follow-up comparing one technique over any other
- Mesh repair is associated with the lowest risk of recurrence (0–33%) compared with simple suture (46–100%) or transposition (0–75%)

- Up to 1/3 of patients undergoing polypropylene mesh repair will suffer a complication. These include recurrence (26%), surgical bowel obstruction (9%), prolapse (3%), wound infection (3%), fistula (3%) and mesh erosion (2%)
- With proper care and attention, the risk of mesh infection should be low. If infection develops, the mesh may need to be removed
- Collagen-based biologic mesh substitutes are expensive but may be considered in patients at higher risk of mesh related complications
- Patients must be warned of failure rates and the significant morbidity and occasional mortality associated with surgery.

Re-siting/transposition

- Re-siting of the stoma is generally associated with poor results and, when considered, should be combined with prophylactic mesh
- The stoma is fashioned in virgin skin
- Usually requires a formal laparotomy with associated complications including incisional hernia at the original stoma site.
- The original stoma site should also be repaired with mesh due to risk of incisional hernia formation

Local repair: mobilisation of mucocutaneous junction

- This may be suitable for small hernias in slim patients
- The mucocutaneous junction is disconnected and dissection close to the stoma is followed down to the pre-peritoneal space
- Mesh may then be placed around the bowel, sutured to the bowel serosa and anchored as an onlay to the transversus abdominus muscle
- Complications include local sepsis and fistula formation, mesh extrusion, inflammation, seroma formation, stoma dehiscence and stenosis.
- Recurrence rate for onlay mesh repair is 15–30%
- A local repair without mesh or using an absorbable or biologic mesh is often performed when performing an emergency repair, for incarcerated/gangrenous parastomal hernia.
- Recurrence rate for primary sutured repair is approximately 70%

Local repair: lateral approach

- An incision is made away from the stoma and dissection carried down to the pre-peritoneal space (Fig. 9.9)
- The hernial sac is identified, reduced and mesh inserted as before
- The advantage of this approach is that the stoma is not disturbed and contamination of the wound and mesh is less likely

Laparoscopic repair: keyhole technique

- This is an increasingly popular approach which also enables concomitant repair of any midline incisional hernias
- A 3-port technique is used although additional ports may be required. The camera port is central and 2×5mm working ports on each side
- The contents of the hernia sac are reduced although the sac itself is left in situ as for the Sugarbaker technique
- A composite mesh (adherent and non-adherent sides) suitable for intraperitoneal placement is used
- Mesh with a keyhole defect is used, aiming to place the mesh at least 5cm beyond the edges of the defect

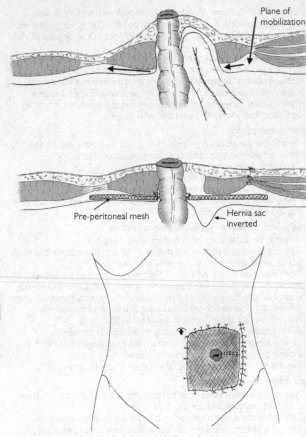

Fig. 9.9 Lateral approach to repair a parastomal hernia.

- The mesh is tacked in place intraperitoneally, with the stoma passing through the centre pre-cut defect. The edges of the keyhole are overlapped and tacked down
- Transfascial sutures are also placed to secure the mesh
- The stoma is not touched, thus reducing the risk of mesh infection
- Risks and complications include:
  - Mesh erosion into adherent bowel. Composite with a non-adherent side reduces the risk of this devastating complication
  - Injury to the stoma or adherent loops of bowel (recognised at the time or delayed presentation). May occur during port insertion or when taking down adhesions. Risk may be lessened by avoiding diathermy when taking down adhesions

- Recurrent hernias may develop over time by herniation alongside the junction of the mesh and the stoma or by prolapse of the mesh itself into the hernial defect
- As with all hernia repairs, recurrence rates increase with time.
- In a recent meta-analysis, the risk of recurrence with open intraperitoneal keyhole repair using mesh was 7% and 11% for a laparoscopic approach.

Sugarbaker technique

- This is the preferred technique for parastomal hernia repair due to reduced recurrence rates
- The technique can be performed open at laparotomy or using a laparoscopic approach
- After reduction of the parastomal hernia the colon is lateralised and sutures are placed between serosa and peritoneum using an absorbable suture
- An intraperitoneal uncut composite mesh (e.g. Proceed®, Ethicon Endosurgery or Parietex® Covidien) is placed in an inlay position covering the lateralised colon and the hernial defect by 5cm in all directions
- Colon passes under the lateral border of the mesh to pass through the abdominal wall
- The edges of the mesh are secured with transfascial non-absorbable sutures.
- In a systematic review, the risk of recurrence with an open Sugarbaker repair was 15% and 12% for a laparoscopic approach.
- In a separate study, compared to other laparoscopic parastomal hernia repair techniques, the Sugarbaker technique is reported to have a lower complication rate (40 vs 70%) and lower recurrence rates at 20 months (16 vs 60%). However, results from longer-term studies are awaited

Stoma prolapse

- Prolapse affects ~2–4% of permanent stomas and is marginally more common in ileostomies. Incidence increases with the length of follow-up
- Affects up to 50% of loop transverse colostomies. The defunctioned distal limb is usually the prolapsed limb.
- Some patients appear to form very few adhesions which may also be a factor
- A parastomal hernia may be present in up to 50% of prolapsed colostomies, which will alter the surgical approach
- Most prolapses are chronic and minor. If they do not interfere with stoma function, surgical correction is not indicated.
- ~10% will present with acute incarceration/strangulation which should be reduced at the earliest opportunity
- Controlled pressure or the application of sugar may reduce oedema to the point where reduction is possible
- If reduction is unsuccessful, the prolapse must be reduced under anaesthetic. Care should be taken to ensure that compromised bowel is not returned to the peritoneal cavity, predisposing to perforation
- The inflammatory reaction associated with an acute prolapse may be sufficient to cause adhesions once it has reduced

- A recurrent prolapse requires surgical repair which can be performed through either resection, revision or resiting
- Resection or revisions are normally carried out locally through the mobilised stoma. Care should be taken not to damage the ostomy site itself. If there is an associated parastomal hernia, this should be repaired at the same time
- Extraperitoneal tunneling or fixing the bowel to the abdominal wall has not been shown to reduce the incidence
- Recurrence following resection is rare. This may require a laparotomy and fixation of the bowel.

Stenosis

- An uncommon complication affecting ~3% of colostomies. It is even less common in ileostomy patients
- Problems may have been evident in the first 24h after surgery (e.g. mucosal or full-thickness ischaemia, mucocutaneous separation)
- Predisposing factors include making the skin incision too large, too many sutures, sutures tied too tightly, local infection and obesity
- Many of these stomas have been formed in unfavourable circumstances and further surgery may be ill advised
- Gentle dilatation should be tried in the first instance
- Local surgery with excision of skin to increase the trephine may help. This may need to be extended down to the fascia if it is also stenosed. This may be very difficult in obese patients
- A laparotomy may be required either to mobilise more colon and refashion the existing stoma or to resect the remaining colon and fashion an ileostomy on the opposite side.

Stoma recession/retraction

Next to parastomal hernia, stoma retraction is the most common complication affecting ~10-15% of stomas. The recession may be intermittent or fixed.

- **Intermittent recession** occurs when the patient lies down or the abdominal muscles are relaxed
  - Usually results from too large a gap in the fascia or inadequate fixation/adhesion formation between the stoma and the abdominal wall
  - Suturing of the bowel to the fascia does not appear to help
  - It may lead to soiling and leakage
- **Fixed recession** is usually 2° to
  - Shortening of the bowel wall through disease (e.g. CD)
  - Excessive stoma tension because of a failure to mobilise the bowel adequately
  - Post-operative weight gain. This may be a factor in patients who were cachectic at the time of the 1° stoma
- Colostomies are affected twice as much as ileostomies
- A degree of retraction affects most colostomies. Therefore, the stoma should be fashioned proud with a little eversion to compensate for this. The patient should be reassured that the appearance will settle with time

- Most cases of stoma retraction can be managed conservatively using specialised convexity appliances
- Refashioning of the stoma may be required if the retraction involves a natural skin crease or has created a skin crease. This decision must balance the morbidity of the current stoma against further surgery
- Intermittent recession can usually be treated by local revisional surgery, whereas fixed recession may require a laparotomy and further bowel mobilisation.

Parastomal fistula

Superficial fistulae may occur at the mucocutaneous anastomosis. They are usually 2° to local trauma and may also occur after rupture of a paracolic abscess which has developed at the site of placement of a serosal hitching suture (used to facilitate eversion of the stoma). In the absence of intrinsic bowel disease, they usually settle.

In patients with CD, deep fistulae originating below the level of the fascia invariably indicate recurrent disease. A full assessment of the entire small bowel is required. and patients usually will require formal reconstruction of the stoma.

Peristomal varices

Varices are abnormal portosystemic vascular connections that develop in response to raised portal pressure.
- They present with stomal bleeding, visible peristomal varices and a dark blue peristomal skin discoloration (Fig. 9.10)
- Other stigmata of portal hypertension may be present.
- The most common causes are
  - Sclerosing cholangitis
  - Alcoholic cirrhosis
  - Extensive metastatic disease of the liver
- Management consists of the following
  - Treat/optimise the underlying medical condition although cure is rarely possible
  - Acute bleeding may be managed with direct pressure and local adrenaline soaks
  - Terlipressin or similar vasopressin analogues used in oesophageal variceal bleeding may be considered
  - Direct injection with sclerosant (e.g. sodium tetradecyl sulphate) may also be considered but is unlikely to give rise to a sustained relieve from bleeding
  - Surgical disconnection of the mucocutaneous junction and re-anastomosis is successful in the short to medium term, but new varices invariably develop
  - Transjugular intrahepatic portosystemic shunting (TIPS) may need to be considered for persistent bleeding.

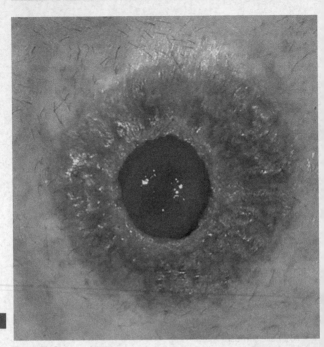

Fig. 9.10 Peristomal varices.

References

Duchesne J, Wang Y, Weintraub S et al. Stoma complications: a multivariate analysis. *Am Surg* 2002;**68**:961–966.

Londono-Schimmer E, Leong A, Phillips R. Life table analysis of stoma complications following colostomy. *Dis Colon Rectum* 1994;**37**:916–920.

Cottam J, Richards K, Hasted A, Blackman A. Results of a nationwide prospective audit of stoma complications within 3 weeks of surgery. Colorectal disease 2007;**9**:834–838.

Prophylactic mesh placement for the PREvention of paraSTOmal hernias: The PRESTO systematic review and meta-analysis.

Pianka F, Probst P, Keller AV, Saure D, et al. *PLoS One* 2017; **12**(2):e0171548.

Patient and appliance-related complications

Patient and appliance-related complications

Although surgery-related complications are well recognized, day to day patient-related morbidity is less well publicized. The large selection of modified stoma appliances, pastes, fillers and barrier creams is a testament to the need for further improvement in stoma formation at the time of surgery. Unfortunately, some surgeons do not recognize the importance of fashioning a good stoma and, at times, the task is delegated to unsupervised, junior members of the surgical team.

The cost in fiscal terms of poor stoma surgery is considerable. It results in the stoma nurse specialist firefighting when their time would be more appropriately spent supporting the patient through their surgery.

Skin problems

Appliance leakage and skin excoriation
- Minor skin excoriation affects up to 25% of ileostomy patients at 2yrs
- Less irritant colostomy contents cause skin problems in 10%
- Skin irritation is treated with barrier creams and pastes to prevent further deterioration
- Skin excoriation and poor appliance adherence predisposes to daytime leakage which affects 20–25% of ileostomy patients and 10–15% of colostomy patients. Although episodes are often minor, they are distressing for the patient particularly if their clothes become soiled
- With good stoma care skin excoriation can be kept to a minimum.

Contact dermatitis
- Patients may develop problems due to appliance-related contact dermatitis
- This may develop suddenly even with an appliance that has been used for years. This may also occur if the manufacturers change the chemical composition of the backing or base plate
- Early recognition and a change in the appliance is necessary
- Severe cases of contact dermatitis may require expert dermatology input
- Early and appropriate use of local steroid cream may quickly bring the inflamed skin under control. Barrier creams may also be used to protect the skin
- Failure to get the situation under rapid control amplifies the vicious cycle of stoma leakage and excoriation which is more difficult to treat and can undermine the confidence of the ostomist.

Nocturnal emptying and leakage
- 95% of colostomists do not need to get up during the night to empty their appliance. 60–70% of ileostomists empty their appliance at least once during the night.
- At 2yrs, ~10% of colostomists and nearly 20% of ileostomists experience soiling of their bed linen or bed clothes
- Although infrequent (occurring every 10–14 days), such episodes are distressing and place a major burden on the patient and their carer.

Pyoderma gangrenosum

- This is a serious condition, where early diagnosis is crucial to preventing further skin breakdown
- The peristomal ulceration with a dusky blue margin should be treated with high dose local and systemic steroids
- At the same time, barrier creams and fillers are used to prevent further breakdown of healthy skin
- If identified and treated early, the stoma can often be saved with little or no permanent scarring
- In severe cases it may be necessary to relocate the stoma. However, there is no guarantee that the process will not start again at the new site.

Perioperative care

Towards safer surgery

Adverse outcomes in surgical operations occur throughout the world. It is increasingly recognised that many such events can be prevented by relatively simple interventions. In 2008, the World Health Organization (WHO) first introduced its "WHO checklist". The importance of multidisciplinary team working was recognised in this checklist. The team, consisting of all members of the theatre nursing, medical and support staff work together as a single unit to ensure a series of simple safety checks are performed both before, during and after surgical operations. This list has undergone several iterations and has been complemented by the introduction of an additional pathway to reduce surgical site infections.

WHO Surgical Safety Checklist

- In a pilot study, mortality and inpatient complication rate was assessed both before and following introduction of the checklist. In total, 7,000 patients participated in the study
  - Mortality ↓ from 1.5% to 0.8% with use of the checklist
  - Inpatient complications ↓ from 11% to 7%
- Several studies have confirmed the profound positive impact of implementation of the WHO checklist (fig 10.1)
- The 19-item checklist is divided into 3 sections
  - Before induction of anaesthesia
  - Before skin incision
  - Before patient leaves the operating room
- With consistent use, all team members become familiar with the relevant checks and the team can work efficiently to go through the list for every patient. This is especially important for emergency operations when simple interventions such as administration of antibiotics may be forgotten

Surgical Site Infections (SSIs)

- SSIs are a cause of significant morbidity and cost to healthcare systems around the world
- In Europe, SSIs affect more than 500,000 people and cost up to €19 billion
- More than 10% of patients who undergo surgery in low- and middle-income countries get an SSI and 2 – 3% of surgical patients in high-income countries get an SSI
- In 2016, WHO produced a guideline with a view to increasing awareness of the burden of SSIs and providing evidence of best practice. The guidelines are categorised into strong and conditional recommendations

Fig 10.1 WHO Surgical Safety Checklist.
Reproduced with permission from WHO surgical safety checklist and implementation manual. Copyright © 2008, World Health Organization.

Strong guideline recommendations

- Patients carrying *S. aureus* on nasal swabs should be treated with intranasal mupirocin 2% ointment +/- body wash with chlorhexidine gluconate
- Mechanical bowel preparation (MBP) alone (without oral antibiotics) should not be used in elective colorectal surgery. A conditional recommendation states preoperative oral antibiotics combined with MBP should be used to reduce the risk of SSI in adult patients undergoing elective colorectal surgery
- In patients undergoing any surgical procedure, hair should not be removed unless absolutely necessary and that being the case, only a clipper should be used. Shaving is strongly discouraged
- Surgical antibiotic prophylaxis should be administered within 2 hours of the operations and before the skin incision
- Surgical hand preparation should be performed before donning sterile gloves using antimicrobial soap/water or an alcohol-based hand rub
- Alcohol-based antiseptic solutions containing chlorhexidine should be used for surgical site preparation
- Adults undergoing a GA should receive 80% fraction of inspired oxygen intraoperatively and for 2-6 hours postop
- Surgical antibiotic prophylaxis should not be continued after completion of the operation

References

Haynes AB, Weiser TG, Berry WR, Lipsitz SR, Breizat AH, Dellinger EP, et al. A surgical safety check-list to reduce morbidity and mortality in a global population. *N Engl J Med* 2009;**360**(5):491–9.

WHO Surgical Safety Checklist. Available at https://www.who.int/patientsafety/safesurgery/checklist/en/

WHO Global guidelines on the prevention of surgical site infection at https://www.who.int/gpsc/ssi-guidelines/en/

Tubes and drains

Nasogastric tubes

- NG tubes cause significant patient discomfort post-operatively
- NG tubes cause increased episodes of post-operative fever
- ↑ pulmonary complications including atelectasis and pneumonia
- NG tubes prolong duration of ileus and delay introduction of oral diet
- No evidence of ↑ anastomotic leak or hernia rates without NG tubes
- ~10% increase in vomiting/bloating without an NG tube.

Prophylactic use of an NG tube is not recommended for elective colorectal surgery.

An NG tube should be used selectively for patients with prolonged vomiting/ileus post-operatively.

Intra-abdominal drains

- Intraperitoneal drains may have an inhibitory effect on healing (Fig. 10.2)
- Drains quickly become encapsulated, leading to ↑ serous exudate
- Intraperitoneal drains may increase the rate of anastomotic leak
- Suction drainage should not be used in the peritoneal cavity
- Collections are more common low in the pelvis due to the surrounding dead space and lack of peritoneal resorption of fluid
- Drainage of low rectal anastomoses does not reduce leak rates
- Only ~5% of leaks are heralded through the drain
- Extraperitoneal drainage does not ameliorate the clinical effects of a leak
- No difference between suction and non-suction drainage in the pelvis.

There is little evidence to support the routine use of intra-/extraperitoneal drainage following elective colorectal resection.

Bladder catheterization

Indications for bladder catheterization include monitoring urine output and avoidance of post-operative urinary retention which can present in up to 50% of patients. Retention may be due to the effect of drugs, damage to pelvic autonomic nerves or loss of anatomical support of the bladder.

- Suprapubic catheterization causes less patient discomfort
- Suprapubic clamping allows easy trial of voiding per urethra
- Rates of UTI may be less with suprapubic catheterization when compared with prolonged use of a urethral catheter
- Early removal of urethral catheters reduces rates of UTI
- Post-operative retention is more common with low rectal cancers

Urinary catheters can be safely removed after 24h following colonic resection. After low anterior resection/abdominoperineal resection, 5 days of bladder drainage is recommended. This can be either urethral or suprapubic depending on preference.

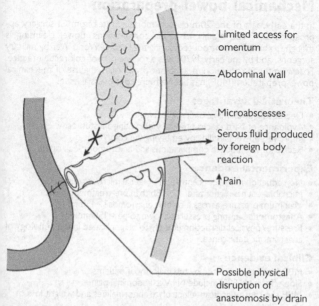

Fig. 10.2 Effect of intra-abdominal drains on healing.

References

Nelson R, Tse B, Edwards S. Systematic review of prophylactic nasogastric decompression after abdominal operations. *Br J Surg* 2005;**92**:673–680.

Urbach DR, Kennedy ED, Cohen MM. Colon and rectal anastomoses do not require routine drainage: a systematic review and meta-analysis. *Ann Surg* 1999;**229**:174–180.

Yeh CY, Changchien CR, Wang JY et al. Pelvic drainage and other risk factors for leakage after elective anterior resection in rectal cancer patients: a prospective study of 978 patients. *Ann Surg* 2005;**241**:9–13.

Perrin LC, Benoist S, Panis Y et al. Optimal duration of urinary drainage after rectal resection: a randomised controlled trial. *Surgery* 1999;125:135–141.

Mechanical bowel preparation

In the early part of the 20th century mortality rates from GI surgery approached 20% due mainly to septic complications. Bowel cleansing is thought to have been introduced during the Second World War by military surgeons, and by the early 1970s was a routine part of colorectal practice. Following the introduction of antibiotic prophylaxis, the use of mechanical bowel preparation (MBP) has been a more controversial issue.

Theoretical advantages
- Decreased intraluminal bacterial counts
- Avoidance of hard faeces physically disrupting anastomoses
- Improved bowel handling by emptying the colon
- Reduction of infective complications and anastomotic leak rates.

Experimental evidence
- No reduction in the concentration of faecal microorganisms
- Microbial counts higher after 12–18h than pre-treatment levels
- Maximum pressure across a colonic anastomosis ~45mmHg
- Anastomotic bursting pressures shown to be >150mmHg
- Pressure/physical disruption unlikely to be implicated in the aetiology of anastomotic dehiscence.

Clinical evidence
- MBP is poorly tolerated by the majority of patients
- Side effects in ~50% include N+V ± abdominal pain
- MBP can cause significant electrolyte abnormalities and weight loss of up to 1kg
- Dehydration typically requires 2–3litres of IV fluid to compensate
- Intraoperative spillage more common with MBP due to fluid bowel content in 50%
- Post-operative diarrhoea may be more common with MBP
- A metanalysis of 21,568 patients from 36 studies compared outcomes for MBP versus no MBP. It concluded there was
  - no difference in anastomotic leak rates
  - no difference in surgical site infections (SSI) or intra-abdominal collections
  - no difference in reoperation rates
  - no difference in hospital length of stay

Combined mechanical bowel preparation & oral antibiotics
- There has been a resurgence in interest in the role of a preoperative regimen of oral antibiotics (OAB) combined with MBP
- Typically, non-absorbed OAP are taken at the time of MBP and combined with IV systemic antibiotics at the time of surgery
- A meta-analysis of 38 randomized trials including 8,458 patients showed that MBP & OAB was associated with the lowest risk of SSI. OAB alone ranked next best and there was no difference between MBP only vs no preparation
- The OAB regimens usually include neomycin combined with erythromycin or metronidazole

Conclusions

- All patients should get a single dose of perioperative IV antibiotics
- MBP alone does not have an impact on risk of infectious complications and should not be used in isolation
- If a low rectal anastomosis with defunctioning ileostomy is being considered, some prefer to give MBP or an enema to empty rectum. However, there is no evidence that this improves outcomes
- Increasingly, consideration should be given to a regimen of MBP & OAP combined with systemic antibiotics for all patients undergoing colorectal surgery

Common agents

Bowel cleansing is still a requirement prior to colonoscopic examination. Adequate hydration is important before and during bowel cleansing whichever agent is used. Osmotic laxatives either draw fluid from the body into the bowel or retain the fluid they are administered with.

Polyethylene glycol

- Examples include Klean-prep® and Moviprep®
- 4litre solution affects tolerability and compliance
- The addition of electrolyte solution makes serious electrolyte disturbance rare
- Newer solutions which include ascorbic acid reduce effective volume to 2litres and may improve taste.

Sodium phosphate solution

- Examples include Fleet Phospho-soda®
- Taken in two 45ml doses 12–24h apart
- Bowel cleansing efficacy and patient compliance may be improved
- May lead to significant shifts in fluid and electrolytes
- Can cause hypernatraemia, hyperphosphataemia, hypocalcaemia and hypokalaemia
- Avoid in patients with cardiac or renal dysfunction.

Compound agents

- Examples include Picolax®
- Combining effects of stimulant and osmotic laxatives
- Sodium picosulphate (stimulant) and magnesium citrate (osmotic) most common

References

Rollins KE, Javanmard-Emamghissi H, Lobo DN (2018) Impact of mechanical bowel preparation in elective colorectal surgery: a meta-analysis. World J Gastroenterol 24:519–536

Toh JWT, Phan K, Hitos K. Association of mechanical bowel preparation and oral antibiotics before elective colorectal surgery with surgical site infection. A Network Meta-analysis. *JAMA Network Open* 2018;**1**(6):e183226

Antibiotic prophylaxis

The infective potential of colonic content was recognized well before colonic resection became commonplace. This bacterial reservoir consisting of high concentrations of aerobic and anaerobic bacteria becomes a potential source of infection after disruption of the mucosal barrier is brought about by surgery.

Criteria for antibiotic prophylaxis

- Reduce rates of post-operative infective complications by administration before contamination or evidence of infection
- Benefits must outweigh the risks of drug toxicity/side effects
- Antibiotics should be site specific, with activity against likely pathogens
- Specificity should reduce selective resistance
- Should maintain antibiotic concentration in the appropriate tissues for the duration of maximum risk.

Mortality rates are 2–3 times higher for patients who develop site-specific infections. It is also known to delay discharge for 1 week on average. The potential benefits of antibiotic prophylaxis are considerable.

Factors influencing antibiotic prophylaxis

- Wound infection is directly related to length of procedure
- Long operations using antibiotics with short half-life lead to more infective complications
- Repeated intraoperative dosing should be considered for long procedures or where there has been significant blood loss
- Surgery below the peritoneal reflection has a significantly higher risk of infective complications than colonic procedures
- Antibiotic prophylaxis reduces the rate of wound infection following colorectal surgery by ~50%
- Prophylaxis also reduces mortality rates by a similar margin
- Antibiotics should be administered <2hrs prior to the start of the operation
- Timing of administration is the most common error
- No improved efficacy between single, triple, or multiple doses
- Exact regimen should be guided by local infection control surveillance
- Most single-agent regimens are inadequate, including metronidazole, gentamicin, or a cephalosporin.

Single dose antibiotic prophylaxis should be administered on induction of anaesthesia. For GI procedures the combination of a cephalosporin and metronidazole or amoxicillin, gentamicin and metronidazole are of equivalent efficacy. Avoidance of cephalosporins may reduce rates of *C. difficile* infection.

References

Song F, Glenny AM. Antimicrobial prophylaxis in colorectal surgery: a systematic review of randomised controlled trials. *Br J Surg* 1998;**85**:1232–1241.

Classen DC, Evans RS, Pestotnik SL, Horn SD, Menlove RL, Burke JP. The timing of prophylactic administration of antibiotics and the risk of surgical-wound infection. *NEJM* 1992;**326**:281–286.

McDonald M, Grabsch E, Marshall C, Forbes A. Single- versus multiple- dose antimicrobial prophylaxis for major surgery: a systematic review. *ANZ J Surg* 1998;**68**:388–395.

Thromboprophylaxis

Venous thromboembolism can occur in up to 30% of colorectal patients without prophylactic measures. Increased rates of DVT following colorectal surgery may be due to increased length of procedure, positioning (Lloyd–Davies/lithotomy), pelvic dissection, malignancy or IBD.

DVT is often asymptomatic. Pulmonary embolism (PE), the most serious complication, can present in ~3% of patients. In 90% of these cases the DVT will have been asymptomatic. DVT can also lead to significant long-term morbidity, with up to 40% of patients suffering from post-thrombotic limb syndrome (chronic pain, swelling ± skin ulceration) within 3yrs. This is unrelated to the position of the DVT or whether it was symptomatic.

For these reasons thromboprophylaxis should be considered in all patients undergoing major colorectal procedures.

Risk factors

- Extent and length of procedure, age >60yrs, malignancy, medical co-morbidity, obesity, immobility, pregnancy, previous history of venous thromboembolism (VTE) or thrombophilia
- Consider stopping hormone preparations (hormone replacement therapy (HRT), combined oral contraceptive (COC)) prior to surgery.

Mechanical prophylaxis

- Graduated compressions stockings (GCS) reduce DVT rates by 50–70%
- GCS reduce venous cross-sectional area, increase blood velocity, and reduce intimal tears related to venodilatation
- Knee-length stockings may have equal efficacy to thigh length and are easier to put on, cheaper and better tolerated
- Intermittent pneumatic compression is of equal efficacy to GCS
- GCS is contraindicated with significant peripheral arterial disease or neuropathy
- Consider a caval filter if recent VTE and anticoagulation is contraindicated.

Pharmacological prophylaxis

- Prophylaxis with heparin reduces rates of DVT and PE by 50–70%
- Combined GCS and heparin has increased efficacy to either used alone
- LMWH and unfractionated heparin have equal efficacy
- LMWH allows once-daily dosing but is more expensive
- LMWH reduces rates of heparin-induced thrombocytopenia (HIT)
  - 50% reduction in platelet count
  - usually seen between day 5 and 10
  - Complication in <1% patients on LMWH
  - Thrombosis is the main risk
  - Oral anti-coagulation with warfarin should be considered
- Higher dose LMWH has greater efficacy than low dose
- Major bleeding complications in <2%, requiring re-operation in <0.2%
- Reversal of LMWH is with protamine but is less effective and difficult to monitor.

Extended prophylaxis after abdominopelvic cancer surgery

- Patients with cancer are at increased risk of VTE as malignancy is associated with a hypercoagulable state
- Abdominal or pelvic surgery for cancer further increases the risk
- VTE is an important cause of mortality in the first 30 days after patients undergo abdominopelvic surgery for cancer
- The risk of VTE is greatest 21 days after surgery
- Several prospective studies have shown that extended prophylaxis after abdominopelvic surgery for cancer can reduce the risk of VTE without increasing the risk of haemorrhagic complications
- UK and US based guidelines now promote the use of extended prophylaxis after major surgery.
- Typically, LMWH is given for at least 4 weeks

References

Agu O, Hamilton G, Baker D. Graduated compression stockings in the prevention of venous thromboembolism. *Br J Surg* 1999;**86**:992–1004.

National Institute of Health and Clinical Excellence. *Venous thromboembolism in over 16s: reducing the risk of hospital-acquired deep venous thrombosis or pulmonary embolism*. London: NICE Guideline (NG89), 2018.

Perioperative nutrition

Introduction

- The reported incidence of malnutrition in hospital in-patients varies between 15 and 40%
- Malnutrition increases the risk of wound dehiscence, respiratory failure, DVT, infectious complications and prolonged hospital stay.

Many studies include both patients in whom nutritional support is mandatory because they cannot take enough orally and those who are treated with nutritional support in addition to oral intake. It would be unethical to randomize the former group to starvation, but this has made the literature difficult to interpret.

It is generally accepted that enteral is superior to parenteral nutrition:

- More physiological
- Simpler
- Cheaper
- Fewer serious complications.

However, more complex approaches to enteral feeding such as PEG, nasojejunal tubes and jejunostomy do carry higher risks, and even the commonly used NG tube feeding can cause death, most often due to tube misplacement. It is important to consider the risks and benefits of any proposed nutritional support in the individual patient.

Goals of perioperative nutritional support

- Attenuate hypermetabolic response
- Reverse loss of lean body mass
- Prevent oxidative stress
- Modulate immune response (glutamine, arginine + omega 3 fatty acids)
- Ensure tight glycaemic control to reduce infectious complications.

Nutritional screening

- Should be performed in all surgical patients by admitting nursing staff, ideally in a pre-operative assessment clinic
- The British Association for Parenteral and Enteral Nutrition has developed the Malnutrition Universal Screening Tool (MUST)
- High risk patients identified by screening should be referred to dietetics or a nutrition support team
- Post-operative nutritional support must be considered for patients who cannot tolerate adequate oral diet for 7–10 days if well nourished and 5–7 days if malnourished.

Pre-operative nutritional support

- Reduced pre-operative fasting times and carbohydrate loading in enhanced recovery programmes
- Severely malnourished patients (weight loss >10% in 6 months) should have 7–10 days pre-operative nutritional support if possible
- Severely malnourished patient will be at risk of re-feeding syndrome and require close monitoring of serum phosphate, magnesium and other electrolyte levels as nutrition is commenced
- Pre-operative nutritional support should be enteral if possible

- Pre-operative PN has been demonstrated to reduce post-operative complications by 10% in malnourished patients but not in those whose nutritional status was deemed adequate.
- Improved mortality has not been demonstrated.

Post-operative nutritional support

- Early enteral feeding is effective and safe in the immediate post-operative period
- Post-operative PN has no effect on complications or mortality rate in non-malnourished patients
- Post-operative enteral nutrition reduces complications and mortality in malnourished/non-malnourished patients undergoing major surgery.

Methods of perioperative nutritional support

- Excess IV fluids should not be given in the post-operative period as this has been shown to increase GI dysfunction and prolong hospital stay.
- Nutritional requirements should be calculated by a dietician. The optimum calorie target is debated but gross under provision of nitrogen and calories is detrimental and overfeeding increases septic complications and liver dysfunction
- If tolerated, oral supplements are as effective at meeting nutritional requirements and reducing complications as enteral tube feeding
- In colorectal surgery, early NG feeding may be used safely provided the patient does not have marked small bowel ileus
- Gastric emptying is often reduced in the critically ill but usually enteral feeding is still possible via a nasojejunal tube
- Parenteral nutrition should only be used if enteral nutrition is impossible, e.g. small bowel ileus, recent onset of high output small bowel fistula with intra-abdominal sepsis, short bowel syndrome
- If PN is essential it should be given via a dedicated line and supervised by a nutrition support team
- Some trials have shown a reduction in complication rates, particularly wound infection and prolonged hospital stay, if enteral immunonutrition is used
- The place of parenteral glutamine supplementation is controversial and should probably only be considered in the critically ill.

References

Weimann A, Braga M, Harsanyi L et al. ESPEN guidelines on enteral nutrition: surgery including organ transplantation. Clin Nutr 2006;**25**:224–244.

Malnutrition Universal Screening Tool Report. BAPEN Publications. ISBN 1 899 467 710X.

Analgesia

After colorectal resection patients will usually require parenteral analgesia at least for the first 48h. The two most common strategies are
patient-controlled analgesia morphine (PCA) and epidural analgesia (EA).
Combination therapy with simple analgesic adjuncts can improve analgesia
and allow reductions in opioid administration.

Thoracic epidurals

LAs and/or opioids are delivered through a fine catheter into the epidural
space. For colorectal procedures thoracic epidural around the T8 level is
important.

Theoretical benefits
- Blocks nociceptive afferents and sympathetic efferent nerves which may
  reduce pain and improve GI motility
- Reduced adrenaline, noradrenaline, adrenocorticotrophic hormone,
  cortisol, aldosterone, and glucose suggest a reduction in the surgical
  stress response.

Clinical endpoints
- EA significantly reduces post-operative ileus
- Evidence suggests EA is superior to PCA morphine
- Combination epidurals with LA + opioid give the best analgesia and
  allow dose reduction due to synergistic effect
- Patient-controlled EA may improve analgesia over continuous regimes
- No difference in hospital stay, morbidity (including respiratory
  complications) or mortality with EA compared with PCA
- No evidence of increase in anastomotic leak rates with use of EA (may
  actually increase splanchnic blood flow).

Complications
- Failure rate can be as high as 20–40%, with the most common reasons
  including failed insertion, inadequate analgesia, and dislodged catheters
- Hypotension can be treated using altered thresholds, fluid boluses or
  vasopressors
- Epidural haematoma/abscess is rare (~1 in 1,000)
- Alteration of anticoagulants/thromboprophylaxis must be carefully
  considered.

PCA morphine

- Opioid of choice (usually morphine) is delivered by IV route
- Safety and efficacy well established, with >20 years experience
- Bolus dose, lockout period and a maximum dose can be set
- Respiratory depression and total dose are reduced compared with IM
  delivery of opioid
- Complications include N+V, pruritis, constipation and sedation.

Alternative approaches

- LA wound catheters have little efficacy for midline wounds but may have a role in transverse wounds
- Transversus abdominus plane (TAP) block has shown promising results although these have not yet been reproduced in other centres
- NSAIDs in the absence of contraindications and acetaminophen are useful adjuncts in an opioid-sparing regime
- Most hospitals will have a local analgesic policy and may have a dedicated pain team.

References

Marret E, Remy C, Bonnet F. Meta-analysis of epidural analgesia versus parenteral opioid analgesia after colorectal surgery. Br J Surg 2007;**94**:665–673.

Jorgenson H, Wetterslev J, Moiniche S, Dahl JB. Epidural local anaesthetics versus opioid-based analgesic regimens for postoperative gastrointestinal paralysis, PONV and pain after abdominal surgery. Cochrane Database Syst Rev 2005;(**3**).

Rigg JRA, Jamrozik K, Myles PS et al. Epidural anaesthesia and analgesia and outcome of major surgery: a randomised trial. Lancet 2002;**359**:1276–1282.

McDonnell JG, O'Donnell B, Curley G, Heffernan A, Power C, Laffey J. The analgesic efficacy of transversus abdominis plane block after abdominal surgery: a prospective randomized controlled trial. Anesth Analg 2007;**104**:193–197.

Laparoscopic colorectal surgery

Laparoscopic colonic resection was first described in the early 1990s but has taken some time to become established within surgical practice, particularly in the UK. Various reasons are attributed to this, including initial concerns about the oncological safety of the technique and the steep initial learning curve. These fears have, however, been overcome by the publication of a number of high profile multicentre RCTs.

Evidence from multicentre RCTs

- Equivalent oncological outcomes to the open approach, i.e. cancer-related survival, LN retrieval, resection margins or recurrence rates
- No ↑ in rate of wound recurrence (<1%)
- Improved short-term outcomes
  - Reduced blood loss
  - Reduced post-operative ileus and earlier resumption of diet
  - Less post-operative pain and reduced analgesic requirements
  - Shorter hospital stay
  - Faster return to normal activities
- Increased theatre costs offset by savings from faster recovery
- Increased operating time
- No definitive difference in long-term outcomes has yet been proven
  - Cosmesis may be improved but trial evidence is lacking
  - Conflicting evidence regarding incisional hernia and post-operative adhesions.

In the light of this evidence confidence has grown, aided in part by the widespread adoption of enhanced recovery programmes (◑ Enhanced recovery p.498). While not exclusive to the laparoscopic approach, these have acted as a 'bridge' in both its inception and propagation within the UK.

Laparoscopic training

Due to the initial technical difficulties encountered, only 'early adopters' embraced the technique. As technology has improved with the advent of high definition optical systems and acceptance of modern training methods, we have seen a quantum leap in uptake of the technique.

- Online resources are available for trainees to improve experience, e.g. websurg (www.websurg.com)
- Simulators allow practice in a virtual environment before moving to the wet labs/cadaver labs to perfect techniques
- Latterly there has been formalization of training with the advent of training fellowships and a national training programme for England (www.lapco.nhs.uk).

Improvements to the facilitation of the technique have allowed the issue of surgical training to be largely overcome. It should always be remembered, however, that these are complex, challenging operations with a long learning curve for those starting without a sound basis in laparoscopic surgery.

National guidelines (UK)

NICE in guidance regarding laparoscopic and laparoscopically assisted resection state that:

- it is recommended as an alternative to open resection for individuals with colorectal cancer in whom both laparoscopic and open surgery are considered suitable
- the decision about which surgical technique is employed should be made after an informed discussion between the patient and the surgeon
- laparoscopic surgery should only be performed by surgeons who have completed appropriate training, and who perform the procedures often enough to maintain competence.

References

The Clinical Outcomes of Surgical Therapy Study Group. A comparison of laparoscopically assisted and open colectomy for colon cancer. *N Engl J Med* 2004;**350**:2050–2059.

Guillou PJ, Quirke P, Thorpe H, Walker J, Jayne DG, Smith AM, Heath RM, Brown JM. Short-term endpoints of conventional versus laparoscopic-assisted surgery in patients with colorectal cancer (MRC CLASICC trial): multicentre randomised controlled trial. *Lancet* 2005;**365**:1718–1726.

Veldkamp R, Kuhry E, Hop WC et al. Colon cancer Laparoscopic or Open Resection Study Group (COLOR). Laparoscopic surgery versus open surgery for colon cancer: short-term outcomes of a randomised trial. *Lancet Oncol* 2005;**6**:477–484.

Abraham NS, Young JM, Solomon MJ. Meta-analysis of short-term outcomes after laparoscopic resection for colorectal cancer. *Br J Surg* 2004;**91**:1111–1124.

National Institute for Health and Clinical Excellence. *Laparoscopic surgery for colorectal cancer (review). (Technology appraisal 105)*. London: NICE, 2006.

Robotic colorectal surgery

The first robotic procedure was performed in 1985 when the PUMA 560 robotic surgical arm was used to perform a brain biopsy. The da Vinci® system was the first to perform a robotic cholecystectomy in 1997 and has been the dominant platform worldwide. The current version of the platform, the Xi system, offers 3D HD imaging with an 8mm scope that can be changed to different ports, rapid laser guided docking, integrated table motion and integrated fluorescence capability to assess blood flow and tissue perfusion.

Over the last decade there has been an exponential increase in robot-assisted surgery, particularly in prostatectomy and gynaecologic surgery. Currently it is estimated that there are 800 robots in Europe and more than 6 million robotic surgeries have been performed worldwide. The first report of a robotic colorectal resection was published in 2002. There has been a slower increase in the number of robotic colorectal procedures and particular interest has focused on robotic rectal cancer surgery.

Potential benefits of robotic surgery

Robotic surgery confers all the advantages of laparoscopic surgery with additional benefits specific to the robotic approach.

- Improved visualisation using a stable 3D high definition platform
  - Enhanced depth perception and greater magnification
  - Precise orientation and adjustment of the camera associated with less fatigue and eye strain
  - Greater definition of anatomic structures may improve safety
- Greater dexterity and range of movement in instruments facilitates surgical accuracy and the technical conduct of operation
  - Enhanced movement in wristed instruments enable 180° of articulation and 540° degrees of rotation
  - Tremor filtering eliminates physiological movement
  - Ultraprecise movement is possible by reducing the ratio of instrument movement in relation to surgeon's wrist movement
  - May translate to improved outcomes for surgery in narrow confined spaces e.g. rectal cancer surgery in the obese male with a narrow pelvis
- Improved ergonomics reduces surgeon fatigue
- Fixed retraction and camera view reduces reliance on experienced assistance
- Some studies have suggested that robotic surgery may be associated with less pain compared even to laparoscopic surgery. This may be related to reduced port movement and instrument torque on the abdominal wall as robotic systems automatically pivot movement at the level of the abdominal wall
- Intra-operative assessment of blood flow can help predict safe healing of gastrointestinal anastomoses

Limitations of robotic surgery

- Lack of tactile feedback is one of the most important drawbacks of current robotic systems
  - Surgeons adapt through conscious and unconscious visual clues e.g. degree of deformation of tissues
  - Researchers are attempting to use similar visual clues to develop computer-generated pseudo-haptic feedback in robotic systems
- The huge capital and ongoing costs of robotic systems have been a substantial bar to the development of robotic colorectal surgery
  - Newer robotic systems offer the promise of lower capital and ongoing costs
  - Procedural costs may be offset by increasing proportions of minimally invasive procedures and further reduction of hospital stay, conversions, complications, and readmission.
- Increased operative time is required to setup and dock the robot.
  - This issue has been addressed with newer and faster robotic systems that dock rapidly and allow changes in table position with automatic adjustment of camera and instrument angles

Training in robotic surgery

The learning curve for an experienced open surgeon progressing to laparoscopic colorectal surgery ranges from 30-100 cases. However, it is only 15-45 cases for an experienced laparoscopic surgeon learning robotic colorectal surgery. There is evidence that a structured program of proctoring and mentoring enables surgeons to rapidly progress in their training while minimizing the risk of adverse outcomes during training.

- Well-structured training programs have been developed in the USA (Fundamentals of Robotic Surgery) and Europe (European Academy of Robotic Colorectal Surgery (EARCS)
- The EARCS program uses a proficiency based structured program of theoretical and practical training modules, hands-on robotic training using computer simulations, and supervised proctoring

Evidence to support robotic colorectal surgery

- Most studies have found comparable short-term clinical outcomes for robotic rectal cancer surgery compared to laparoscopic surgery. These include blood loss, length of stay and postoperative complications.
- In 2017, the Robotic vs. Laparoscopic Resection for Rectal Cancer (ROLARR) trial reported its results. This important, large multi-national study was criticised on a number of counts but most importantly, because it was underpowered to demonstrate a significant difference in its primary end-point of a difference in conversion rates between the two arms. Secondary end points included quality of TME, CRM positivity, complications, quality of life at 6 months, mortality and bladder/ sexual function. It noted that
  - No significant difference in conversion rates for robotic versus laparoscopic surgery (8.1% versus 12.2%)
  - No difference in secondary end points

- A trend towards reduced conversion rates in obese patients and in males with lower 1/3 tumours
- Given the increased cost, it was concluded that robotic rectal cancer surgery could not be justified
- A 2018 meta-analysis of 5 randomised trials comparing robotic versus laparoscopic rectal cancer surgery, reported
  - No difference in quality of surgery markers such as quality of TME specimen, CRM positivity rates or lymph nodes harvested
  - No difference in complications such as mortality and anastomotic leak rate
  - Reduced risk of conversion to open surgery
  - Increased operative time

Despite these results, many surgeons point to the fact that technology has moved on and the outcomes of surgery with the latest Xi version are even better than the Si version (which was used for most of the preceding studies).

They also point out that some studies have shown improved nerve preservation, less pain, shorter length of stay and lower conversion rates. Lower conversion rates are an especially important in those who would benefit most for a minimally invasive approach i.e. obese, male patients with lower 1/3 cancers. It seems that robotic rectal cancer surgery is here to stay and increasing experience and better technology will better outcomes.

The future

- The "Robot-assisted Surgery and Laparoscopy-assisted Surgery in patients with Mid or Low Rectal Cancer (COLRAR)" trial finished recruiting in December 2018. Primary outcomes will be quality of the TME specimen and secondary outcomes include complications, pelvic nerve preservation and 5 year survival figures. It is expected to provide definitive answer regarding the benefit if any of robotic rectal surgery
- Several novel robotic systems are either in development or have recently been launched. Some systems are based on the robotic-laparo-endoscopic single-site surgery (R-LESS) concept such as the Sport surgical system from Titan robot. Others have focused on developing a low cost modular design such as the CMT Versius® robotic system, which is small, portable and can be moved easily to different operating theatres.

References

Jayne D, Pigazzi A, Marshall H, et al. Effect of Robotic-Assisted vs Conventional Laparoscopic Surgery on Risk of Conversion to Open Laparotomy Among Patients Undergoing Resection for Rectal Cancer: The ROLARR Randomized Clinical Trial. Jama 2017;**318**:1569–80.

Prete FP, Pezzolla A, Prete F, et al. Robotic Versus Laparoscopic Minimally Invasive Surgery for Rectal Cancer: A Systematic Review and Meta-analysis of Randomized Controlled Trials. Ann Surg 2018;**267**:1034–46

Enhanced recovery after surgery

Introduction

Enhanced recovery after surgery (ERAS) is an idea popularized by Prof. Henrik Kehlet (Denmark). The aim of the approach is to attenuate the surgical stress response and reduce end organ dysfunction through an integrated recovery pathway. This pathway should incorporate perioperative strategies with a proven evidence base to reduce hospital stay following surgery and allow a quicker return to baseline function. While the success of a single strategy in isolation may be limited, as part of a multimodal rehabilitation regime the potential benefits are significant.

Introduction of an enhanced recovery protocol requires multidisciplinary support. It can be applied to a wide range of surgical procedures and does not require patient selection. Using a typical enhanced recovery protocol outlined below, significant improvements in perioperative recovery can be achieved.

Preadmission care

- Extended preadmission information, education, and counselling
- Preoperative optimization
  - Optimise medical conditions. Consider medical risk assessment including cardiopulmonary exercise testing if higher risk
  - Encourage smoking cessation for at least four weeks
  - Avoid alcohol abuse (preoperative abstinence for four weeks)
- Prehabilitation
  - May expedite recovery of functional capacity and reduce complications
  - May be of particular benefit in less fit patients
- Preoperative nutritional care
- Management of anaemia
  - Anaemia is a risk factor for complications and mortality
  - Transfusion may also have a negative impact on outcomes
  - Oral or IV therapy should be considered in anaemic patients

Preoperative optimisation

- Prevention of post-operative nausea and vomiting (PONV)
  - Use a multimodal approach to identify risk factors and administer single or multiple agent prophylactic antiemetics as appropriate
  - Early administration of different salvage antiemetic drugs if PONV occurs
- Avoid routine preoperative sedative medication
- Single dose preoperative antibiotics
- Skin preparation with chlorhexidine-alcohol
- Mechanical bowel preparation (see page 482)
- Avoid unnecessary preoperative fasting and ensure patients are normovolaemic on arrival to theatre
  - 6 hours fasting for solids: 2 hours fasting for liquids
  - Preoperative carbohydrate drinks taken up to 2 hours before induction of anaesthesia

Intraoperative optimisation

- Short acting anaesthetic agents should be used
- High inspired oxygen concentration
- Intraoperative fluid optimisation
  - Aim for perioperative near-zero fluid balance
  - Goal-directed fluid therapy (GDFT) may be considered where large fluid shifts are expected or co-morbidity is significant
- Intraoperative normothermia should be maintained
  - Avoid intraoperative hypothermia. Use active warming
- Use a minimally invasive approach if feasible
  - Laparoscopic or robotic approach is associated with a fast recovery, fewer complications, and a reduced requirement for post-operative analgesia
- Avoid post-operative nasogastric tubes and intra-abdominal and pelvic drains

Postoperative optimisation

- Use an opiate-sparing analgesic regimen
  - Multimodal analgesia combined with spinal/epidural analgesia or TAP blocks
- DVT prophylaxis
  - Use compression stockings in hospital
  - LMWH in hospital. Consider extending to 28 days in patients with cancer or pelvic surgery
- Aim for net near-zero fluid and electrolyte balance
  - Use balanced salt/hypotonic crystalloid solutions. Avoid 0.9% saline
- Balanced anti-emetic regimen
- Earlier removal of urinary catheter
- Optimise post-operative nutritional care
  - Oral diet from day one with regular protein-rich drinks
  - Consider immunonutrition
- Prevent post-operative ileus
  - Adopt a multimodal approach
  - Limit opiates (minimally invasive surgery will reduce the need for post-operative analgesia and opiates)
  - Bowel simulation with laxatives, chewing gum, coffee etc
- Active mobilisation following a structured program from day 1

Outcomes

There is good evidence to recommend many of these interventions. However, it is not possible to individually test the contribution of all these measures. When taken as a whole, significant improvements in perioperative recovery can be achieved when using an ERAS protocol as outlined above. Some of the proven benefits include

- Reduced postoperative ileus
- Shorter hospital stay
- Reduced post-operative morbidity
- Less reduction of lean body mass

- Improved post-operative exercise performance
- Less fatigue
- Earlier resumption of normal activities
- Reduced healthcare costs
- No increased burden on primary care
- With fast-track surgery hospital stays of 2–3 days following colorectal resection are achievable.

References

Basse L, Hjort J, Dorthe RN, Billesbolle P, Werner M, Kehlet H. A clinical pathway to accelerate recovery after colonic resection. *Ann Surg* 2000;**232**:51–57.

MacKay G, Molloy RG, O' Dwyer PJ. Fast-track colorectal surgery and perioperative outcomes. *Semin Colon Rectal Surg* 2008;**19**:16–19.

Gustafsson UO, Scott MJ, Hubner M et al. Guidelines for perioperative care in elective colorectal surgery: Enhanced Recovery After Surgery (ERAS) Society recommendations: 2018. *World J Surg* 2019: **43**: 659–695

General complications

The best management of complications is prevention where possible. When complications do occur, they are often part of a cascade, with prolonged hospital stay and poorer outcome as the end result.

Wound infection

Infection of the wound after surgery is commonly referred to as a surgical site infection (SSI) and may be *superficial incisional* (skin/subcutaneous tissue), *deep incisional* (fascial/muscle layers) or *organ or space infection*.

SSIs account for ~15% of nosocomial infections, affecting ~5% of patients following operation, with higher rates for colorectal surgery (10–15%). Morbidity related to SSIs is varied, including higher rates of re-operation, prolonged hospital stay, increased healthcare costs, functional impairment, poor cosmetic outcome, and psychological disturbance.

Pathogenesis
- Dependent on the interaction between contamination of the wound with microorganisms and the host immune response
- Contamination is most frequently by endogenous organisms, with pathogenicity important in determining eventual outcome
- Inoculation may be during the procedure or in the post-operative course prior to complete wound healing.

Risk factors

↑ *risk of endogenous contamination*
- Surgical site, e.g. clean, clean-contaminated, contaminated, dirty
- Remote site infection/colonization, e.g. methicillin-resistant *Staphylococcus aureus* (MRSA)
- Prolonged pre-operative stay, pre-operative shaving

↑ *risk of exogenous contamination*
- Prolonged operation time, poor aseptic technique.

Reduced immune response
- ↑ age, diabetes, malignancy, malnutrition, chemotherapy, immunosuppressives, intraoperative haemorrhage, emergency surgery, FB, tissue damage/ischaemia, obesity, smoking.

Prevention
- If hair removal is required, this should be with electric clippers using a single-use head immediately prior to surgery
- Antibiotic prophylaxis has previously been discussed (➋ Antibiotic prophylaxis p.484) and is recommended for all patients undergoing colorectal surgery
- Full sterile technique is used with sterile gloves, gowns, and drapes. Double gloving is recommended for deep-cavity surgery
- Skin antisepsis using povidone–iodine or chlorhexidine solution
- Maintain perioperative temperature, oxygenation and euvolaemia
- Close blood glucose control is important for diabetic patients
- Positive pressure theatre ventilation, appropriate air filtration and reducing movement in and out of theatre play a role
- A sterile wound dressing should be considered for the first 48h, with any dressing change carried out using aseptic technique.

Management
- Frequently wound discharge does not represent active infection but simply tissue exudate or delayed healing. Inappropriate antibiotic prescribing is common
- Adequate drainage is often all that is required, which may be facilitated by removal of sutures/skin clips
- Cellulitis/signs of systemic sepsis may require administration of antibiotics with a spectrum appropriate for the most likely pathogens and guided by local microbiology advice. An attempt should be made to culture causative organisms to direct antibiotic therapy.
- Management of open wounds may require input from the local tissue viability service.

Wound dehiscence

Superficial wound dehiscence describes a separation of the wound above the musculoaponeurotic level and is a common complication of abdominal wounds. It may be related to wound infection, haematoma, seroma, delayed wound healing and suture failure. Fascial dehiscence is a less frequent (~1%) but more serious post-operative complication.
- Risk factors are similar to those for wound infection, including increasing co-morbidity and abdominal distension
- Surgical technique is thought to be the most important determinant.

Prevention
- Optimization of medical co-morbidities, nutritional status and advising smoking cessation represent good practice, although effect on reducing risk of dehiscence is unclear
- Expedient surgery, secure haemostasis, antibiotic prophylaxis, normothermia and tissue oxygenation may contribute to ↓ risk of dehiscence
- The single most important factor is wound closure technique with mass closure using appropriate suture material, evenly spaced bites, without undue tension and a suture to wound ratio of 4:1.

Management
- Fascial dehiscence occurs at a mean of day 8 and may be heralded by a pink serosanguinous discharge
- Evisceration should be controlled with saline or povidone–iodine soaked swabs and an adhesive binding
- Resuscitation, IV antibiotics and prompt return to theatre should be arranged
- Simple technical failure may simply be re-sutured
- Interrupted sutures alone or in combination with a continuous suture may be preferred to limit the effect of sutures cutting out
- Failure associated with sepsis or raised intra-abdominal pressure may require staged secondary closure using absorbable mesh to maintain the abdominal contents or management as an open laparostomy
- Mortality of 25% reflects the level of co-morbidity and systemic upset often associated with the condition.

Haemorrhage

- Commonly subgrouped into 1° (<48h) and 2° (>48h) post-operative haemorrhage
- Primary causes include inadvertent visceral injury (e.g. spleen, liver), slipped ligature, suture/staple line bleeding or from unsealed vessels following post-operative vasodilatation (re-warming and resuscitation) or release of positive pressure (laparoscopy)
- Secondary haemorrhage is related to infection and vessel erosion
- There is no substitute for meticulous intraoperative haemostasis
- If difficult to control, e.g. pelvic bleeding, consider packing to allow time for resuscitation and reversal of coagulopathy. Packs can be removed after 24–48h
- Haemorrhage should be excluded in patients displaying hypotension in the post-operative period.

Chest infection/atelectasis

- Post-operative respiratory compromise includes ↓forced expiratory volume in 1s (FEV_1), ↓forced vital capacity (FVC), ↓functional residual capacity (FRC) and less effective clearance of airway secretions
- Airway closure leads to ventilation/perfusion mismatch, atelectasis and predisposes to infection
- Risk factors include smoking, COPD, ↑ age, obesity, and upper abdominal incisions
- Smoking cessation and pre-operative optimization of respiratory function should be considered where time permits
- Deep breathing exercises and incentive spirometry may reduce risk
- An enhanced recovery regime should be used where possible to optimize analgesia and encourage early mobilization (Ↄ Enhanced recovery p.498)
- Signs of established infection include tachypnoea, pyrexia, productive cough, cyanosis, coarse crepitations and bronchial breathing typically presenting around the 3rd post-operative day
- Management consists of upright positioning, humidified oxygen, chest physiotherapy with sputum samples for microbiology and antibiotics as per hospital protocol for hospital-acquired pneumonia. Nebulized saline and bronchodilators may also be required
- Acute segmental/lung collapse due to mucus plugging may require bronchoscopy and bronchial lavage.

DVT/PE

- DVT and PE are discussed with thromboprophylaxis (Ↄ Thromboprophylaxis p.486).

Urinary tract infection/retention

- UTI is a common post-operative complication closely related to route and duration of catheterization (risk ↑ 3–10%/day)
- Urinary catheters should be removed after <48h where possible to reduce risk of UTI
- Common pathogens include *E. coli* (65–80%), *Proteus*, *Klebsiella*, *Enterobacter*, *Candida*, enterococci, *Pseudomonas*, and coagulase-negative staphylococci
- Dysuria, frequency, urgency, and sensation of incomplete emptying may be presenting features. There may be lower abdominal or loin pain. In the elderly, acute confusion is sometimes the only sign
- Investigation is by urinalysis looking for nitrites and leucocytes and culture of a midstream specimen of urine (MSSU)
- Treatment is empirical until antibiotic sensitivities are available
- Catheterization and retention have previously been covered (→ Tubes and drains p.480).

Acute confusion

- More common in patients >65yrs (incidence 5–26% after abdominal surgery)
- Associated with ↑ morbidity, ↑ hospital stay, ↑ use of rehabilitation services and possibly long-term post-operative cognitive dysfunction
- Common causes include:
  - Hypoxia, e.g. oversedation, respiratory compromise
  - Sepsis
  - Drugs, e.g. opiates, polypharmacy
  - Acute alcohol withdrawal
  - Electrolyte disturbance
  - Unrecognized dementia
  - An underlying complication should be actively excluded by history examination, blood work-up, electrocardiography (ECG), CXR, urinalysis and MSSU
- Management involves treatment of the underlying condition. Sedation and psychiatric evaluation may be required.

Post-operative hepatic dysfunction, renal failure and cardiovascular abnormalities may complicate the perioperative course but are not covered in detail in this text.

Post-operative ileus

After surgery, the GI tract takes time to recover coordinated propulsive activity. This delay in functional recovery is often referred to as post-operative ileus. The speed of recovery varies for different parts of the alimentary tract (Fig. 10.3). Ileus prolonged past 3 days is sometimes called paralytic ileus but may be part of the same condition. Ileus is common after colorectal surgery but can be associated with a wide range of procedures, orthopaedic trauma and retroperitoneal pathology.

Complications of post-operative ileus
- Abdominal pain, N+V
- Abdominal distension, absent bowel sounds, delayed defecation
- Reluctance to mobilize
- Delayed introduction of oral diet
- Prolongation of hospital stay with increased cost.

Pathophysiology
- Multifactorial and incompletely understood
- Inhibitory reflex arcs with afferents from somatic, visceral, and parietal fibres
- Parasympathetic, sympathetic, and intrinsic nervous systems involved
- Inflammatory mediators, endogenous and exogenous opioids play a role
- Parietal peritoneum thought to be particularly important.

Factors influencing ileus
- No clear evidence that handling of the intestines affects ileus
- Duration of ileus not related to extent, site, or duration of operation
- Early oral diet and mobilization do not affect duration
- NG tubes and opioid analgesia prolong ileus
- Fluid excess can prolong ileus through GI mucosal oedema
- Epidural analgesia is the most effective intervention to reduce ileus
- Minimally invasive surgery and pre-operative counselling may reduce ileus
- Peripherally selective opioid antagonists may have a role
- Laxatives, erythromycin, metoclopramide, neostigmine, and cholecystokinin have shown either equivocal or negative results.

Treatment of ileus
- Prevention using epidural + opioid-sparing analgesia, fluid optimization and an enhanced recovery protocol ± minimally invasive surgery
- Treatment is supportive and may include a 'drip and suck' regime
- Return of bowel sounds is NOT a good predictor of resolution of ileus/tolerance of oral diet
- Early oral diet is tolerated by the majority of patients post-operatively.

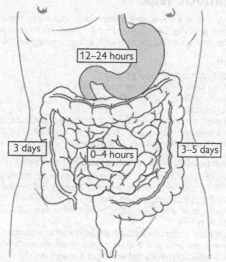

Fig. 10.3 Duration of post-operative ileus.

References

Graber JN, Schulte WJ, Condon RE, Cowles VE. Relationship of duration of postoperative ileus to extent and site of operative dissection. *Surgery* 1982;**92**:87–92.

Bredtmann RD, Herden HN, Teichmann W *et al.* Epidural analgesia in colonic surgery: results of a randomised prospective study. *Br J Surg* 1990;**77**:638–642.

Neudecker J, Schwenk W, Junghans T, Pietsch S, Bohm B, Muller JM. Randomised controlled trial to examine the influence of thoracic epidural analgesia. *Br J Surg* 1999;**86**:1292–1295.

Basse L, Madsen JL, Billesbolle P, Bardram L, Kehlet H. Gastrointestinal transit after laparoscopic vs open colonic resection. *Surg Endosc* 2003;**17**:1919–1922.

Anastomotic leak

Anastomotic leak is a devastating complication and a significant cause of morbidity and mortality following colorectal surgery. Incidence ranges from 1 to 20% depending on criteria used, with an average rate of 3–6%.

Definition

Definitions of anastomotic failure include:
- Generalized peritonitis requiring reoperation
- Faecal discharge from the wound/drain
- Localized abscess
- Extravasation of contrast on CT or water-soluble contrast enema in an otherwise asymptomatic patient. The incidence of radiological leak is higher than the rate of clinically apparent anastomotic failure.

Factors associated with anastomotic breakdown

Knowledge of associated risk factors is important to help surgical decision-making, and in particular when to form a defunctioning stoma. A defunctioning stoma reduces both the rate of symptomatic leakage and the consequences of a leak, including re-operation rate (➲ Classification and indications p.444).

- The single most important factor associated with anastomotic breakdown is the level of the anastomosis. Anastomoses below the peritoneal reflection have a higher rate of leakage. A defunctioning stoma should be considered for low anastomoses
- Patient-related risk factors include medical co-morbidity (↑ American Society of Anesthesiologists (ASA) score), advanced age, smoking, alcohol use, malnutrition, vitamin deficiency (particularly vitamin C), steroid use, male sex, obesity
- Operative factors include infection in the operative field, tension on the anastomosis, an inadequate blood supply to either proximal or distal end, prolonged operation time and intraoperative blood transfusion
- Blood supply at an anastomosis is reduced in the normal situation. If it is further compromised by hypotension, hypovolaemia or platelet aggregation this may increase the chance of breakdown
- The effect of neoadjuvant treatment on anastomotic failure is unclear, with contradictory evidence in the published literature. A majority of surgeons perform a diverting stoma after TME in patients treated with neoadjuvant chemoradiotherapy.
- Factors not associated with reduced anastomotic leak include: mechanical bowel preparation, hand-sewn vs stapled anastomosis, open vs laparoscopic surgery, omental wrapping of anastomoses, surgical drains, early feeding, and epidural analgesia.

Presentation

- The patient may simply fail to progress. There may be a persistent ileus, tachycardia, ↑ CRP or leucocytosis. A high index of suspicion is vital to facilitate early and aggressive management
- <50% of anastomotic leaks present with classical abdominal pain, peritonitis, fever and leucocytosis
- Leakage may be heralded by apparently unrelated cardiac symptoms
- Mean time to diagnosis is day 7.

Investigation

- The value of investigations depends on the clinical picture
- If the picture is clearly one of dehiscence with a rapidly deteriorating patient, time should not be wasted on investigations. The patient should be taken back to theatre for repeat laparotomy
- If the picture is unclear or the patient is not progressing, CT may identify free intraperitoneal air or leakage of rectal contrast in a patient with a left-sided anastomosis. Alternatively, water-soluble contrast enema may be carried out (Fig. 10.4).

Management

Management is determined by the general condition of the patient, the severity of the leak and the preference of the surgeon.

Generalized peritonitis

- These patients may be profoundly unwell. Appropriate resuscitation with fluids, oxygen and IV antibiotics should be instituted. It may be necessary to admit the patient to intensive care for optimization prior to returning to theatre
- The safest course of action in the unstable patient is to exteriorize both the proximal and distal ends, if sufficient length can be achieved distally
- Careful and thorough lavage of the abdomen should remove gross contamination
- In less severe cases laparotomy and washout with a diverting stoma may allow salvage of the anastomosis.

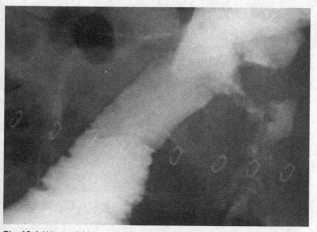

Fig. 10.4 Water-soluble enema showing an anastomotic leak.

Localized leak/failure to progress

- If there is radiological evidence of a leak in a patient with localized signs, slow progress and in the absence of systemic sepsis, a conservative approach with fluids, IV antibiotics and nutritional support may allow resolution. Repeated reassessment of the clinical picture is vital
- A small leak below the peritoneal reflection may produce a pelvic abscess. Radiological drainage may allow satisfactory resolution
- Endoscopic debridement and lavage combined with self-expanding plastic stents, fibrin glue or vacuum devices have been described for less severe leaks. This may be in combination with radiological drainage. Little evidence is available with regard to efficacy.

Outcome

- Studies suggest anastomotic leak may increase local recurrence and reduce cancer-specific survival in rectal cancer
- Mortality ranges from 15 to 40%
- Poorer functional outcomes include anastomotic stricture, fistulae, urgency, and incontinence
- Fewer than half of patients have reversal of their stoma following operation for anastomotic failure.

References

den Dulk M, Marijnen CAM, Collette L et al. Multicentre analysis of oncological and survival outcomes following anastomotic leakage after rectal cancer surgery. *Br J Surg* 2009;**96**:1066–1075.

Tan WS, Tang CL, Shi L, Eu KW. Meta-analysis of defunctioning stomas in low anterior resection for rectal cancer. *Br J Surg* 2009;**96**:462–472.

Adhesions

Adhesions represent a significant post-operative complication following abdominal surgery, and as yet the perfect preventative strategy remains elusive. Formation of adhesions is thought to affect ~95% of patients after open colorectal surgery and in ~5% leads to readmission to hospital. Of those readmitted, 30–60% require further surgery with an even higher risk of subsequent admissions. Readmission is most common in the first year after surgery. Following this period, the rate is steady over the next decade. Certain procedures are associated with higher rates of adhesions, e.g. 25% rate of SBO following IPAA.

Clinical consequences

- SBO
  - Adhesions account for 40% of all bowel obstruction and ~70% of SBO
- Female infertility
  - 20–40% of secondary female infertility
- Chronic abdominal pain
- Difficult re-operative surgery
  - Prolonged operating time including access, ↑ blood loss and ↑ visceral injury.

Aetiology

- Adhesion formation is a response to peritoneal injury, tissue ischaemia or presence of foreign material
- Immediately after injury there is increased vascular permeability with fluid leakage from injured surfaces
- Infiltration of inflammatory cells with release of pro-inflammatory cytokines and activation of complement and coagulation cascades
- This leads to deposition of fibrin on the injured peritoneal surface, causing serosal surfaces to coalesce
- Fibrinolysis should occur within 72hs. If it does not occur within 5–7 days post-injury, fibrinolytic activity is reduced. The fibrin matrix becomes organized, with deposition of collagen and gradual formation of fibrous adhesions.

Preventative measures

Surgical technique

- Careful tissue handling with avoidance of serosal injury where possible
- Minimizing contamination and secure haemostasis
- Avoidance of foreign materials, e.g. starch, talc, gauze, excess suture material
- Preventing tissue desiccation
- Try to exclude important structures from areas where adhesions will inevitably form
- Use of minimal access techniques causes less peritoneal injury and may lead to the formation of fewer adhesions.

Synthetic agents

- A number of different prophylactic interventions have been investigated with aims of inhibiting fibrin and fibroblast deposition, separation of surfaces and controlling adhesion formation by splinting or plicating small bowel
- Barrier agents include 4% icodextrin solution (Adept®, Baxter, Deerfield, IL, USA) and hyaluronate–carboxymethylcellulose membrane (Seprafilm®, Genzyme, Cambridge, MA, USA)
- Use of barrier agents may reduce extent and severity of adhesions but does not appear to influence incidence of SBO
- There is some evidence to suggest use of these substances may be related to a higher rate of anastomotic failure.

Management of adhesions

- Management of SBO has previously been reviewed (→ Small bowel obstruction p.418)
- Likelihood of adhesions should be considered prior to re-operative surgery, and history of previous procedures, incisions, complications, and intra-abdominal sepsis should be elicited
- Where possible re-operative surgery should be delayed for at least 3 months from the previous procedure
- Extra theatre time should be scheduled to avoid pressure
- Previous incisions should be extended into virgin territory to gain access to the peritoneal cavity
- Diathermy, scissors, or scalpel may be used to divide adhesions depending on the situation and preference
- Traction on the tissues is important to display the correct plain of dissection
- Limiting the extent of adhesiolysis may be appropriate depending on the aim of surgery. In re-operation for IBD or malignancy full abdominal assessment is more likely to be required
- Laparoscopic adhesiolysis may result in fewer subsequent adhesions.

Reference

Ellis H. Postoperative intra-abdominal adhesions: a personal view. *Colorectal Dis* 2007;**9**(Suppl 2):3–8.

Incisional hernia

Incisional hernia is a common complication of colorectal surgery, occurring in 10–20% of patients.

- Up to 2/3 are small, reduce easily and have minimal or no symptoms
- Of the remaining 1/3, some will cause pain which is worse on coughing or while taking exercise
- Some will become larger and irreducible and may go on to develop thinning and ulceration of the overlying skin
- ~1–2% present acutely with SBO or strangulation.

Management

Patients with small reducible hernias can be reassured and advised to return to their doctor if they develop symptoms. The principles of repair of symptomatic incisional hernias fall into the following categories: sutured repair; sutured repair with onlay mesh; sutured repair with sublay mesh; inlay mesh and laparoscopic repair (Fig. 10.5).

Sutured repair

- This usually involves closing the fascial edges of the defect after adequate mobilization with a continuous non-absorbable suture such as No.1 polypropylene
- Suture sites should be ~1cm apart and 1cm lateral from the fascial edge
- Such repairs are associated with high recurrence rates up to 30% at 5yrs and 60% at 10yrs.

Sutured repair with onlay mesh

- The defect is closed as described for sutured repair but in addition a mesh, usually polypropylene, is placed on the rectus sheath overlapping the repair by 5cm all around the defect
- The edge of the mesh is sutured to the sheath with continuous or interrupted No.1 polypropylene (Fig. 10.5)
- In addition, the mesh is secured to the sheath on either side of the repair usually with interrupted sutures placed ~1cm from the edge of the repair. This is to prevent herniation of abdominal contents between the rectus sheath and mesh should the repair break down
- Wound complications of seroma, haematoma and infection are common (20%) and may be reduced by placing closed suction drains anterior to the mesh for 48h.

Sutured repair with sublay mesh

- The mesh is placed posterior to the rectus muscle bilaterally resulting in a three-layer repair (Fig. 10.5)
- The posterior rectus sheath is closed with a continuous non-absorbable suture, the mesh is secured laterally with interrupted absorbable sutures with at least a 5cm overlap at either side of the defect and the anterior rectus sheath is then closed, again with a continuous suture
- This is probably the gold standard open repair with low wound complication rates and long-term recurrences of <10%.

(a)

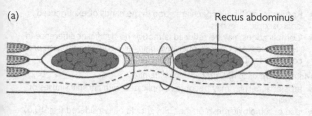

Rectus abdominus

(b)

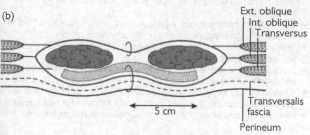

Ext. oblique
Int. oblique
Transversus

Transversalis
fascia

Perineum

5 cm

(c)

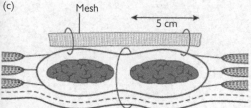

Mesh

5 cm

Fig. 10.5 Open techniques for incisional hernia repair.

Inlay repair
- If fascial closure cannot be achieved mesh is sutured to the edges of the fascia circumferentially to close the defect
- This is regarded as the least effective mesh repair, and the component separation method (CSM) should be considered in these circumstances.

Laparoscopic repair
- Suitable for incisional hernias 4–10cm including those with multiple defects
- As mesh is placed intraperitoneally a composite prosthesis is recommended. This usually consists of an anti-adhesive barrier coated onto a polypropylene or polyester mesh
- Mesh is secured with sutures and titanium or absorbable tacks
- A double crown technique with an inner and outer ring of tacks may be used
- Usually the defect is left open and overlapped by 5cm

- Results from this approach are good in the hands of experienced laparoscopic surgeons
- Complications may be reduced, although no significant difference in recurrence rates or post-operative pain have consistently been proven compared with the open technique.

Management of complicated incisional hernias
- Incisional hernias may become complicated with chronic sinuses or fistulae
- Use of a biologic mesh or the CSM should be considered (Fig. 10.6)
- The CSM is also effective for patients with large defects (>15cm) and when combined with a mesh repair is associated with low recurrence rates (<15%)
- CSM reduces complications, e.g. respiratory compromise from 'loss of domain' by increasing the volume of the peritoneal cavity
- Skin and subcutaneous tissue are dissected off anterior rectus sheath and external oblique widely
- External oblique aponeurosis is divided longitudinally lateral to rectus, and external oblique is separated from internal oblique muscle laterally
- If fascial closure in the midline is still difficult due to tension, posterior rectus sheath can be separated from muscle and anterior rectus sheath
- Drains are placed anterior to the fascial closure to reduce seroma.

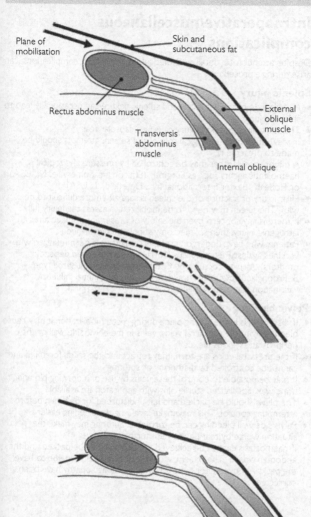

Fig. 10.6 Component separation technique.

Intraoperative/miscellaneous complications

Despite attention to detail and meticulous technique, complications can arise during a procedure.

Splenic injury

- Mobilization of the left colon and splenic flexure can occasionally lead to splenic injury
- This is usually a traction injury causing a capsular tear
- In view of the immunological role of the spleen, attempts should be made to preserve it
- A minor capsular tear may be controlled by pressure and topical haemostatic agents such as Surgicel® (Ethicon Inc.,Somerville, NJ, USA) or FloSeal® (Baxter International Inc., Deerfield, IL, USA)
- Hilar injury or fracture of the spleen is rare and more difficult to deal with. The spleen may need to be mobilized to assess the injury fully
- If there is any concern over the safety of preserving a spleen after an iatrogenic injury, then splenectomy should be performed
- Patients who have undergone splenectomy should be immunized with vaccines against *Pneumococcus* (10yrly booster required depending on titers), *Meningococcus* type C and *Haemophilus influenzae* type B. Prophylactic penicillin should be considered. Annual influenza vaccination may also be helpful.

Pelvic bleeding

- If dissection is in the wrong plane during rectal mobilization it may cause bleeding from the presacral veins, veins in the pelvic side wall or the periprostatic venous plexus
- If the presacral veins are torn, they retract into the sacral foramina and cannot be controlled by diathermy or suturing
- It may be possible to control these veins by use of a drawing pin and bone wax. Specialized sterile pins with applicator are available
- The pelvis should be packed and left undisturbed for 5–10min before attempting control. This may make localizing the bleeding easier
- Pelvis side wall bleeding can be torrential. Suturing may make the situation worse by tearing the veins further
- If haemostasis cannot be achieved the pelvis should be packed and the abdomen closed. The patient should return to theatre in 48h to have the packs removed after hypovolaemia and coagulopathy have been corrected.

Trocar site bleeding

- Inadvertent injury to vessels within the abdominal wall during port insertion can cause bleeding from the port site
- Blood will run down the trocar and drip into the operative field
- Temporary control may be achieved by angling the trocar against the abdominal wall
- Haemostasis may be achieved by compressing the abdominal wall, or suturing the port site
- The injury may not be apparent until the trocar is removed. All ports should be removed under direct vision
- Bleeding from a port site after the port has been removed can be controlled by suturing to encompass the entire port site

Duodenal injury

- Dissection of a locally advanced cancer around the duodenum may lead to inadvertent duodenal injury
- This should be carefully repaired primarily, and patched with jejunum
- If the injury is of sufficient severity, there may be a need for a tube-duodenostomy.

Ureteric injury

- Ureteric injury is discussed in detail later (➔ Ureteric injury/reconstruction p.632).

Missed cancer

- With the advent of CRC screening, patients coming to surgery have small cancers which can be difficult to detect
- All cancers should be tattooed to facilitate easy identification at laparoscopy or laparotomy
- Without tattooing, at operation it may not be possible to identify the cancer positively
- If the patient has been fully bowel prepped, on-table colonoscopy should be employed to identify the lesion positively
- If the patient has not been prepped, on-table lavage may need to be performed to allow accurate localization of the lesion
- If the pathology post-operatively does not identify a cancer within the specimen, the case needs to be carefully reviewed through the MDT
- Initial pathology must be confirmed. CTs should be reviewed and the patient should undergo repeat colonoscopy at the earliest opportunity.

Common operations

Appendicectomy

Indications
- Appendicitis.

Preparation
- IV antibiotics according to local guidelines
- Rehydration with balanced IV fluids
- Thromboembolism prophylaxis.

Position
- Supine.

Incision
- The abdomen should be palpated, with the placement of incision directed by any palpable mass or thickening
- Lanz incision is preferred (Fig. 11.1a). A small initial wound can easily be extended depending on difficulty.

Procedure
- External oblique is divided in the line of its fibres. Internal oblique and transversus abdominus are split by opening a scissors and using Langenbeck retractors (Fig. 11.1b). Peritoneum is opened between artery forceps taking care not to pick up bowel. The wound can be extended medially or laterally to improve exposure, even dividing rectus if necessary
- Peritoneal swabs sent for culture rarely influence management
- Identify the caecum and follow the taenia coli which converge on the base of the appendix. Avoid grasping forceps where possible, as these may traumatize bowel. Gentle finger dissection of inflammatory adhesions may be necessary to deliver the appendix. If delivery is difficult, consider improving exposure
- The mesoappendix should be ligated at the level of the base of the appendix
- Appendix base should be divided between clamps and ligated with 2/0 polyglactin or similar absorbable suture. Crushing the base is unnecessary but consider a transfixion suture technique. Ensure the entire appendix is removed
- It is not usually necessary to bury the base of the appendix unless there is concern about the quality of the tissues. If deemed appropriate, insert an absorbable seromuscular purse-string suture to the caecum, 1cm from the base. The stump should be invaginated before securing the knot
- The RIF should be lavaged with warm saline if turbid free fluid or pus is found in the peritoneal cavity. Drainage is not necessary after appendicectomy.
- If the appendix is normal exclude an MD. The presence of pus or free fluid suggests significant pathology. In this situation either extend the wound to look for alternative diagnoses or perform a midline laparotomy (remember perforated peptic ulcer).

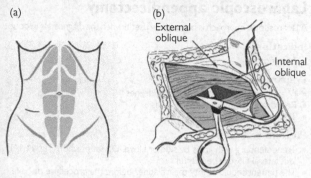

Fig. 11.1 Lanz incision. This is centered on McBurney's point (a). The external oblique is opened in the direction of its fibers and the internal oblique and transversus abdominus separated by opening a scissors and using Langenbeck retractors (b).

Closure

- The wound is closed in layers with an absorbable suture. If approximating sutures are placed in the internal oblique these should be loose. A mass closure technique can also be employed
- The skin is closed with a subcuticular suture and infiltrated with LA.

Post-operative care

- Fluids and diet can be offered immediately
- Multidose antibiotics are not usually necessary, but post-operative antibiotics should be considered in the presence of an appendix abscess or where the appendix was gangrenous or there was frank perforation.

Post-operative complications

- Wound infection
- Intra-abdominal abscess
- Haemorrhage
- Ileus/small bowel obstruction
- Incisional hernia
- Faecal fistula.

Laparoscopic appendicectomy

A laparoscopic approach is particularly useful when the diagnosis is in doubt.

Indications
- Appendicitis

Preparation
- IV antibiotics according to local guidelines
- Rehydration with balanced IV fluids
- Thromboembolism prophylaxis.

Position
- Trendelenburg with arms by side or Lloyd–Davies position (Fig. 11.14). Left lateral tilt may be helpful
- The patient should empty their bladder before the procedure or have an in/out catheter.

Incision
- A 10mm subumbilical incision is used to insert first port using an open technique. A pneumoperitoneum is induced
- A 30° laparoscope should be considered, especially if the surgeon is familiar with its use
- If a 10mm laparoscope is used, further 5mm and 10mm ports are placed under direct vision (Fig. 11.2). If a 5mm laparoscope is used, a 5mm port can be substituted instead of the 10mm port
- Alternative port placements are possible. The most important principle is that the camera port lies between the two working ports.

Procedure
- After laparoscopy has been performed the caecum is retracted cranially with atraumatic graspers which should help locate the appendix
- The appendix is grasped gently by the tip and a window is made in the mesoappendix at its base
- The mesoappendix is dissected off close to the appendix using diathermy. The mesoappendix can be endo-looped to ensure haemostasis (Fig. 11.3). Alternatively, laparoscopic clips can be used before division.
- The base is ligated with 2 endo-loops and the appendix is transected
- An alternative method is to divide the mesentery and then the appendix with a laparoscopic stapler, but this is more expensive
- Lavage and suction should be carried out if there is free fluid or pus
- Lavage fluid can be sent for culture and sensitivity
- The appendix can be removed either by placing it in the 10mm port and removing the port or by placing it in a retrieval bag.

Closure
- The fascia of the 10mm port site is closed using the purse-string suture, making sure to check for complete closure
- Skin wounds can be closed with subcuticular sutures, tissue glue, skin clips or steristrips according to preference
- Infiltrate wounds with LA.

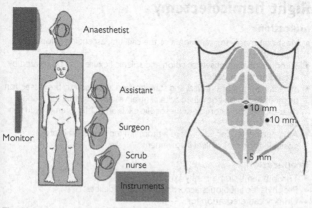

Fig. 11.2 Laparoscopic appendicectomy setup.

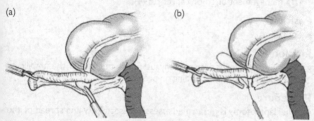

Fig. 11.3 The appendix is retracted distally and a hole dissected in the mesoappendix (a). After division of the appendicular vessels, two endo-loop sutures are placed around the base and the appendix divided between the sutures (b).

Post-operative care

- Fluids and diet can be introduced without delay.

Post-operative complications

- As for appendicectomy
- Haemorrhage
- Visceral injury
- Port site hernia.

Right hemicolectomy

Indications
- Most commonly for carcinoma of the caecum, ascending colon and hepatic flexure
- Tumours of the transverse colon and splenic flexure may be treated by extending the resection
- Increasingly, a more radical and standardised approach to the dissection of the mesocolon combined with central vascular ligation and node clearance called a complete mesocolic excision (CME) is employed for cancer resections
- Also performed for CD where a more limited resection is often possible for terminal ileal involvement

Preparation
- Thromboembolism prophylaxis
- Prophylactic antibiotics according to local guidelines
- Urinary catheterization for 24–48h
- Pre-operative staging should be complete where possible
  (➜ Management of colon cancer p.344).

Position
- Supine.

Incision
- Transverse right-sided laparotomy just above the level of the umbilicus or a midline incision depending on preference.

Procedure
- A full laparotomy is performed assessing resectability and spread of the tumour
- The small bowel is packed in the left side to reveal the root of the small bowel mesentery and transverse mesocolon
- The right colon is retracted into the wound by the assistant standing on the left side taking care not to manipulate the tumour or disturb any adhesions around it
- The operator standing on the right side divides the lateral peritoneal attachments of the right colon with diathermy along the white line of Toldt
- Dissection is continued around the caecum and appendix to mobilize the TI
- Developing the plane between mesocolon and retroperitoneum enables identification of the right ureter and gonadal vessels
- The duodenum is then dissected off posterior surface of right mesocolon; sharp dissection may be preferred to avoid thermal injury
- When performing a CME, a meticulous dissection between the visceral and parietal fascia, along the line of Toldt, enables mobilisation of the entire mesocolon
- The suspensory omental attachments to the hepatic flexure can be divided with diathermy, ligating larger vessels

- Points of transection of the bowel are identified at the junction of proximal 1/3 and distal 2/3 of transverse colon and TI
- The anterior peritoneum of the right mesocolon may be scored with diathermy along the intended plane of resection
- The ileocolic, right colic and hepatic branch of the middle colic arteries are ligated and divided. The ileal branches are divided close to the bowel to maintain good supply to the small bowel end.
- When performing a CME, a central division of the entire arterial supply of the right colon is performed. The ileocolic artery and vein & right colic vessels (if present) are divided close to their origins from the superior mesenteric artery and vein.
- The middle colic artery and vein are ligated at a point close to their origin from the superior mesenteric artery and Trunk of Henle, respectively. All lymphatic and nodal tissue to the right of this central vascular pedicle which has been ligated is removed en bloc with the intact colon/mesocolon
- Anastomosis is performed using either a stapled or sutured technique
- For a sutured anastomosis soft bowel clamps are placed on ileum and transverse colon with crushing clamps on the side for resection. The ileum and transverse colon are divided on the crushing clamps which are removed with the specimen. An end-to-end anastomosis can be performed using interrupted serosubmucosal sutures using 3/0 polyglactin or polydioxanone (Fig. 11.4)
- Alternatively, the colonic end may be closed. An end-to side anastomosis is formed between ileum and a colotomy made along the anti-mesenteric border of transverse colon using the same sutured technique
- For a stapled side-to side (functional end-to-end) anastomosis, the anti-mesenteric borders of transverse colon and ileum are brought together. Openings are made to introduce the blades of a linear cutting stapler and anastomosis is performed. The enterotomies are approximated with Babcock's and excluded by completion of the anastomosis using a non-cutting linear stapler. The right colon is resected by dividing the bowel on the stapler with a scalpel (Fig.11.5)
- Alternatively, the transverse colon and ileum can be divided separately with a linear cutting stapler performing the anastomosis as before
- One or two interrupted seromuscular sutures are placed distal to the staple line to take tension off the anastomosis. Any bleeding from the staple line can be under-run
- The mesenteric window can be closed with interrupted superficial absorbable sutures or left open if the defect is wide
- Drainage is not advised.

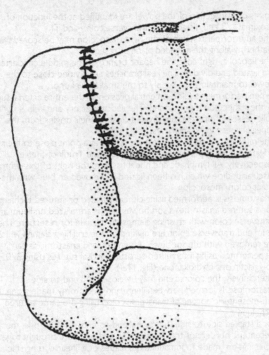

Fig. 11.4 Sutured ileocolic anastomosis.

Reproduced with permission from McLathchie, G and Leaper, D (Eds.) (2006). *Operative Surgery*, 2nd edition. Oxford, UK: Oxford University Press

Closure

- Mass closure with looped polydioxanone or nylon is followed by skin clips or a subcuticular suture.

Post-operative care

- An enhanced recovery protocol should be employed (➔ Enhanced recovery p.498).

Post-operative complications

- Anastomotic leak
- Wound infection
- Haemorrhage
- Post-operative ileus
- Incisional hernia.

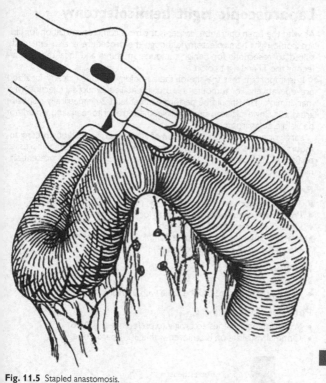

Fig. 11.5 Stapled anastomosis.

Laparoscopic right hemicolectomy

As with the open operation, cancer is the most common indication for laparoscopic right hemicolectomy although the procedure is also eminently suited to resections for benign tumours, strictures and localized CD affecting the TI and right colon.

It is important that the site of the pathology has been clearly localized pre-operatively. For tumours, this usually entails submucosal injection with marking ink. This should be performed in at least 2 diametrically opposite areas as a single injection site may lie in the retroperitoneum and would not be visible at laparoscopy.

Large or bulky tumours, infiltration of adjacent organs and obstructing tumours should be viewed as relative contraindications. Associated abscesses or fistulae or laparoscopic surgery in obese patients may also present significant technical challenges.

Preparation

- Thromboembolism prophylaxis
- Prophylactic antibiotics according to local guidelines
- Urinary catheterization for 24–48h
- Pre-operative staging should be complete where possible (➔ Management of colon cancer p.344).

Position

- Supine
- The patient is secured to the table with both arms at sides.

Port positions

- Port positioning varies according to preference (Fig. 11.6)
- Optimal visualization is achieved with a 30° laparoscope.

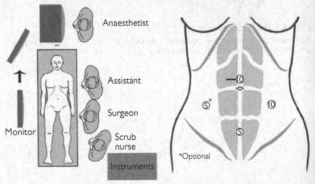

Fig. 11.6 Theatre setup and port placement. The upper midline 10mm port is extended to remove the specimen.

Procedure

- A full laparoscopy confirms the position of the tumour and local infiltration or metastatic disease is excluded
- The ileocolic artery (ICA) is identified by elevation and lateral/caudal traction on the ileocaecal junction (Fig. 11.7)
- The retroperitoneal plane is entered by incising the peritoneum just below the ICA. The retroperitoneal structures (duodenum, gonadal vessels and ureter) are reflected posteriorly
- The artery and vein are divided close to the superior mesenteric vein using endoscopic staplers, clips or an appropriate energy source
- Dissection is continued superiorly to the root of the middle colic artery and vein. The right branch of this vessel may also be divided
- For principles of a complete mesocolic excision, see chapter on open right hemicolectomy (⮕ Right hemicolectomy p.526)
- The entire right colon can now be mobilized anteriorly away from the retroperitoneal structures including the duodenum
- The peritoneal reflection at the inferior border of the caecum and the TI mesentery is incised, opening a window into the retroperitoneum
- The omentum is mobilized from the transverse colon, allowing access to the hepatocolic ligament, which is incised, thereby making a further window into the preceding retroperitoneal dissection
- The only remaining attachment of the right colon is the lateral peritoneal attachments which are divided
- The right colon is delivered, extending the upper midline port site and using a wound protector (e.g. Alexis Retractor® Allied Medical, CA, USA). This incision lies over the base of the middle colic pedicle to ensure maximum mobility of the transverse colon
- The specimen is resected and an ileocolic anastomosis fashioned
- The anastomosis is returned to the abdomen
- A pneumoperitoneum is re-established and a washout performed.

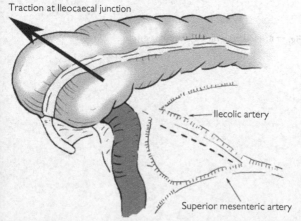

Traction at Ileocaecal junction

Ileocolic artery

Superior mesenteric artery

Fig. 11.7 Traction on the ileocaecal junction identifies the ileocolic artery.

Closure

- The wound extraction site is closed with a continuous polydioxanone suture as a mass closure
- Skin wounds can be closed with subcuticular sutures or tissue glue
- Infiltrate wounds with 0.25% bupivacaine and 1/200,000 adrenaline.

Post-operative care

- An enhanced recovery protocol should be employed (➔ Enhanced recovery p.498).

Post-operative complications

- As for appendicectomy.

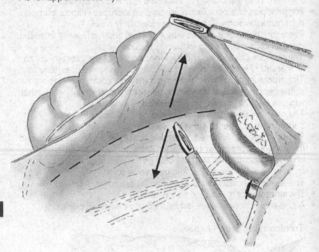

Fig. 11.8 Mobilization in the retroperitoneal plane.

Left hemicolectomy

Indications
- Tumours of the splenic flexure, descending and sigmoid colon
- Complicated diverticular disease.

Preparation
- Thromboembolism prophylaxis
- Prophylactic antibiotics and blood cross-matched according to local guidelines.
- Phosphate enemas may be given for bowel preparation
- Urinary catheterization for 24–48h
- Pre-operative staging should be complete where possible (➔ Management of colon cancer p.344).

Incision
- Midline laparotomy.

Position
- Supine with legs split or Lloyds–Davies (Fig. 11.14)
- Reverse Trendelenburg may be used for splenic flexure mobilization.

Procedure
- A full laparotomy is performed assessing resectability and spread of the tumour
- The small bowel is packed in the RUQ to reveal the mesentery of the left colon and the rectum entering the pelvis
- The left colon is retracted into the wound by the assistant standing on the right side, taking care not to manipulate the tumour or disturb any adhesions around it
- The operator standing on the left side divides the lateral peritoneal attachments of the left colon with diathermy along the white line of Toldt
- Dissection is continued from the rectosigmoid junction toward the splenic flexure
- Developing the plane between mesocolon and retroperitoneum the left ureter and gonadal vessels should be identified and protected
- The greater omentum is dissected off the transverse colon and the lesser sac is entered, continuing the dissection toward the splenic flexure. If the tumour is close to the splenic flexure the omentum can be resected with the specimen
- The peritoneum around the splenic flexure is divided and the mobilization is completed. The capsule of the spleen can be torn by either a retractor in the LUQ or traction on adhesions to the tip of the spleen. After careful mobilization haemostasis should be confirmed.
- The left colon is retracted into the wound and the peritoneum is scored along the intended plane of resection
- The inferior mesenteric artery is ligated proximal to the origin of the left colic artery. The inferior mesenteric vein is ligated close to the pancreas. The left branch of the middle colic artery may be ligated depending on tumour position (Figs 11.9 and 11.13). The inferior mesenteric artery may be preserved with ligation of the left colic in cases where age or co-morbidity make it preferable to avoid a rectal anastomosis.

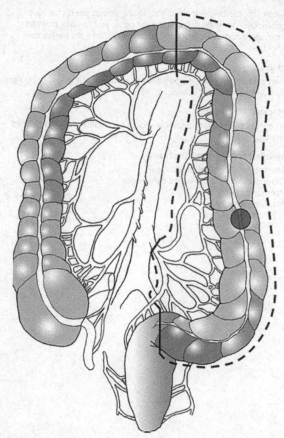

Fig. 11.9 Resection lines for colon and inferior mesenteric artery during a left hemicolectomy for cancer.

- The rectum is divided with a linear stapler. The transverse colon is divided taking care to ensure that there is arterial bleeding in the marginal artery
- A purse-string suture is inserted into the divided proximal colon (2/0 polypropylene) and the anvil of a circular stapler is secured. This is brought to lie in the pelvis without tension
- A stapled end-to end anastomosis is performed by transanal passage of a circular stapler. Check that doughnuts are complete
- A sutured end-to-end anastomosis with interrupted serosubmucosal 3/0 polyglactin or polydioxanone can also be performed depending on preference

- A leak test can be performed insufflating air into the rectum with a sigmoidoscope while submerging the pelvic anastomosis in water
- Drainage is not necessary for anastomoses above the peritoneal reflection

Closure

- Mass closure with looped polydioxanone or nylon is followed by skin clips or a subcuticular suture.

Post-operative care

- An enhanced recovery protocol should be employed (➲ Enhanced recovery p.498).

Post-operative complications

- Anastomotic leak and pelvic sepsis
- Wound infection and wound dehiscence
- Haemorrhage
- Post-operative ileus
- Incisional hernia.

Hartmann's procedure

This was first described by Hartmann in 1921. It was the operation of choice for carcinoma of the upper and middle third of the rectum before the advent of safe anterior resection.

The principles of the operation are resection of 1/3 to 1/2 of the rectum and sigmoid colon, with the formation of a left-sided colostomy and closure of the rectal stump.

Indications

- Faecal peritonitis secondary to perforated sigmoid colon either from diverticular disease or a perforated cancer where gross peritoneal contamination makes primary anastomosis hazardous
- Elective rectal cancer resection in patients where the additional risk and morbidity associated with a low rectal anastomosis is deemed to be unacceptably high
- Elective cancer resection patients in whom the risk of local recurrence is deemed high.

Preparation

- Emergency patients should be fully resuscitated
- Urinary catheterization
- Thromboembolism prophylaxis
- Prophylactic antibiotics and blood cross-matched according to local guidelines
- Pre-operative review by stoma therapist when possible and appropriate site for a stoma marked.

Position

- Lloyd–Davies position in order to facilitate lavage of the rectal stump
- Supine position with legs split also provides adequate access to the rectum and may reduce the risk of compartment syndrome

Incision

- Lower midline. May need to be extended above the umbilicus.

Procedure

- Careful laparotomy to identify site of perforation/pathology. The sigmoid may be obviously inflamed with adherent loops of small bowel, uterus, fallopian tubes, ovaries, bladder or omentum
- Divide the lateral peritoneal reflection of the sigmoid colon. Mobilize medially to identify the left ureter and gonadal vessels
- It may be difficult to identify the ureter at the pelvic brim due to inflamed, thickened and oedematous tissues. In this situation, dissection should be continued in a cephalad direction and, once the ureter is identified, traced distally into the pelvis
- The sigmoid mesentery will be shortened due to inflammation, making access difficult. It is therefore best to perform a high tie on the inferior mesenteric artery and vein, even if the condition is known to be due to benign disease

- The mesentery of the proximal bowel is divided, taking care to ensure that there is a good arterial blood supply. The bowel is divided with a linear stapler
- Dissection is carried into the upper mesorectal plane until healthy rectum is reached
- The mesorectum is divided between clips and ties and the rectum transected using a linear stapler. It may also be oversewn
- The apex of the rectal stump may be marked with a non-absorbable suture (e.g. polypropylene) to aid subsequent identification
- Ensure the left colon has adequate mobility to fashion a colostomy. It may be necessary to mobilize the left colon and splenic flexure fully
- A trephine is then formed through the previously marked colostomy site and the stapled proximal colon delivered through it (Fig. 11.10)
- Perform a thorough lavage to remove gross contamination
- Ensure haemostasis.

Closure

- Mass closure with looped polydioxanone or nylon is followed by skin clips or a subcuticular suture
- The skin may be left open if there has been gross faecal contamination
- The stoma should be created by suturing the opened colon to the skin using an absorbable suture.

Post-operative care

- Many patients will require a stay in intensive care or a surgical high dependency unit
- If performed for peritonitis, antibiotics should be continued, the choice based on microbiology results and local antibiotic protocols
- Oral fluids and diet should be encouraged, but nutritional support may be required in the critically ill patient.

Complications

- Pelvic sepsis
- Subphrenic collection
- Ischaemia or retraction of the stoma
- Wound infection, dehiscence and incisional hernia.

Reversal of Hartmann's procedure

GI continuity can be restored if the patient so desires and provided they are sufficiently fit. Reversal should not be scheduled within 3 months of the initial surgery and ideally at least 6 months after the primary operation in order to allow a reduction in adhesions.

Preparation

- Bowel preparation is unnecessary
- Urinary catheterization
- Thromboembolism prophylaxis
- Prophylactic antibiotics and blood cross-matched according to local guidelines
- The rectal stump should be lavaged to remove any inspissated mucus.

Position

Lloyd–Davies position or supine with legs split

Incision

- The previous midline incision is carefully re-opened and a careful adhesiolysis undertaken if required.

Procedure

- The rectal stump should be located in the pelvis and mobilized to allow safe performance of an anastomosis. The rectal mobilization can be difficult and may be helped by the insertion of a rigid sigmoidoscope
- Once sufficient rectal mobilization has been achieved, the stoma is mobilized clear of the abdominal wall. It is important to ensure adequate length of colon is mobilized to allow anastomosis without tension. If necessary, the splenic flexure can be mobilized if this has not already been done
- A hand-sewn or stapled anastomosis can be fashioned. The circular stapling gun is passed through the rectal stump. It may not be possible to pass the gun to the apex of the stump as a result of atrophy and scarring. Care should be taken not to split the rectal stump by overenthusiastic efforts to insert the gun. It may be necessary to bring the spike of the stapling gun though the anterior wall of the rectum (i.e. distal to the old stapled transection point)
- The anastomosis is leak tested by submerging under lavage fluid and gently inflating the bowel with air via a rectal catheter
- A loop ileostomy can be fashioned if there is concern about anastomotic breakdown.

Closure

- Mass closure with looped polydioxanone or nylon is followed by skin clips or a subcuticular suture
- The skin may be left open if there has been gross faecal contamination.

Post-operative care

- These patients may require high dependency care in the early post-operative phase
- An enhanced recovery protocol should be employed (➔ Enhanced recovery p.498).

Post-operative complications

- Anastomotic leak and pelvic sepsis
- Wound infection and dehiscence
- Haemorrhage
- Incisional hernia
- Post-operative ileus.

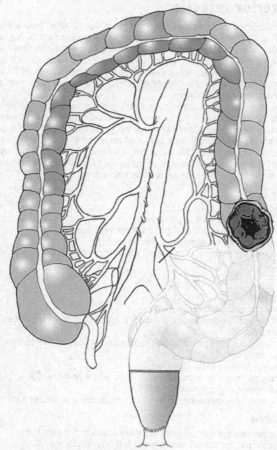

Fig. 11.10 Hartmann's resection.

Anterior resection

When appraising the various surgical options for curative treatment of rectal cancer, consideration is given to individual patient factors (e.g. age and morbidity), presentation (elective or emergency) and the site and stage of the cancer. The majority will be suitable for radical resection although ~1/3 will have non-resectable metastatic disease at presentation. APER and anterior resection are the two most common procedures performed for the treatment of rectal cancer.

The term 'low' anterior resection refers to the operation where the entire rectum is mobilized, the rectum is transected below the point where the mesorectum peters out just above the pelvic floor (i.e. a TME is performed) and the anastomosis is fashioned below the level of the peritoneal reflection (Fig. 11.11). A TME should be performed for cancers of the lower 2/3 of the rectum. For tumours of the upper 1/3 and rectosigmoid junction, the rectum may be transected 5cm below the tumour.

Indications

- Rectal cancer
  - Not invading into the sphincters
  - Where an adequate (1–2cm) distal margin is possible
  - In a patient with adequate sphincter control
- Diverticular disease and its complications (e.g. stricture or colovesical fistula)
- Rectal stricture.

Preparation

- Thromboembolism prophylaxis
- Prophylactic antibiotics and blood cross-matched according to local guidelines
- Phosphate enema or full bowel preparation may be considered if loop ileostomy is likely
- Urinary catheterization for 24–48h
- Pre-operative staging should be complete where possible (⊖ Management of colon cancer p.344)
- Pre-operative review by a stoma nurse to counsel and site for a stoma.

Position

- Supine with legs split provides adequate access to the perineum and rectum for stapled anastomoses and may reduce the risk of compartment syndrome
- Alternatively, Lloyd–Davies (modified lithotomy) to provide access to the perineum (Fig. 11.14)
- Hips and knees should be flexed at 45° and the hips abducted just enough to allow access to the perineum
- The calves and feet should lie at the same level or above the knees in order to facilitate venous drainage.

Incision

- Midline incision
- A low transverse incision may be preferred.

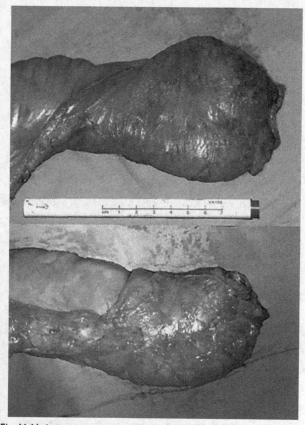

Fig. 11.11 An intact mesorectum with no defects is seen.

Procedure

- A DRE and rigid sigmoidoscopy are performed to confirm site, size and mobility of the tumour
- The rectum is washed out with water and povidone–iodine.

Abdominal mobilization

- A full laparotomy is performed assessing resectability and spread of the tumour
- The small bowel and caecum are packed away to the right side of the abdomen
- The sigmoid and left colon are retracted anteromedially and the left lateral peritoneal attachments incised with diathermy

- The dissection is continued medially and in a cephalad direction, taking care to follow the white line of Toldt. The correct plane is avascular
- During the medial mobilization, the left ureter and gonadal vessels are identified and preserved
- The IMA is identified and divided at a point 1cm from its origin on the aorta, thereby reducing the potential for damage to the hypogastric nerve plexus lying on the aorta. Alternatively, it can be divided immediately distal to its first branch (left colic artery)
- The inferior mesenteric vein is divided more proximally just lateral to the junction of the 4th part of the duodenum and jejunum. The vein is usually the limiting factor in mobility and a high ligation ensures maximum mobility (Fig. 11.13)
- The splenic flexure is mobilized by releasing the greater omentum for the transverse colon. This dissection is continued laterally after entering the lesser sac
- After mobilizing around the apex of the splenic flexure, the dissection joins the previous plane of mobilization at the left colon
- The left colon/sigmoid is divided with a linear stapler at a suitable point. Ensure that there is brisk arterial bleeding from the marginal vessel on the proximal aspect of the point of division before ligation. There should be good length to reach into the pelvis for the anastomosis.

Pelvic dissection
- The pelvic dissection is commenced by lifting the rectum forward and anteriorly
- The previous incision at the lateral peritoneal attachments of the sigmoid is extended to run over the pelvic brim and continued into the pelvis, taking care to incise the peritoneum just beyond the edge of the mesorectum (for cancer cases)
- On the right side of the rectum the peritoneum is similarly incised with diathermy, extending anteriorly at the base of the bladder/pouch of Douglas to join with the left side
- When dividing the peritoneum at the anterior peritoneal reflexion, the incision should be towards the rectal side for posterior tumours and benign conditions whereas the incision should extend as far onto the bladder as necessary for anterior tumours in order to obtain a satisfactory margin
- The rectal mobilization begins by entering into the plane behind the mesorectum and in front of the presacral fascia and the hypogastric nerve plexus
- Although diathermy is the most commonly used method of mobilization, alternatives such as sharp scissors dissection with meticulous haemostasis or alternative energy sources (e.g. harmonic scalpel) can be used. A bloodless field offers the best chance to identify and preserve the hypogastric and pelvic nerve plexus
- The correct fascial plane is mostly avascular and the surface of the mesorectum posteriorly should be smooth with no defects (Fig. 11.11)
- As dissection is continued distally around the curve of the sacrum, Waldeyer's fascia (rectosacral ligament) is divided, giving access to the pelvic floor

- The lateral dissection also follows the line of the mesorectum until the lateral ligaments are encountered (containing autonomic nerves and, occasionally, a middle rectal vessel). These are divided, although care should be taken to avoid excessive medial traction during the division as this can tent up the pelvic plexus which can be damaged at this point (Fig. 11.16)
- The anterior dissection follows the plane behind Denonvilliers' fascia which will prevent damage to the periprostatic nerve plexus lying behind the seminal vesicles. However, for anterior tumours, the fascia is incised and the plane lies in front of this fascia. On occasion it may be necessary to resect the seminal vesicles themselves in order to achieve satisfactory cancer clearance
- In women, the rectovaginal septum is separated, although it may be necessary to perform an *en bloc* resection of the posterior wall of the vagina for locally advanced anterior tumours
- The pelvic dissection is complete when the anorectal ring is reached on all sides
- If possible, the rectum is cross clamped below the tumour and the rectum irrigated again prior to cross stapling with a linear stapler.

Anastomotic techniques
- A double-stapled technique is usually used for low anastomoses
- A single circular stapler may be used if the distal rectal stump is divided directly and not cross-stapled. A hand-inserted purse-string suture or a Furness clamp can be used to insert the purse-string
- The anastomosis may also be fashioned with a hand-sutured technique (usually a single layer)
- For ultralow anastomosis, the colon may be anastomosed to the anus/distal rectal stump by fashioning the anastomosis from the perineal end through the anus
- For low anastomoses, consideration should be given to fashioning a colonic pouch to improve post-operative bowel function
- A defunctioning loop ileostomy should be considered.

Closure
Abdominal incision
- Some surgeons will leave a low-pressure suction drain deep in the pelvis and brought out through the abdominal wall
- A mass closure of the abdominal wound is performed with looped polydioxanone or nylon followed by skin clips or a subcuticular suture.

Post-operative care
- An enhanced recovery protocol should be employed (⊃ Enhanced recovery p.498).

Post-operative complications
- Anastomotic leak and pelvic sepsis
- Sexual and bladder dysfunction
- Post-operative haemorrhage and ileus
- Wound infection, dehiscence and incisional hernia.

Laparoscopic anterior resection

Indications

- Cancer of the rectum or distal sigmoid is the most common indication for resection (see indications for open anterior resection)
- Diverticular disease and its complications (e.g. stricture or colovesical fistula).

Relative contraindications

Although there are no absolute contraindications to a laparoscopic approach, the following factors are associated with a higher risk of conversion, which may also be associated with a poorer short- and long-term outcome.

- Obesity
- Previous open abdominal/pelvic surgery
- Locally advanced cancer
- ASA grade III/IV
- Inexperienced surgeon
- Lower 1/3 cancers.

Pre-operative preparation

- Thromboembolism prophylaxis
- Full bowel preparation although a phosphate enema alone may be considered
- Prophylactic antibiotics according to local guidelines
- Urinary catheterization for 24–48h
- Preoperative by a stoma nurse to counsel and site for a stoma
- Pre-operative staging should be complete where possible (➔) Management of colon cancer p.344).

Operative setup

- Draw out landmarks including midline and any scars
- Modified Lloyd–Davies position or supine with legs split
- Arms tucked in by the side
- Ensure all cables and gas tubing are tidy to ensure ease of movement around operating table by the surgical team.

Port placement

There is no perfect way to set up ports for this or any laparoscopic colorectal procedure. A suggested routine is shown in Fig. 11.12. The following principles apply to all laparoscopic colorectal cases

- Operator and assistant, camera and screen should be aligned
- The camera should be placed between the operator's two main working ports
- A 30° laparoscope should be used
- Rather than placing the ports as close as possible to the working area, consider placing ports as far away as is practicable (within the limitations of the length of the laparoscope and the instruments). This ensures a wide angle of view and makes for an easier operation
- Bring all the cables and gas supply off the table on the side of the pathology and the monitors, e.g. for an anterior resection the cables come off the left side of the table. The operator and assistant therefore have the whole of the right side free to move about
- Bring cables off at the point of rotation of the table. This minimizes movement of the cables when performing steep head-down or -up tilt.

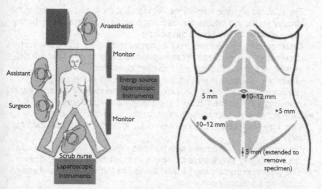

Fig. 11.12 Theatre setup and port positioning for a laparoscopic anterior resection. A 12mm Hassan port inserted at umbilicus using an open cut down unless a very short lower abdomen, then placed more superiorly. Pneumoperitoneum established and further two 5mm ports and a 12mm port in the right iliac fossa to be utilized for transection of the rectum.

Procedure

- A DRE and rigid sigmoidoscopy are performed to confirm site, size and mobility of the tumour
- The rectum is washed out with water and povidone–iodine
- As with any laparoscopic colon resection, confirm level of pathology with colonoscopy and ensure that the bowel is tattooed on two opposing sites just below the lesion. This is less relevant for mid and low rectal cancers
- Full laparoscopy and assessment of the tumour
- Position patient with head-down tilt with left side up to allow small bowel to fall from the pelvis; precipitous tilt not always required but always be aware of thermal injury to surrounding structures
- Divide the right lateral pelvic peritoneum with assistant holding the rectum over to the left. Divide this widely from sacral promontory down to the depth of the pelvis
- Proceed in the mesorectal plane medial to lateral to identify the ureter first and then the gonadal vessels
- Once the ureter is identified, proceed to skeletonize the inferior mesenteric artery and divide as a high tie using your energy source of choice, staples or Hem-o-lok® clips (Weck Closure Systems, NC, USA)
- Continue mobilization laterally underneath the left colon and cranially to show inferior mesenteric vein. Divide the structure but beware of encroaching too laterally on the mesentery and damaging the marginal vessels
- The lateral peritoneal reflection could now be divided and splenic flexure taken down completely
- Pick a point in the rectum to divide (distal to the tattoo). Divide the mesorectum using energy source of choice and then transect the rectum with an endoscopic stapler inserted via the RIF port

- Try to avoid multiple staple lines. Aim for 2 at most and ensure that the circular staple gun excises the bisecting portion of the staples by having the spike exit the rectum at this point
- Cross-stapling of the lower rectum can be technically difficult. In such circumstance, consideration can be given to performing a Pfannenstiel incision and cross-stapling as for an open operation
- Utilize a lower midline wound and insert a wound protector (Alexis retractor, Allied Medical, CA, USA) before exteriorizing the bowel and resecting the specimen. Ensure good length and vascularity
- Exercise caution with obese patients as the mesentery tears easily. One may also use a Pfannenstiel or an LIF incision or even an umbilical incision
- Proximal bowel is prepared with purse-string suture and the anvil of a circular staple gun is inserted. Bowel is then returned to the abdomen
- The wound protector can be used to seal the extraction wound and re-establish a pneumoperitoneum
- Anastomosis is performed laparoscopically
- Check bowel orientation for twists
- Air leak test with lavage and check for haemostasis
- Placing a drain is a matter of individual choice, although most surgeons place a drain in lower 1/3 anastomoses

Closure

- The fascia of the 12mm port sites may be closed under direct vision
- Extraction wound is closed using polydioxanone or nylon to fascia
- Skin wounds can be closed with steristrips, subcuticular sutures or tissue glue
- Infiltrate wounds with LA

Post-operative care

- An enhanced recovery protocol should be employed (➔ Enhanced recovery p.498).

Post-operative complications

- As for open anterior resection
- Haemorrhage
- Visceral injury
- Port site hernia

Additional notes

- Avoid shoulder restraints as they can cause brachial plexus injury
- Ensure orientation and keep energy source in view at all times
- If the disease is more advanced than expected, starting with the splenic flexure mobilization may be appropriate and an easier start point
- Position table with head-up tilt and left side up
- Identify the duodenojejunal flexure and divide the peritoneum beneath the inferior mesenteric vein (Fig. 11.13)
- Proceed in the avascular plane in a medial to superolateral direction but beware the pancreas which is easily lifted
- Once dissection has been carried out superolaterally, lift the gastrocolic omentum and dissect the colon free from medial to lateral

- Enter into the lesser sac and continue around the splenic flexure
- On occasion, the medial approach is hampered by the small bowel obscuring the view, despite steep head-down tilt. In this circumstance, divide the lateral reflection early to aid retraction on the colon and begin lateral to medial
- Beware the wide AP pelvis as it may present difficulties when passing the circular stapling gun up through the rectum. Ensure that the rectum is adequately mobilized below the point of vision in order to avoid the risk of injury/splitting
- Try to ensure that the assistant plays a passive role. Overhelpful assistants may hinder smooth progress during laparoscopy by lifting and dropping structures.

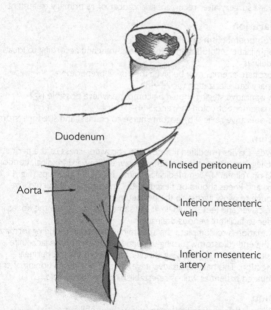

Fig. 11.13 Access to the retroperitoneum. This can be gained by incising the peritoneum between the duodenojejunal flexure and the inferior mesenteric vein.

Abdominoperineal excision of the rectum

APER was the classic radical operation for rectal and anal cancer first described by Miles in 1908. Low anterior resection for rectal cancer and chemoradiotherapy for anal cancer have now resulted in a reduction in the requirement for APER.

Indications

- Rectal cancer
  - Invading into the sphincters
  - Where a distal margin is impossible
  - In a patient with very poor sphincter control
- Rectal cancer recurrence after anterior resection
- Salvage surgery after recurrent anal cancer or as primary treatment

Preparation

- Thromboembolism prophylaxis
- Prophylactic antibiotics and blood cross-matched according to local guidelines
- Phosphate enemas may be given for bowel preparation
- Urinary catheterization for 24–48h
- Pre-operative staging should be complete where possible (⊃ Management of colon cancer p.344)
- Pre-operative review by a stoma nurse to counsel and site for a stoma.

Position

- Lloyds–Davies (modified lithotomy) to provide access to the perineum. The legs are supported with Lloyd–Davies (Steward Medical, London, UK) or Yellofin® (Allen Medical Systems, MA, USA) stirrups (Fig. 11.14)
- Hips and knees should be flexed at 45° and the hips abducted just enough to allow access to the perineum
- The calves and feet should lie at the same level or above the knees in order to facilitate venous drainage
- A variation is to complete the abdominal dissection including formation of the end colostomy, turning the patient into the prone jack-knife position (Fig. 11.28) allowing excellent exposure for the perineal dissection. This has the disadvantage of requiring repositioning of the intubated patient as well as re-establishing the sterile field.

Incision

- Midline incision, often limited to below the umbilicus
- A low transverse incision may be preferred.

Procedure

The traditional APER is an open procedure performed synchronously by an abdominal and perineal surgeon, but the abdominal and pelvic dissection may also be performed laparoscopically employing the same principles. The specimen is then removed through the perineal incision.

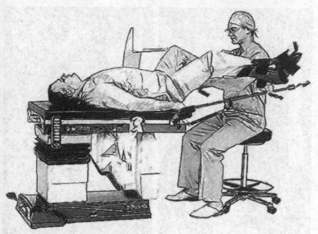

Fig. 11.14 Lloyd–Davies (modified lithotomy) position. This enables the perineal dissection.

The aim of the procedure is to remove the rectum, levator ani muscles and anus as a continuous cylinder and to avoid 'coning' in at the termination of the mesorectum. If one follows the anatomical plane of the mesorectum there is a risk of coming too close to the rectal muscle wall and compromising a potentially curative operation. The specimen should not show 'waisting' at the termination of the mesorectum, just above the levator ani muscles (Fig. 11.15).

Abdominal mobilization

- A full laparotomy is performed assessing resectability and spread of the tumour
- The sigmoid and left colon are mobilized as for anterior resection, preserving the ureters and gonadal vessels
- Ligation of the superior rectal or inferior mesenteric artery is performed and the sympathetic nerves are identified and preserved
- The left colon/sigmoid is divided with a stapler at a suitable point at a right angle to its blood supply with ligation of the mesenteric vessels
- The well vascularized left colon is brought out at the pre-marked stoma site in the LIF
- The stoma is matured with an absorbable suture once the abdominal wound has been closed.

Pelvic dissection

- The pelvic dissection is commenced by lifting the rectum forward and anteriorly
- The previous incision at the lateral peritoneal attachments of the sigmoid is extended to run over the pelvic brim and continued into the pelvis, taking care to incise the peritoneum just beyond the edge of the mesorectum (for cancer cases)

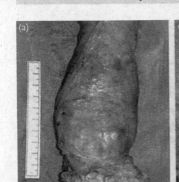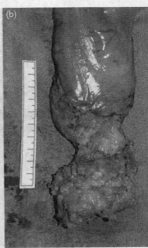

Fig. 11.15 Abdominoperineal resection specimen. In a, the mesorectum is intact and a continuous cylinder of tissue extends below to the anus. In b, there is 'waisting' at the end of the mesorectum where the dissection is too close to the muscle of the rectal wall.

- On the right side of the rectum, the peritoneum is similarly incised with diathermy, extending anteriorly at the base of the bladder/pouch of Douglas to join with the left side
- When dividing the peritoneum at the anterior peritoneal reflexion, the incision should be towards the rectal side for posterior tumours and benign conditions whereas the incision should extend as far onto the bladder as necessary for anterior tumours in order to obtain a satisfactory margin
- The rectal mobilization then begins by entering into the plane behind the mesorectum and in front of the presacral fascia and the hypogastric nerve plexus
- Although diathermy is the most commonly used method of mobilization, alternatives such as sharp scissors dissection with meticulous haemostasis or alternative energy sources (e.g. harmonic scalpel) can be used. A bloodless field offers the best chance to identify and preserve the hypogastric and pelvic nerve plexus
- The correct fascial plane is mostly avascular and the surface of the mesorectum posteriorly should be smooth with no defects (Fig. 11.11)
- As dissection is continued distally around the curve of the sacrum, Waldeyer's fascia (rectosacral ligament) is divided giving access to the pelvic floor
- The lateral dissection also follows the line of the mesorectum until the lateral ligaments are encountered (containing autonomic nerves and, occasionally, a middle rectal vessel). These are divided, although care

should be taken to avoid excessive medial traction during the division as this can tent up the pelvic plexus which can be damaged at this point (Fig. 11.16)

- The anterior dissection follows the plane behind the fascia of Denonvilliers which will prevent damage to the periprostatic nerve plexus lying behind the seminal vesicles. For anterior tumours, the fascia is incised and the plane lies in front of this fascia. On occasion it may be necessary to resect the seminal vesicles themselves in order to achieve satisfactory cancer clearance
- In women, the rectovaginal septum is separated, although it may be necessary to perform an *en bloc* resection of the posterior wall of the vagina for locally advanced anterior tumours
- Care must be taken not to extend this pelvic dissection too low as there is a tendency to follow the mesorectum as it thins out into the muscle tube of the rectum at the anorectal ring. Ideally, the perineal operator should incorporate the levators and the entire anorectal ring to remove a cylinder of tissue (Fig. 11.15a).

Perineal dissection

- A purse-string suture is applied to occlude the anus
- An elliptical incision is made starting at the perineal body anteriorly, extending laterally to the ischiorectal spines and ending posteriorly at the tip of the coccyx
- The skin, ischiorectal membrane and fat are incised, exposing the levators. The perineal surgeon then coordinates the dissection in the pre-coccygeal plane
- The anococcygeal ligament in the posterior midline is opened and the perineal surgeon then places a finger to retract the levator muscle down into the operative field. The levators are then divided circumferentially as a wide margin.
- The anterior dissection is often completed after the resection specimen has been everted out to the perineal surgeon
- In cases of suspected anterior infiltration into the vagina, the posterior vagina and perineal body should be resected *en bloc*.

Closure

Abdominal incision

- The omentum can be mobilized on the left gastroepiploic pedicle or the caecum mobilized and dropped into the pelvis to exclude the small bowel in an attempt to prevent subsequent adhesive obstruction
- Most surgeons will leave a low-pressure suction drain deep in pelvis and brought out through the abdominal wall
- Abdominal wound: mass closure with looped polydioxanone or nylon followed by skin clips or a subcuticular suture.

Perineal incision

- Primary closure. The edges of the levators or ischiorectal fat are closed with absorbable sutures and the perineal wound is closed
- Reconstruction. If the patient is in the lithotomy position, a rectus abdominus flap may be used. If the perineal dissection has been performed in the prone jack-knife position, a gluteus maximus flap is recommended. These procedures can significantly reduce perineal wound morbidity.

Post-operative care

- An enhanced recovery protocol should be employed (→ Enhanced recovery p.498).

Post-operative complications

- Wound infection and wound dehiscence
- Unhealed perineal wound (↑ risk if patient has had pre-operative RT)
- Haemorrhage
- Post-operative ileus
- Incisional hernia and parastomal hernia.

References

Miles WE. A method of performing abdomino-perineal excision for carcinoma of the rectum and of the terminal portion of the pelvic colon (1908). *CA Cancer J Clin* 1971;**21**:361–364.

Salerno G, Daniels I, Heald RJ, Brown G, Moran BJ. Management and imaging of low rectal carcinoma. *Surg Oncol* 2004;**13**:55–61.

Christian CK, Kwaan MR, Betensky RA, et al. Risk factors for perineal wound complications following abdominoperineal resection. *Dis Colon Rectum* 2005;**48**:43–48.

Surgery for acute colitis

The surgical technique when operating on patients with toxic colitis and toxic megacolon is similar. Even greater care needs to be exercised when handling an acutely dilated toxic colon. In such circumstances, the wall of the colon may become paper thin and every effort must be made to avoid iatrogenic perforation.

Indications

- Toxic colitis or toxic megacolon (➜ Severe acute colitis and toxic megacolon p.186).

Preparation

- Emergency patients should be fully resuscitated
- Urinary catheterization
- Thromboembolism prophylaxis
- Prophylactic antibiotics and blood cross-matched according to local guidelines
- Immunosuppressives therapy should be reviewed. Steroids should be continued in the perioperative period for patients at risk of adrenal insufficiency (≥20mg prednisolone equivalent daily for ≥3 consecutive weeks in the preceding year). Hydrocortisone 100mg IV is commonly given at induction and then 8hly for at least 24h
- Pre-operative review by stoma therapist when possible and appropriate site for a stoma marked.

Position

- Lloyd–Davies position in case access to the rectum is required.

Incision

- Midline laparotomy.

Procedure

Subtotal colectomy and end ileostomy

- In cases of toxic megacolon, colonic decompression may be necessary before any attempt is made to proceed with resection. The bowel should be quarantined away from the rest of the abdominal cavity contents prior to insertion of a wide-bore needle attached to suction tubing
- Mobilization of the colon starts in the RIF at the caecum
- The TI is divided close to the ileocaecal valve. The terminal branches of the ICA are divided as they enter the caecum, leaving intact the main trunk and its arcade with the terminal branches of the SMA. This leaves open the option of dividing the terminal branch of the SMA and using the ICA to supply the TI when fashioning an ileal pouch. Although rarely necessary, this manoeuvre can be helpful if there is concern about the ileal pouch reaching the anal canal when fashioning an ileal pouch at subsequent surgery
- The branches of the middle colic artery are best divided close to the colon wall, again avoiding mobilization at the root of the mesentery

- Particular care needs to taken when mobilizing the splenic flexure as this is the area of the colon where localized perforations are most likely to occur
- If omentum is adherent to the colon, this should be resected *en bloc* rather than attempting to mobilize it from the colon
- The IMA is left intact and the left colic and sigmoid branches are divided individually close to the colon
- The rectum itself is left undisturbed and no attempt is made even to incise the peritoneal reflexion of the upper rectum. The benefit to limiting mobilization of the rectum, retroperitoneum and IMA is readily apparent when the patient undergoes completion proctectomy at a later date. Not only is dissection easier, but of greater importance is the fact that the inferior hypogastric nerve plexus will also be undisturbed, reducing the likelihood of inadvertent damage
- The colon is divided at a point in the sigmoid that will allow the distal end to reach the anterior abdominal wall. Although a linear stapler may be used, the colon may be so friable that staples readily cut out. It is therefore advisable to oversew this staple line.

Rectal stump management

The inflamed oedematous rectal stump may be managed in a number of different ways:

- It may be left to lie *in situ* within the peritoneal cavity. Although this is satisfactory, some patients will develop a leak from the stump, leading to a pelvic abscess (Fig. 11.16). At best, this will delay recovery and make subsequent surgery more difficult. A soft, large-bore rectal drain placed for several days through the anus will allow the rectal stump to decompress and may reduce the risk of intraperitoneal stump blowout
- Alternatively, the closed rectal stump is brought up to the level of the subcutaneous fat at the lower end of the wound. The fascia is closed around it and skin closed over the end so that the stapled end lies within the subcutaneous space. This technique offers the advantage of avoiding a mucus fistula. If the staple line does break down, it will simply lead to a subcutaneous abscess, which can be drained under LA. A rectal stump drain may be placed through the anus
- Another option is to fashion a formal mucus fistula which may be brought out through the lower end of the wound. Although it is perhaps the safest option, a mucus fistula can be difficult to manage and many patients find it more troublesome than the ileostomy
- In rare instances when the colon is so inflamed that consideration cannot be given to stapling or suturing the rectum or sigmoid, the divided open distal end is brought out through the lower end of the wound, leaving at least 7–10cm protruding beyond skin level. This is wrapped in gauze and no attempt is made to fashion a mucous fistula initially. The protruding sigmoid colon is subsequently amputated once it has become adherent. This stump is usually ready for amputation between 5 and 7 days after the initial surgery. A formal mucus fistula is then fashioned.

Intra-abdominal rectal stump

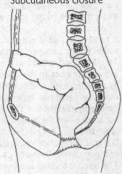

Subcutaneous closure

Mucus fistula

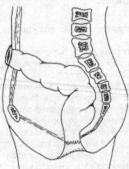

Ultralow Hartmann's

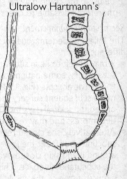

Fig. 11.16 Options for management of the rectal stump in patients undergoing colectomy for toxic colitis.

Total proctocolectomy and end ileostomy

- Rarely performed in ill patients with toxic colitis, as it is associated with excessive mortality and morbidity
- May be considered in less toxic patients unsuitable for subsequent IPAA (e.g. CD, advanced age or incontinence)
- Proctectomy in the acute setting is associated with an increased risk of bleeding, damage to the autonomic nerves and pelvic sepsis
- A less radical alternative is a conservative proctocolectomy or ultralow Hartmann's procedure which leaves a small rectal stump *in situ*.

Blowhole colostomy and loop ileostomy

- With improved medical therapy, better antibiotics and more sophisticated perioperative management, the indications for this procedure have greatly diminished. Indications include multiple sealed perforations with adherent small bowel loops, pregnancy and critically ill patients in whom a lesser procedure may be appropriate

- Usually performed through a small lower midline incision
- A suitable loop of TI, 40–50cm from the ileocaecal valve, is brought out through a pre-marked site in the RIF. This should not interfere with formation of an ileal pouch at a later stage
- This wound is closed and a second small vertical incision (midline/paramedian) is made over the transverse colon, the position of which is identified by a plain AXR with a coin in the umbilicus or directly at the time of fashioning the loop ileostomy
- The incision is extended down through the peritoneum
- The seromuscular layer of the colon is sutured directly to the parietal peritoneum, which quarantines the incision from the peritoneal cavity
- The colon is decompressed with needle suction prior to formally opening the colon and suturing the bowel edges to the skin or subcutaneous fat, depending on how far it will reach
- No attempt is made to pull the colon into the wound as this will lead to tearing and perforation of the dilated, thin-walled colon
- Detoxification is rapid in most patients and a formal colectomy is usually performed 4–6 months after this procedure.

Post-operative care

- Fluids and diet can be introduced without delay
- Nutritional supplementation may be required
- Antibiotics may be continued in septic patients/peritoneal contamination
- Steroids should be tapered dependent on pre-operative dose and duration.

Post-operative complications

- Wound infection
- Intra-abdominal abscess
- Rectal stump leak
- Haemorrhage
- Ileus/small bowel obstruction
- Retraction or ischaemia of the stoma
- Incisional hernia.

Restorative proctocolectomy

Indications
UC is the most common indication for RPC. It is also commonly used for patients with familial polyposis coli. Rarely, it may be considered for patients with slow transit constipation and a megarectum (Box 11.1).

Preparation
- Thromboembolism prophylaxis
- Prophylactic antibiotics and blood cross-matched according to local guidelines
- Urinary catheterization for 24–48h
- Pre-operative review by a stoma nurse to counsel and site for a stoma.

Incision
- Midline laparotomy.

Position
- Lloyds–Davies (Fig. 11.14).
- Reverse Trendelenburg may be used for splenic flexure mobilization.

Procedure
RPC involves removing the entire colon and rectum. A completion proctectomy and IPAA follows on from a subtotal colectomy after emergency surgery and is similar in technique, other than the fact that the colon has already been removed.

Both procedures can be performed laparoscopically. In addition to potential benefits in terms of a faster recovery, fewer adhesions and wound related problems, there is also some evidence that a laparoscopic approach may have a lesser impact on fertility compared to open surgery.

Abdominal mobilization
- A full laparotomy is performed assessing the small bowel to exclude CD and assess if an ileal pouch will reach the pelvic floor
- The small bowel is packed in the left side to reveal the root of the small bowel mesentery and transverse mesocolon
- The operator standing on the right side divides the lateral peritoneal attachments of the right colon with diathermy along the white line of Toldt, continuing around the caecum, appendix and TI

Box 11.1 Indications for restorative proctocolectomy

Ulcerative colitis
Ongoing symptoms despite maximal medical therapy
Failure to tolerate medication due to side effects
Growth retardation/failure to thrive (adolescents/teenagers)
Dysplasia or cancer
Toxic colitis (usually treated with initial subtotal colectomy and subsequent completion proctectomy and ileal pouch)
Familial polyposis coli

Severe constipation and a megarectum

- Developing the plane between mesocolon and retroperitoneum, the right ureter and gonadal vessels should be identified and protected
- The duodenum is dissected off the posterior surface of right mesocolon and sharp dissection may be preferred to avoid thermal injury
- The suspensory omental attachments to the hepatic flexure can be divided with diathermy and ligation of larger vessels
- Care is taken to preserve the ICA by dividing its terminal branches close to the caecum. This allows for the possibility of dividing the terminal branches of the SMA to gain length
- The TI is divided either between clamps or with a linear stapler close to the caecum
- Dissection is continued across the transverse colon, dividing branches of the middle colic artery close to the colon
- The greater omentum is dissected off the transverse colon and the lesser sac is entered, continuing the dissection toward the splenic flexure. If the omentum is attached to the colon with inflammatory adhesions, the omentum should be resected with the specimen
- The left colon and rectum are then mobilized by initially packing the small bowel in the right upper quadrant to reveal the mesentery of the left colon and the rectum entering the pelvis
- The operator standing on the left side divides the lateral peritoneal attachments of the left colon with diathermy along the white line of Toldt, continuing from the rectosigmoid junction toward the splenic flexure
- The plane between mesocolon and retroperitoneum, left ureter and gonadal vessels is developed, identifying these structures
- The peritoneum around the splenic flexure is divided and the mobilization is completed. Care should be taken to avoid splenic capsule injury which can be either by a retractor in the LUQ or traction on adhesions to the tip of the spleen
- The left colon is retracted into the wound and the peritoneum is scored along the intended plane of resection
- Mesenteric windows are made on either side of the IMA which is ligated well away from the aorta in order to avoid damage to the hypogastric nerves.

Pelvic mobilization

- The pelvic dissection is commenced by lifting the rectum forward and anteriorly
- The previous incision at lateral peritoneal attachments of the sigmoid is extended to run over the pelvic brim and continued into the pelvis, taking care to incise the peritoneum on the mesorectal side of the edge of the mesorectum
- Alternatively, a close rectal mobilization may be performed although it is associated with an increased risk of blood loss
- On the right side of the rectum, the peritoneum is similarly incised with diathermy, extending anteriorly at the base of the bladder/pouch of Douglas to join with the left side
- When dividing the peritoneum at the anterior peritoneal reflexion, the incision should be made on the rectal side

- The rectal mobilization then begins by entering into the plane behind the mesorectum and in front of the presacral fascia and the hypogastric nerve plexus
- Although diathermy is the most commonly used method of mobilization, alternatives such as sharp scissors dissection with meticulous haemostasis or alternative energy sources (e.g. harmonic scalpel) can be used. A bloodless field offers the best chance to identify and preserve the hypogastric and pelvic nerve plexus
- The correct fascial plane is mostly avascular and the surface of the mesorectum posteriorly should be smooth with no defects (Fig. 11.11)
- As dissection is continued distally around the curve of the sacrum, Waldeyer's fascia (rectosacral ligament) is divided, giving access to the pelvic floor
- The lateral dissection also follows the line of the mesorectum until the lateral ligaments are encountered (containing autonomic nerves and, occasionally, a middle rectal vessel). These are divided close to the rectum, although care should be taken to avoid excessive medial traction during the division as this can tent up the pelvic plexus which can be damaged
- The anterior dissection follows the plane behind the fascia of Denonvilliers close to the rectum which will prevent damage to the periprostatic nerve plexus lying behind the seminal vesicles
- As the distal rectum is reached, a much closer plane on the rectal wall is the goal, particularly anteriorly in order to minimize the risk of nerve injury
- The pelvic dissection is complete when the anorectal ring is reached on all sides
- The surgeon double gloves and places a finger in the anus in order to assess the digital limit of dissection both anteriorly and posteriorly. The aim is to cross-staple the distal rectum at a point 2cm above the dentate line in order to leave the transition zone intact. This may improve continence (Fig. 11.17).
- The specimen is removed and the pelvis is packed while attention is directed towards fashioning an ileal pouch.

Fashioning an ileal pouch
- In order to ensure good pouch mobility, ensure the small bowel mesentery is fully mobilized right up to the duodenum/pancreas. The mesenteric window between the SMA and ICA is also excised
- A number of different pouch forms have been successfully used including S, J, H and W configurations
- The S pouch gives additional length but is associated with impaired pouch evacuation. The W pouch may be associated with a reduced frequency of defecation. The ease and speed of a double-stapled technique employing a J pouch has led to its widespread use
- A point 15cm from the end of the TI is identified and grasped with a forceps. Previously, a 20cm J pouch was thought best. However, increasingly, shorter length pouches are fashioned (12 – 15 cm) which are thought to give rise to fewer evacuation difficulties, a problem that can develop as the pouch increases in size with time.

(a)   (b)

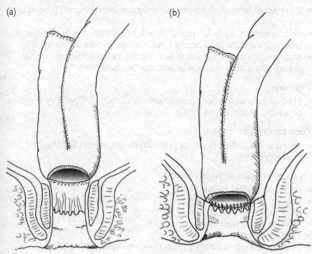

Fig. 11.17 Different methods to fashion an IPAA. A double-stapled technique leaves the anal transition zone intact and may be associated with better pouch function (a). A mucosectomy and hand-sewn anastomosis removes all the colonic mucosa, is felt to reduce the long-term risk of cancer in the rectal stump but may be associated with an increased likelihood of faecal leakage (b).

- By placing this point on traction, potential tethering points on the mesentery can be identified
- With care, transverse 2cm incisions are made 1cm apart on the peritoneum overlying the anterior and posterior aspect of the SMA
- The small intestine is opened at the proposed apex of the pouch and a 100mm linear stapler inserted.
- The pouch is constructed with 2–3 firings of the stapling gun. Maximum length and minimum tension are achieved by constructing the pouch with the mesentery lying posteriorly.
- A hand-inserted 2/0 polypropylene purse-string suture is inserted around the enterotomy which is used to secure the anvil of a circular stapling gun
- The gun is placed per rectum and the spike directed through or just behind the staple line. The head and anvil of the gun are connected after ensuring correct orientation of the pouch
- In women, extreme care is taken to ensure that the vagina lies well clear of the staple line
- Tension is again assessed before firing the gun
- Check that donuts are complete. A leak test can be performed by insufflating air into the pouch with a catheter while submerging the pelvic anastomosis under water
- Two atraumatic low-pressure suctions drains are placed in the pelvis

- If the pouch is to be defunctioned, an appropriate loop of TI close to the pouch is identified
- Two different sutures are placed in order to identify the proximal and distal ends and the loop brought out in a pre-marked RIF stoma site
- After closure of the abdominal wound, the stoma is matured with an absorbable suture. A stoma bridge may be considered.

Closure
- Mass closure with looped polydioxanone or nylon followed by skin clips or a subcuticular suture.

Post-operative care
- An enhanced recovery protocol should be employed (→ Enhanced recovery p.498).

Post-operative complications
- Anastomotic leak/pelvic sepsis
- Wound infection and dehiscence
- Haemorrhage
- Post-operative ileus
- Incisional hernia
- Pouch-specific problems (→ Ileal pouch complications p.176).

Radical pelvic surgery

Radical pelvic surgery

- The surgical options available for locally advanced and locally recurrent rectal cancer (LRRC) are dependent on the area of recurrence and the extent of disease. The procedures available range from standard abdominoperineal resection to total pelvic exenteration with composite sacrectomy (➔ Recurrent rectal cancer p.370)
- These operations carry a significant morbidity but with careful patient selection an R0 resection can result in improved quality of life and 5yr survival of 35% to 50% for LRRC.

Preparation

Patient selection is paramount. MDT review of patient and imaging is important to confirm resectability of the tumour and absence of metastatic disease, provide a guide to the surgical operative plan and ensure the patient's fitness for major surgery. The magnitude of the operation and potential complications are discussed in depth with the patient and family.

- Pre-operative review by a stoma nurse to counsel and site for a stoma
- Thromboembolism prophylaxis
- Prophylactic antibiotics and blood cross-matched according to local guidelines
- Urinary catheterization
- The need to involve other specialties should be anticipated and may include urology, plastic surgery orthopaedics, neurosurgery or radiotherapists.

Position

- Lloyds–Davies (Fig. 11.14). Particular care with positioning is required to avoid upper and lower limb nerve injury, compartment syndrome and/or venous thrombosis during prolonged procedures
- Bilateral ureteric stents are normally inserted.

Incision

A midline incision is usually made. Transverse incisions are generally avoided because they compromise the placement of stomas and the blood supply of the rectus muscle, which may be required in the perineal reconstruction.

Procedure

- The abdomen is entered and adhesions are carefully divided
- A full laparotomy looking for evidence of extrapelvic tumour is performed. Particular attention is paid to the liver, omentum, peritoneum, retroperitoneum and any area of prior dissection. The presence of extrapelvic disease is a contraindication to radical resection apart from rare exceptions where a synchronous pelvic recurrence and liver resection may be performed
- The small bowel is packed into the upper abdomen to facilitate pelvic exposure
- Dissection begins at the level of the aortic bifurcation to enter a virgin fascial plane which aids in the posterior dissection to the level of the pelvic floor

- The ureters are identified along their entire course to their insertion into the bladder, to avoid injury and to ensure adequate length if an ileal conduit is required
- The operation performed then depends on the pattern of recurrence and the fixation of the recurrent tumour
- There is no standard classification for staging advanced primary rectal cancer or LRRC. However, many surgeons use the following classification which is based on the anatomic region of the pelvis involved with the tumour

Central (tumour confined to pelvic organs and soft tissue. No adherence to bone or major vessels)

These tumours have the best prognosis as it is usually possible to achieve a clear margin. Depending on the site, *en bloc* total or partial resection of adjacent organs may be required.

In females, the resection may require only an *en bloc* excision of the posterior wall of the vagina and reconstruction. If the upper vagina or lower uterus is involved more extensively, *en bloc* hysterectomy and posterior vaginectomy are necessary. The uterus usually affords some protection, avoiding a cystectomy. Males with an anterior recurrence usually require partial cystectomy, total cystectomy or cystoprostatectomy.

If a completion APER is required, the resection is similar to a standard extralevator APER, but the pelvic fibrosis induced by prior surgery and radiotherapy can obliterate normal planes (➔ Abdominoperineal excision of the rectum p.550). The distinction between fibrosis and tumour can be impossible and if there is any question about the nature of the tissue, particularly when it would threaten resectability or alter the surgical approach, a frozen section should be performed.

Sacral/posterior recurrence

Tumour invades the presacral space to abut or invade the sacrum and or coccyx. These usually require an abdominoperineal resection and composite sacrectomy. The proximal extent of the sacral resection limited to S2–3. The operation involves 4 distinct parts:

- The anterior dissection
- The posterior dissection
- The use of IORT if required
- The perineal reconstruction.

Anterior dissection

- The pelvic dissection in the posterior plane is performed to the level of proximal tumour involvement of the sacrum. This allows early confirmation that the tumour does not extend above S2–3
- The rectum is mobilized in the anterior and lateral planes, leaving sacral fixation as the only point of attachment
- Bilateral ligation of the internal iliac arteries and veins may be performed at this point to reduce blood loss during sacrectomy
- The rectum is mobilized anteriorly and laterally, the stomas are created and the abdominal incision is closed
- The patient is repositioned in the prone jack-knife position

Posterior dissection
- A posterior midline incision from the region of the last lumbar vertebra to the coccyx is made and the gluteal muscles are freed
- The pudendal and sciatic nerves are identified and preserved
- The sacrum is then transected and the dural sac is closed.

Lateral/pelvic sidewall involvement

These are the most difficult group as disease can involve the bony pelvis, ureters, iliac vessels and sciatic nerves. These are technically challenging operations where the risk of a positive margin is higher

- The dissection may be started in a plane lateral to the common and external iliac vessels. Internal iliac vessels are ligated.
- If the external iliac vessels are involved, these are resected en bloc medially with the tumour mass
- Posterior dissection will lead to the lumbar-sacral trunk and sacral nerve roots and nearby piriformis and obturator muscles
- The sacral nerve, bony ischium, sacrotuberous and sacrospinous muscles can all be resected en bloc with acceptable morbidity

Reconstruction

Resections for recurrent disease often result in a wide defect, rendering primary closure impossible. Most patients will also have received pre-operative RT which increases perineal wound morbidity. Myocutaneous flaps using gracilis, gluteus or rectus abdominus are often used as they significantly reduce perineal wound complications and morbidity compared with primary closure.

References

Warrier SK, Heriot AG, Lynch AC. Surgery for Locally Recurrent Rectal Cancer: Tips, Tricks and Pitfalls. *Clin Colon Rectal Surg.* 2016;**29**(2):114–122.

Heriot AG, Tekkis PP, Darzi A, Mackay J. Surgery for local recurrence of rectal cancer. *Colorectal Dis* 2006;**8**:733–747.

Sagar P, Gonsalves S, Heath R, Phillips N, Chalmers A. Composite abdominosacral resection for recurrent rectal cancer. *Br J Surg* 2009;**96**:191–196.

Rectal prolapse: rectopexy

Rectopexy aims to restore normal anatomy and hence relieve rectal prolapse and restore function. This procedure includes several options; the surgeon's choice is often guided by personal preference rather than good quality evidence. The variety of described techniques reflects the fact that the ideal operation has yet to be developed.

Patients with rectal prolapse are frequently elderly; it is vital to establish that they are sufficiently healthy to withstand an abdominal procedure. The relative safety of a less invasive, perineal procedure should be considered.

Indications

- Full-thickness 1° or recurrent rectal prolapse
- Full-thickness internal intussusception, particularly if associated with symptoms of FI, SRUS or obstructed defecation.

Preparation

It is important actively to question the female patient about associated urinary dysfunction and vaginal prolapse. Symptoms may be present in 20–30% of females and require investigation and a multidisciplinary approach.

- Proximal pathology is excluded as appropriate to the patient's age and symptoms
- In consenting to surgery, patients should be informed of the relative risks of prolapse recurrence and post-operative constipation
- Thromboembolism prophylaxis is given
- Full bowel preparation is not necessary
- Prophylactic antibiotics and blood cross-matched or group and save according to local guidelines.

Position

- Surgery is ordinarily undertaken under GA in the supine position with a degree of head-down tilt.

Incision

- Lower abdominal midline or Pfannenstiel incision
- Alternatively, a laparoscopic approach may be utilized, with the potential advantage of a more rapid post-operative recovery.

Procedure

Rectal mobilization

- Dissection commences at the pelvic brim, immediately to the left of the sigmoid mesentery and developed in the presacral plane, posterior to the mesorectal fascia, down to the distal rectum, thus exposing the levator ani muscles
- The mesentery is then divided on the right side of the rectosigmoid junction and continued down into the pelvis and posteriorly to join the mobilization from the left side
- The operative view is likely to be good since a typical patient will be an elderly female with a wide pelvis and lax tissues
- The pelvic autonomic nerves and ureters are identified and preserved

- Tissues immediately lateral to the distal rectum may contain potentially important neurovascular bundles and these should not be divided; the bundles will have been stretched sufficiently to allow the prolapse to be reduced without their division
- Anteriorly, the dissection should not open the rectovaginal septum
- In males, the anterior dissection stops at the seminal vesicles.

Rectal fixation

- The mobilized rectum may be fixed at a variety of sites with a number of different materials
- Some surgeons place a series of sutures along the length of the posterior mesorectum, to the curve of the presacral fascia, thus restoring an approximation of normal anatomy
- Alternatively, one can place 2 or 3 sutures between the lumbosacral disc and the right side of the mesorectum, without penetrating the rectal wall, to create a degree of 'bowstringing' and hold the mobilized rectum higher in the pelvis (Fig. 11.18)
- Care is taken to avoid trauma to the fragile presacral veins
- The rectum is only fixed on one side to prevent the creation of an obstructing, narrow ellipse in the bowel lumen
- Fixation should be performed with a non-absorbable suture such as a polypropylene or braided nylon suture
- Other fixation materials include alternative suture material, polypropylene mesh and polyvinyl acetate sponge
- There is no good evidence that any one material is superior to the others, but there is potential for mesh or sponge to erode intestine, harbour chronic infection or produce adhesions
- Increasing anxiety regarding the use of mesh in prolapse procedures has led to a decline in use and procedures such as laparoscopic ventral mesh rectopexy (LVMR) are now only infrequently performed.
- It is possible to hitch uterus to anterior abdominal wall for additional support, but this technique may impair urinary bladder capacity.

Sigmoid resection

- Rectopexy may be complicated by severe, chronic post-operative constipation
- Resection rectopexy (i.e. simultaneous sigmoid colectomy and prolapse repair) may reduce the incidence of this complication
- Sigmoid colectomy should be reserved for patients with no evidence of diarrhoea, FI or anal sphincter weakness (where a degree of post-operative constipation may actually be desirable)
- A primary anastomosis is fashioned after sigmoid resection
- Splenic flexure is not mobilized since doing so would increase colonic mobility and theoretically encourage prolapse recurrence.

Closure

- Mass closure with looped polydioxanone or nylon.

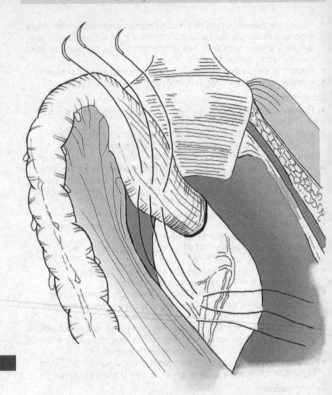

Fig. 11.18 Placement of sutures between the lumbosacral disc and the right side of the mesorectum. Care is taken not to catch any of the hypogastric nerve plexus which crosses the pelvic brim at this point.

Post-operative care

- An enhanced recovery protocol should be employed (➔ Enhanced recovery p.498).
- It can take several days for a return of bowel function. This be frustrating when all other aspects of the recovery have been uneventful; laxatives may be necessary in these circumstances.

Post-operative complications

- Wound infection and dehiscence
- Haemorrhage
- Post-operative ileus
- Urinary retention
- Post-operative constipation
- Incisional hernia
- Anastomotic leak (if a resection rectopexy has been performed)
- Recurrent prolapse.

Results

Continence is usually improved with any procedure for rectal prolapse as the mechanical effect of the prolapse on the sphincter complex is removed and the sphincters are no longer by-passed. Recurrence of prolapse after abdominal procedures ranges from 2 to 10%.

Rectal prolapse: perineal procedures

Perineal procedures for rectal prolapse are associated with less perioperative morbidity than abdominal procedures but are generally more prone to recurrence. They are usually reserved for:
- Patients unfit for an abdominal procedure
- Well informed young males who wish to reduce the risk of sexual dysfunction.

Indications
- Full-thickness 1° or recurrent rectal prolapse
- Full-thickness internal intussusception, particularly if associated with symptoms of FI, SRUS or obstructed defecation.

Preparation
It is important actively to question female patients about associated urinary dysfunction and vaginal prolapse. Symptoms may be present in 20–30% and require investigation and a multidisciplinary approach.
- Proximal pathology is excluded as appropriate to the patient's age and symptoms
- Bowel preparation is not necessary
- Thromboembolism prophylaxis
- Prophylactic antibiotics and blood cross-matched or group and save according to local guidelines
- Urinary catheterization.

Position
- Prone or lithotomy position under general or spinal anaesthesia.

Incision
- Circumferential incision of the rectum 1–2cm proximal to the dentate line either full-thickness or submucosal depending on procedure.

Procedures
Delorme's procedure (Fig. 11.19)
Delorme's procedure (mucosal sleeve resection and muscle imbrication) is one of the most commonly performed perineal procedures. It is well tolerated.
- The prolapse is reproduced and the submucosal plane infiltrated with 1 in 200,000 adrenaline
- Dissection commences 1cm proximal to the dentate line
- The submucosal plane is entered circumferentially
- The dissection then proceeds proximally to the apex of the prolapse, dissecting the mucosa off the underlying muscle tube
- Eight imbricating braided absorbable sutures are placed vertically to plicate the redundant muscle
- The excess mucosa is trimmed and circumferential mucosal apposition obtained with interrupted absorbable sutures.

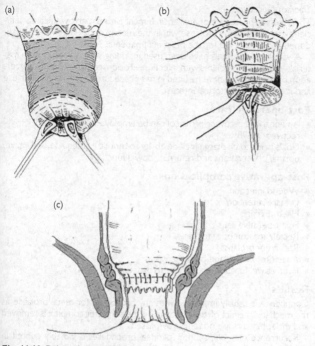

Fig. 11.19 Delorme's procedure.

Altemeier's procedure

Altemeier's procedure (perineal proctosigmoidectomy) may be combined with an anterior levatorplasty.

- The prolapse is delivered and a full-thickness incision sited anteriorly 1–2cm proximal to the dentate line
- The hernial sac is entered, taking care not to injure small bowel
- The incision is continued circumferentially
- The mesorectum is divided sequentially, pulling down the redundant rectum and sigmoid, until no more redundant colon is apparent
- At this point the levators are exposed anteriorly and can be opposed with 2 or 3 sutures
- Anterior levatorplasty may decrease recurrence and improve continence
- The redundant colon is divided hemicircumferentially
- Stay sutures are placed between the colon and divided anal canal
- The proximal division is completed and all the sutures placed under direct vision before sequential ligation
- Coloanal anastomosis can also be carried out using a circular stapler.

Thiersch procedure

The Thiersch procedure of anal encirclement aims to narrow the anus sufficiently to maintain the prolapse within the rectum. It has largely been abandoned and is reserved for the most unfit patients.

A variety of materials have been used including wire, various suture materials and mesh. Problems with infection, erosion, recurrence and incarceration of the prolapse have resulted in this procedure having very limited use and it is largely of historical interest.

Post-operative care

- An enhanced recovery protocol can be employed (→ Enhanced recovery p.498)
- Goals prior to discharge include ability to mobilize, adequate oral intake, normal observations and return of bowel function.

Post-operative complications

- Wound infection
- Urinary retention
- Haemorrhage
- Post-operative ileus
- Rectal/anastomotic stricture
- Recurrent prolapse
- Anastomotic leak and pelvic sepsis
- Poor bowel function due to due to proctectomy.

Results

Continence is usually improved with any procedure for rectal prolapse as the mechanical effect of the prolapse on the sphincter complex is removed and the sphincters are no longer by-passed.

Recurrence of prolapse after perineal procedures is variably quoted in the literature. Some of this is accounted for by variation in technique and duration of follow-up. Recurrence rates are higher after Delorme's procedure and are in the order of 7–22%. Quoted figures for Altemeier's procedure are ~5–15%.

Recurrent prolapse

The number of operations described for rectal prolapse is testament to the fact that all procedures carry an appreciable recurrence rate. The options for further surgery for recurrent prolapse depend on the patient's condition and the primary procedure. For example, those with a recurrent prolapse following resection rectopexy are not considered suitable for Altemeier's procedure due to the risk of leaving an ischaemic segment of colon between the two anastomoses. It is possible to repeat a Delorme's procedure but scarring from the primary operation can make surgery difficult. In these circumstances, consideration should be given to performing Altemeier's procedure.

Reference

Tou S, Brown SR, Malik AI, Nelson RL. Surgery for complete rectal prolapse in adults. *Cochrane Database Syst Rev* 2008;(**4**):CD001758.

Rectocele repair

Some degree of rectocele can be found in most females. Appropriate patient selection for surgery is paramount. A diagnosis can be reached in most patients with a good history and clinical examination. Defecating proctography may demonstrate trapped contrast in the rectocele.

Rectocele is a benign condition in which the potential benefits of an operation may be outweighed by risk of surgery. Pre-operative trials of biofeedback are safe and may successfully relieve some patients' symptoms. It is important actively to question female patients about associated urinary dysfunction and vaginal prolapse. A transanal approach offers the chance to address anorectal problems such as haemorrhoids.

Indications

Repair is reserved for patients with obstructed defecation who digitate their vagina or support their perineum to achieve rectal emptying.

Preparation

- A phosphate enema is given prior to surgery and the rectum and vagina washed out with povidone–iodine prior to operation
- Thromboembolism prophylaxis
- Prophylactic antibiotics according to local guidelines.

Position

- Prone jack-knife position is best for a transanal approach (Fig. 11.28)
- Lithotomy is best for a transvaginal approach and either position can be used to perform the repair via a transperineal approach.

Procedure

The aim of repair is to reinforce the rectovaginal septum. This is achieved by dissecting the space between the rectal and vaginal walls and plicating the thinned muscularis propria of the rectum and the puborectalis portion of the levator ani muscle towards the midline using multiple longitudinal rows of interrupted sutures to create a buttress.

- When performing a transanal approach a suitable anal retractor (Hill–Ferguson or Pratt) gives good access in the prone position
- Anterior rectal mucosa is infiltrated with 1/200,000 adrenaline
- The rectal mucosa from the level of the dentate line is incised proximally in a linear fashion
- Stay sutures are used to pick up divided mucosa, thereby improving access and, as the dissection continues, drawing the rectovaginal septum down into the wound facilitating more proximal mobilization
- The mucosal edges are undermined laterally with sharp and blunt dissection to allow access to the thinned muscularis propria of anterior rectal wall/rectocele
- Vertical absorbable plicating sutures are placed through exposed muscularis propria to incorporate deeper connective tissues of the rectovaginal septum. On occasion, it may be more appropriate to use transverse plication sutures
- A finger in the vagina can help to push the rectocele into the operative field and is also used to ensure that plicating sutures do not go full thickness through into the vagina

- Redundant rectal mucosa is removed prior to closure with a continuous suture
- LA is infiltrated (0.25% bupivacaine + 1/200,000 adrenaline).

Post-operative care

- Patients are encouraged to mobilize and commence normal diet
- Goals prior to discharge include ability to mobilize, adequate oral intake, normal observations and return of bowel function.
- Faecal impaction must be avoided to prevent disruption of the repair. Laxatives should be prescribed and occasionally gentle rectal irrigation via a soft catheter may be necessary.

Post-operative complications

- Wound infection
- Urinary retention
- Haemorrhage
- Suture line dehiscence although this rarely causes significant problems
- Rarer and potentially more serious complications including rectovaginal fistula, haemorrhage and trauma to an unsuspected enterocele should be avoided with careful surgical technique.

Outcome

- Rectocele repair should initially relieve obstructed defaecation in the majority of appropriately selected patients. Benefits may be short-lived since the repair only approximates muscle rather than fascia and so lacks strength. Symptomatic recurrence of rectocele is common
- A significant proportion of patients experience post-op dyspareunia.

Alternative procedures

- A transvaginal or transperineal approach can be used. Transperineal approach also offers the opportunity to plicate the pelvic floor
- An alternative to traditional rectocele repair is the STARR procedure (Stapled transanal rectal resection)
- A patient with diffuse pelvic floor weakness, whose rectocele co-exists with a rectal prolapse or intussusception, might be more appropriately managed with rectopexy (→ Prolapse: rectopexy p.570)
- Recent techniques have utilized implantation of non-absorbable, synthetic mesh or acellular porcine dermis to reinforce the rectovaginal septum. Such techniques provide a tension-free repair that may be securely anchored to the pelvis and is not liable to stretch. Experience with such techniques is currently limited and there is concern regarding risk of infection and erosion of prosthetic material.
- Dissection of the cranial portion of the rectovaginal septum may be undertaken laparoscopically
- Rectocele repairs are relatively uncommon procedures; therefore, the opportunity to conduct large-scale comparative studies of different therapies has been limited.

Transanal endoscopic microsurgery

TEM was developed by Buess in the 1980s. The classic system comprises an operating sigmoidoscope with an integrated microscope (4× magnification), insufflation/irrigation system and instruments that are used to excise rectal lesions (Fig. 11.20). Lesions may be excised in the submucosal plane or by full-thickness excision of a disc of bowel wall. More recent systems for transanal endoscopic surgery include the TEO platform (Karl Storz, Tuttlingen, Germany) and the GelPOINT Path (Applied Medical).

It is important to perform a careful assessment of suitability for TEM prior to proceeding to resection. MRI, ERUS +/- biopsy may clarify whether invasive tumour is present in a villous adenoma and may demonstrate the depth of invasion through the bowel wall in a small carcinoma (Fig. 11.21). The majority of surgeons aim to stay below the peritoneal reflection when performing TEM, thus avoiding the risk of perforation in submucosal excision and the need for repair of the defect after full-thickness excision. Leaders in the field, such as Buess, may be prepared to undertake anterior resection by a combination of the laparoscopic and TEM approaches.

Indications
- Villous adenomas of rectum considered too large for snaring via the colonoscope
- Early rectal cancers

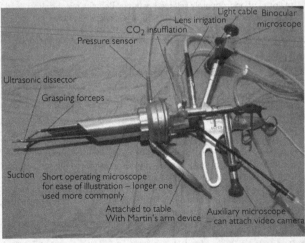

Fig. 11.20 TEM instrumentation.

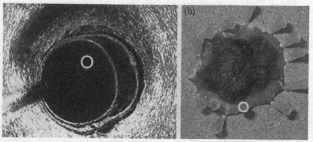

Fig. 11.21 Endorectal ultrasound of a uT0 rectal lesion (a) and the operative specimen showing a partial thickness excision of a villous adenoma (b).

Practicalities

- Initial EUA with ERUS may give more adequate assessment than clinic or flexible endoscope examination. Knowledge of the precise site of the lesion is helpful for appropriate patient positioning (lesion below the oblique end of the operating sigmoidoscope). For some platforms such as the GelPOINT Path most lesions can be approached with the patient in lithotomy position.
- Consider the site of the peritoneal reflection in relation to the lesion and the sex and body habitus of the patient. MRI can help determine the relationship of the lesion to the peritoneal reflection.
- There is a significant learning curve for the technique in which the instruments can be difficult to manipulate because they run in parallel down the sigmoidoscope. Gel port platforms allow greater range of movement but at the expense of stability when approaching higher lesions.
- The use of an ultrasonic dissector helps improve control of bleeding and hence visibility
- Closure of full thickness defects may reduce complication rates but without clear evidence a selective approach to closure is also appropriate
- Specimens should be pinned out on a corkboard for accurate pathological assessment of the peripheral and deep margins (Fig. 11.22).

Complications

- Many patients are pyrexial on the first post-operative night, presumably due to bacteraemia
- Inadvertent perforation of the rectum is more common in anterior lesions in females and may require laparotomy
- Both primary and secondary post-operative haemorrhage may occur but are relatively rare. Operative intervention is rarely necessary.
- Septic complications are rare but may be very troublesome.

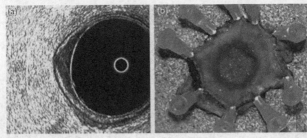

Fig. 11.22 Endorectal ultrasound of a uT1 with a breach of the submucosa and the rectal lesion (a) and the operative specimen showing a full-thickness excision of a uT1 cancer (b).

Long-term results

- Recurrence of villous adenomas is associated with histological involvement of the resection margins
- Caution should be exercised in local excision for carcinoma with the aim of cure. Recurrence rates are 29% for T2 carcinomas treated by local excision alone. 10–20% of T1 carcinomas locally excised recur over 5yrs. However, in patients with significant co-morbidity the risk of recurrent tumour after TEM may be judged to be less than the risk of low anterior resection and therefore TEM may be the best option
- Anal sphincter function is temporarily reduced after TEM
- Some patients will develop benign rectal strictures, usually after extensive resections.

References

Buess, G, Kipfmuller K, Iblad R et al. Clinical results of transanal endoscopic microsurgery Surg Endosc 1988;**2**:245–250.

Suppiah A, Maslekar S, Alabi A, Hartley JE, Monson JR. Transanal endoscopic microsurgery in early rectal cancer: time for a trial? Colorectal Dis 2008;**10**:314–329.

Haemorrhoidectomy

Indications

- Ongoing rectal bleeding and/or prolapse despite avoidance of straining and an adequate intake of fluid and fibre
- Failure or intolerance of less invasive procedures such as banding or injection.

Preparation

- Proximal pathology should be excluded as appropriate for the patient's age and symptoms
- Informed consent should be obtained and risks and expected results clearly explained and documented
- Prophylactic antibiotics according to local guidelines
- Phosphate enemas may be given for bowel preparation.

Operative choices

The main options are excisional haemorrhoidectomy and stapled haemorrhoidopexy. The choice of procedure depends on the patient's main symptom, the surgeon's experience and the patient's preference. Stapled haemorrhoidopexy is usually reserved for patients with 2nd and 3rd degree haemorrhoids refractory to less invasive interventions. Excisional haemorrhoidectomy is indicated for symptomatic 3rd and 4th degree haemorrhoids and in patients failing outpatient procedures.

Position

- Procedures can be performed in lithotomy or prone jack-knife position.

Procedures

Excisional haemorrhoidectomy
- The anal verge, anal canal and haemorrhoids are assessed before and after insertion of an anal retractor
- Tissue to be excised is marked with diathermy to ensure mucocutaneous bridges can be preserved between each haemorrhoidal excision
- The external component of the largest haemorrhoid is grasped and downward and medial traction applied
- The assistant keeps an Eisenhammer or similar anal retractor within the anal canal to allow good views and to keep the internal sphincter under gentle tension, allowing it to be identified
- Diathermy excision with meticulous haemostasis proceeds from the external component medially, visualising and preserving the internal anal sphincter
- The proximal pedicle can be sealed with diathermy or ligated (Fig. 11.23)
- The procedure is repeated for the other haemorrhoids
- Haemostasis is ensured at the end of the procedure
- A bilateral pudendal block is performed with levobupivacaine or similar long acting LA.

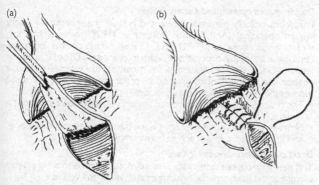

Fig. 11.23 Closed haemorrhoidectomy. The mucosa and haemorrhoid pedicle are raised with diathermy or sharp dissection, taking care to avoid damage to the underlying internal sphincter (a). The wound is closed with a running stitch (b).

Variations in technique include leaving the resultant defect open (Milligan–Morgan haemorrhoidectomy) or closing the defect (Ferguson haemorrhoidectomy). With the open method the wounds are left to heal by 2° intention which takes 4–8 weeks. Some studies have shown decreased healing times with the closed method, but this has not been a consistent finding.

Excision has also been carried out with newer devices such as LigaSure vessel sealing system (Covidien, Mansfield, MA, USA) or the ACE harmonic scalpel (Ethicon Endosurgery, Cincinnati, OH, USA). The additional cost and lack of clear evidence supporting improved outcomes have so far limited their widespread adoption. A recent Cochrane review concludes that LigaSure haemorrhoidectomy was better tolerated and resulted in significantly less immediate post-operative pain without any adverse effect on complications, recovery or continence. The long-term risk of recurrence is not yet known.

Stapled haemorrhoidopexy

The aim of the procedure is to excise redundant mucosa at the apex of the haemorrhoids, to divide the arterial supply and fix the remaining haemorrhoidal tissue in the upper anal canal. Most commonly performed using the PPH03 kit (Ethicon Endosurgery, Cincinnati, OH, USA).

- The circular anal dilator (CAD) is secured in place and a purse-string suture (polypropylene) placed 4cm above the dentate line
- Care should be taken to ensure that the lumen is not occluded and that the purse-string suture is not full thickness
- The circular stapler is inserted with the head fully open
- The purse-string is secured around the stem of the gun and the stapler closed and fired
- A circumferential strip of mucosa and submucosa is excised
- The staple line is checked for haemostasis and to ensure it is circumferential, intact and above the dentate line.

Doppler-guided haemorrhoidal artery ligation

Procedure typically performed using the HALO® (haemorrhoidal artery ligation operation) (AMI Feldrich Austria) or THD® (transanal haemorrhoidal devascularisation) (THD S.p.a. Corregio, Italy) devices. Both systems use a disposable proctoscope which incorporate a Doppler probe to facilitate Doppler-guided ligation of the haemorrhoidal arteries above the dentate line. A concomitant plication of prolapsing haemorrhoidal tissue reduces the risk of haemorrhoidal prolapse.

• The procedure is usually performed under GA but may be carried out under LA
• Short-term results are encouraging when the main symptom is bleeding and in the absence of 4th degree haemorrhoids.

Direct current electrotherapy (eXroid®)

This newly introduced technology uses a disposable probe to apply a direct current to the haemorrhoid, inducing thrombosis of the vessels.

• It is usually performed as an outpatient procedure. Sedation or local anaesthetic are not usually required
• Patient positioned in the left lateral position. A single use negatively charged disposable dual probe is used to apply current to the base of the haemorrhoid pedicle.
• Current is increased to a maximum of 16 milliamps or until patient experiences discomfort.
• Each haemorrhoid pedicle is treated for an average of 10 minutes.
• Early results are encouraging although longer term follow up and randomised trials comparing treatments are required.

Post-operative care

• Laxatives are prescribed to prevent constipation
• Studies report less pain if metronidazole is administered for 5–7 days
• The procedure may be carried out on a day case or 23h stay basis, ensuring the patient is able to pass urine prior to discharge.

Complications

• Haemorrhage, 1° or 2°
• Retention of urine
• Pain
• Delayed wound healing
• Recurrence
• Anal stenosis
• Impaired continence
• Pelvic sepsis
• Staples within the anal canal.

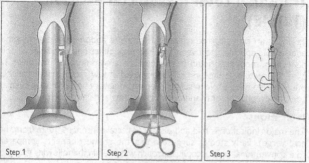

Fig. 11.24 Doppler-guided haemorrhoidal artery ligation. In Step 1, the anoscope with embedded Doppler ultrasound identifies the haemorrhoidal arteries. This directs placement of suture via an aperture in the anoscope to ligate the haemorrhoidal arteries (Step 2). In Step 3, tissue is plicated to treat haemorrhoidal prolapse.

Results

Both excisional and stapled haemorrhoidectomy were deemed safe by a recent Cochrane meta-analysis. Excisional haemorrhoidectomy appears to be associated with less frequent recurrence or need for further intervention. Stapled haemorrhoidopexy is less painful, allowing quicker resumption of normal activities. Given the premise that the most important outcomes in haemorrhoid surgery are recurrence and prolapse, excisional haemorrhoidectomy remains the gold standard.

References

Jayaraman S, Colquhoun PH, Malthaner R. Stapled versus conventional surgery for hemorrhoids. *Cochrane Database Syst Rev* 2006;(**4**):CD005393.

Nienhuijs S, de Hingh I. Conventional versus LigaSure hemorrhoidectomy for patients with symptomatic Hemorrhoids. *Cochrane Database Syst Rev* 2009;(**1**) CD006761.

Transanal total mesorectal excision (TaTME)

TaTME is an emerging technique that combines abdominal and a transanal endoscopic approach to overcomes technical difficulties with laparoscopic dissection, mobilization and transection and anastomosis of the lower 1/3 of the rectum. It has primarily been used in low rectal cancer patients but may also have a role in surgery for inflammatory bowel disease such as completion proctectomy and proctocolectomy and ileal pouch.

Indications

The major indication is mid and distal 1/3 rectal cancers (< 10cm from the anal verge). Early studies suggested that the greatest benefits compared to a conventional laparoscopic approach was seen in the following groups

- Narrow pelvis
- Prostatic hypertrophy
- Visceral obesity or body mass index (BMI) > 30 kg/m²
- Tumour diameter > 4cm
- Distorted tissue planes due to neoadjuvant radiotherapy
- Difficult recognition of the distal resection margin
- Tumors < 10cm from anal verge

However, it seems that many surgeons have adopted the technique for more proximal rectal cancer which is a concern as the technique involves complete mesorectal excision with concomitant impact on bowel function.

Contraindications

TaTME is a complex operation and perhaps the most important contraindication is inadequate training. Ideally the procedure should be undertaken by colorectal surgeons who have significant experience in laparoscopic or robotic TME, transanal minimally invasive surgery or intersphincteric resection and have an annual case volume of at least 20 procedures. The two-team approach is required with one surgical team performing the laparoscopic abdominal component and the second surgical team performing the perineal component. The following are considered to be relative contraindications to the procedure.

- Clinical T3 tumours with margins < 1 mm from the endopelvic fascia
- Tumours with ingrowth into the internal sphincter or levator ani
- T4 tumours

Preparation

- Fully informed consent
- Review of radiology and endoscopic confirmation of the site of the tumour
- Full bowel preparation
- Prophylactic antibiotics according to local guidelines
- Thromboembolism prophylaxis
- Although the procedure can be performed by a single team, a two-team approach enables shorter operation times, improved visualisation and better traction and counter-traction

- Appropriate equipment should be to hand including a 3-D laparoscope or extended length 5mm laparoscope for the perineal end (to avoid clashes between the laparoscope and working instruments).
- Ideally a continuous CO2 insufflation device with integrated smoke evacuation system (AirSeal System Surgiquest, Milford, US)

Patient position

- Lithotomy

Operative technique

- The operation starts with a standard laparoscopic insertion of ports and mobilisation of the splenic flexure, left colon and division of inferior mesenteric artery
- The perineal team can simultaneously start. The rectum is irrigated with a tumoricidal. A transanal access platform such as the GelPort (Applied Medical, California, US) is used to insert a purse-string to occlude the rectum below the tumour. This is a critical point of the operation and failure of the purse-string can compromise both the technical conduct of the operation and the oncological outcome.
- Using diathermy, a circumferential mucosal tattoo is placed before the rectum is circumferentially incised through mucosa and full thickness of the muscle wall
- Dissection is continued proximally in the avascular TME plane to meet the abdominal operator.
- The specimen may be extracted transanally or if large, through a Pfannenstiel incision.
- A purse-string is inserted into the divided distal rectal stump using either the transanal platform or directly transiently for very low resections
- The head of a circular stapling device is inserted into the proximal divided bowel either transiently or via an abdominal incision if the specimen was removed through the abdomen
- The fully mobilised left colon containing the head of the stapler is passed into the pelvis and a circular stapling gun used to fashion and end-to-end a circular stapled anastomosis.

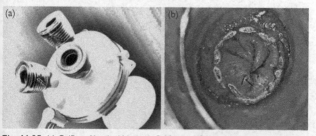

Fig. 11.25 (a) GelPort (Applied Medical, California, USA) used to perform perineal end of a TaTME; (b) Circumferential mucosal diathermy tattoo after insertion of a rectal purse-string below the tumour.

Complications

All of the usual complications to a laparoscopic low anterior section can occur after a TaTME procedure. In addition, the following complications are specific to the TaTME component of the procedure

- Urethral injury has been described in up to 10% of cases. The membranous urethra is particularly at risk if the prostate has been pulled posteriorly or the dissection plane is to anterior
- As with a laparoscopic TME and anastomotic leaks can occur but do not appear to occur more frequently with TaTME
- Conversion rates to open surgery vary from 0 to 10%
- During the perineal mobilisation of the rectum, there is a 1-5% risk of significant bleeding due to in inadvertent dissection into the side wall of the pelvis. Dissection beyond the correct plane can also lead to damage to the autonomic nervous laterally and sacral venous plexus posteriorly.

Reference

Vignali A, Elmore U, Miline M et al. Transanal total mesorectal excision (TaTME): current status and future perspectives Updates Surgery Innov 2008;**15**:105–109.

Pilonidal surgery

Indications

- Drainage of an acute pilonidal abscess
- Definitive surgery for a primary or recurrent pilonidal sinus (➔ Pilonidal sinus p. 282).

Preparation

- Thromboembolism prophylaxis
- Prophylactic antibiotics according to local guidelines.

Position

- Drainage of an abscess can be performed with the patient in the lateral or prone position
- Definitive surgery is usually performed with the patient in the prone jack-knife position and the buttocks taped apart (Fig. 11.26).

Drainage of pilonidal abscess

- May be performed under LA or GA
- A longitudinal 2cm paramedian incision is made over the area of maximum erythema and thinning of the skin
- Midline incisions create additional natal cleft skin defects in the vicinity of the primary sinus whereas a more lateral cut could necessitate excision of an inappropriately large area of skin at later definitive surgery
- Hairs should be curetted out of the abscess cavity and a swab sent for bacteriological culture
- De-roofing of the abscess cavity is not required
- The wound should only be packed superficially to hold the skin edges apart
- Definitive management of pilonidal sinus is best undertaken at a later date, after any abscess has been drained.

Definitive surgery

A number of operations have been described for patients with pilonidal sinus. The evidence base to guide the choice of procedure is weak, with few well-designed, comparative studies. Surgery may be undertaken under GA or LA as an inpatient or day case. Primary wound closure techniques may avoid the inconvenience of prolonged dressings.

When obtaining consent, patients should be aware of the relative risks of wound dehiscence, sinus recurrence and cosmetic deformity. A single dose of IV antibiotics, providing aerobic and anaerobic organism cover, should be given at the start of the procedure.

Operations that produce a wound that lies off the midline have a lower incidence of wound failure or sinus recurrence. These procedures include Karydakis flap, Bascom's original procedure, Bascom's cleft lift, Limberg flap, V–Y advancement and Z-plasty.

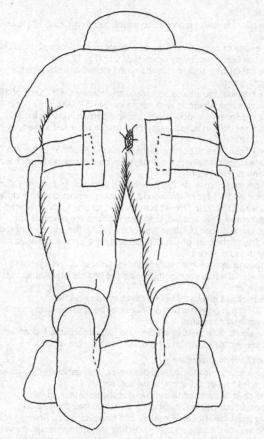

Fig. 11.26 Prone jack-knife position. For patients undergoing elective pilonidal sinus surgery.

Karydakis flap

- The pilonidal cavity is probed to establish its longitudinal and lateral limits
- An ellipse of tissue is outlined to encompass the entire pilonidal sinus and the lateral secondary opening or scar (Fig. 11.29a)
- The lateral edge should extend beyond the most lateral secondary opening or scar
- The edges of the area to be excised are infiltrated with 20mls of 1% lidocaine hydrochloride with adrenaline 1 in 200,000
- The medial edge is incised with a scalpel perpendicular to the skin and down to, but not through, the thoracolumbar fascia overlying the sacrum
- The ellipse's lateral border is incised at an angle of 45° to the skin to meet the medial incision, thus removing the sinus and associated openings (Fig, 11.29b)
- A 1cm thick, 2cm wide flap is mobilized with cutting diathermy along the entire medial edge of the wound. In patients whose disease is close to the anus, particular care is taken to avoid trauma to the sphincters
- Interrupted, 2/0, braided, absorbable sutures are placed at 1cm intervals between the deep limit of the medial flap and the longitudinal midline of the base of the elliptical cavity, the buttock tapes are released and the sutures tied
- A second layer of interrupted sutures is placed at 1cm intervals between the free edge of the medial flap and the lateral aspect of the wound
- Haemostasis is secured with spray coagulating diathermy
- A 10 French gauge suction drainage may be used selectively but is generally not required
- The skin is closed with a subcuticular, 3/0, absorbable, monofilament suture. Adhesive skin strips and a dry dressing are applied.

Bascom's original procedure

- The primary midline pilonidal pits are excised, removing each pit within an individual, small (~2mm) rhomboid cut
- The cavity is curetted to remove granulation tissue and hair
- The subcutaneous pilonidal cavity is drained laterally via a 2cm longitudinal paramedian incision, 2cm lateral to the midline
- The wall of the abscess cavity opposite the lateral drainage incision is incised across its base, allowing it to be lifted to the opposite site of the cavity and sutured to the bridge of skin between the midline pits and the lateral drainage wound. This provides a buttress of fibrous tissue deep to the primary pit wounds
- The midline pit wounds are closed with a subcuticular, 4/0, non-absorbable suture
- The lateral wound is left open but not packed.

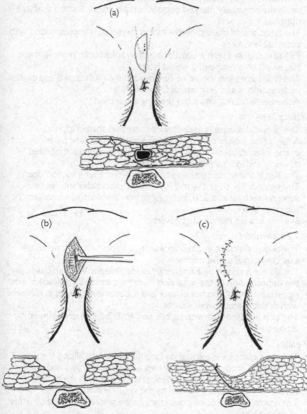

Fig. 11.27 Karydakis flap. An ellipse of tissue to incorporate any secondary tracts is marked out (a). The ellipse is excised, taking care to incise the medial incision straight down to the thoracolumbar fascia and the lateral incision at an angle of 45° towards the midline (b). A 2cm full-thickness flap is elevated from the medial side which facilitates closure of the wound in two layers (c).

Bascom's cleft lift

- The normal line of contact of the patient's buttocks is marked prior to surgery
- An ellipse of skin incorporating the primary pilonidal pits is drawn with its longitudinal axis 2cm lateral to the midline and this is excised
- The underlying cavity and secondary openings are scrubbed clean with gauze but not excised

- A 7mm thick flap of skin is raised bilaterally from the excision's edge up to the previously marked buttock contact points. Suction drainage is optional.
- The tapes are released then the subcutaneous fat is approximated with absorbable sutures
- The skin is closed with a subcuticular, non-absorbable, monofilament suture which is removed 2 weeks later
- The final suture line should lie 2cm beyond the most cranial and caudal midline defects and 2cm lateral to the midline
- Adhesive skin strips and a dry dressing are applied.

Limberg flap
- The pilonidal disease is excised via a rhomboid-shaped incision
- A flap of equivalent dimensions of the excised area (and based on one of the inferior, lateral edges of the excised rhomboid) is mobilized down to and including the gluteal fascia
- The flap is transposed medially to fill the defect over a suction drain
- The wounds are closed with 2/0, braided, absorbable sutures to subcutaneous fat and 2/0, interrupted non-absorbable, monofilament suture to skin
- Skin sutures are removed at 2 weeks.

V–Y advancement
- The pilonidal sinus is excised via a vertical ellipse with its longitudinal axis 2cm lateral to the midline
- The defect is closed by a unilateral fasciocutaneous V–Y flap based on the opposite side of the natal cleft from the excision's longitudinal axis
- Approximation of the fascial layer and subcutaneous tissues is achieved with braided, absorbable sutures
- The skin is closed with interrupted non-absorbable, monofilament sutures.

Z-plasty
- The sinus complex is excised via longitudinal midline ellipse
- A 'Z-shaped' incision comprising two equilateral triangles and incorporating skin and subcutaneous fat is made, with the middle section of the 'Z' being formed by the sinus excision wound
- The apices of the resulting two triangles are placed at the lateral limits of the incision
- The wound is closed with interrupted non-absorbable sutures to skin.

Post-operative care
- Most procedures can be performed as a day case although, for extensive sinuses and flaps which may necessitate drainage, an overnight stay should be considered.

Post-operative complications

- Wound dehiscence
- Flap necrosis
- Wound infection
- Haemorrhage
- Recurrent sinus formation.

Reference

Velasco AL, Dunlap WW. Pilonidal disease and hidradenitis. *Surg Clin North Am* 2009;**89**:689–701.

Lateral sphincterotomy

Lateral sphincterotomy aims to relax the sphincter complex sufficiently to allow improved blood supply to heal the fissure. Informed consent should include risk of impairment of continence. 2° causes should be excluded in patients with unusual/multiple fissures.

Indications

- Chronic fissure in ano unresponsive to non-surgical treatment
- No impairment of continence
- Caution should be exercised in females, particularly of child-bearing age or with a complicated obstetric history and in patients with chronic diarrhoea
- Pre-operative anorectal physiology may be useful in selected patients.

Preparation

- A phosphate enema is administered before surgery.

Position

- Lithotomy position.

Procedure

An Eisenhammer or similar anal retractor is used to put the sphincter complex under gentle stretch, allowing appreciation of the intersphincteric plane. The procedure can be performed open (through an incision) or closed (through a stab wound) with no apparent difference in fissure healing and patient satisfaction, although impaired continence may be more common after open sphincterotomy.

Open sphincterotomy

- A 0.5cm radial incision is made over the intersphincteric groove, which lies ~0.5cm from the anal verge (Fig. 11.28)
- Incision can be made on the left or right lateral anal canal. Posterior or anterior sphincterotomies are avoided to prevent keyhole deformity
- An artery forceps is inserted into the intersphincteric groove with tip pointed medially, taking care that external sphincter (red/brown) is lateral and internal sphincter (pale/white) is on the medial side
- The forceps tip is guided to the depth of the desired sphincterotomy. Division to dentate line is reported to be more effective in achieving healing
- The tip of the artery forceps is directed medially to the mucosa thereby delivering the internal sphincter. This is divided under direct vision with diathermy. The internal sphincter does not contract when touched with diathermy whereas the external sphincter does
- Pressure is placed on the wound for 5min to ensure haemostasis
- The wound is left open and infiltrated with LA and adrenaline.

Closed sphincterotomy

- The intersphincteric groove is identified as for open sphincterotomy
- The pointed tip of a size 11 scalpel blade is inserted into the groove with the blade in a circum-anal orientation
- The blade is advanced to the depth of the desired sphincterotomy

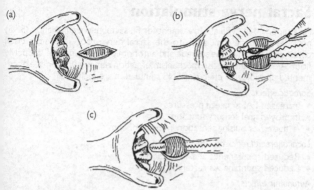

Fig. 11.28 Open lateral internal sphincterotomy. A radial incision over the intersphincteric groove (a). An artery forceps delivers the internal sphincter (b) and this is divided with diathermy (c).

Adapted with permission from Beck, D and Wexner, S (Eds.) (1998). *Fundamentals of Anorectal Surgery*, 2nd edition. London, UK: Elsevier.

- The cutting edge is turned medially and internal sphincter carefully divided, taking care not to cut through mucosa. A finger in the anal canal will help direct the depth of the cut
- Direct digital pressure is applied for haemostasis and to disrupt any residual fibres at the sphincterotomy site
- Infiltration with LA as for open sphincterotomy.

Post-operative care

- Faecal impaction must be avoided and laxatives should be prescribed
- Analgesia is prescribed on an as-required basis; patients often describe marked decrease in pain after the procedure
- Lateral sphincterotomy is usually performed on a day case basis.

Postoperative complications

- Early complications, e.g. haemorrhage, abscess and pain are uncommon
- Late complications include
  - Delayed wound healing
  - Persistent fissure
  - Recurrent fissure, usually due to an inadequate sphincterotomy
  - Impaired continence: wide range reported in the literature but incontinence affecting quality of life is reported to occur in <3%.

Alternative procedures

- Botulinum toxin injection (➔ Anal fissure p.288)
- Anal stretch has been abandoned due to an unacceptable rate of sphincter injury and impaired continence
- Balloon dilatation has been suggested as a more controlled alternative with less risk of occult sphincter injury; long-term data are lacking
- Rotation or advancement flaps have been reported to be efficacious at least in the short term (Fig. 6.5).

Sacral nerve stimulation

First reported in 1995 as a treatment for FI, sacral nerve stimulation (SNS) provides electrical stimulation to the sacral nerve roots, the most distal common location of the somatic and autonomic nerve supply of the pelvic floor. Although the precise mechanism of action remains unclear, the documented physiological effects of SNS stimulation are multiple.

Somatic effects
- Increased EAS squeeze pressures
- Improved anal sensory function
- A 'flutter' or pulsing sensation in the perineum.

Local anorectal reflex arc effects
- Reduced spontaneous anal relaxations
- Reduced spontaneous rectal motility.

Autonomic effects
- Reduced rectal sensory and urge thresholds
- Improved rectal balloon expulsion time
- Increased rectal mucosal blood flow.

Possible conversion of fast twitch type II EAS fibres to slow twitch type I fibres effects
- Increased sphincter contraction duration.

Indications

The recommended indications for SNS are continuing to expand. The cost of the procedure however has limited its application in some centres.

Faecal incontinence
- ≥1 episode FI per week as evidenced by a continence dairy
- <180° defect in the EAS
- <75yrs of age
- Failed conservative management including stool bulking agents, pelvic floor physiotherapy/biofeedback and amitriptyline where indicated for rectal hypersensitivity.

Contraindications

- Sacral abnormality preventing lead placement (e.g. spina bifida)
- Major perineal anatomical deformity (e.g. cloacal defect)
- Skin conditions affecting the insertion site
- Bleeding diathesis
- Psychological instability
- Medical condition requiring MRI
- Cardiac pacemaker or implantable defibrillator
- Pregnancy

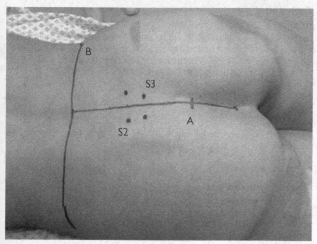

Fig. 11.29 SNS bony landmarks. The coccygeal promontory lies at (A), the iliac crest (B), and S3 lies midway between the two.

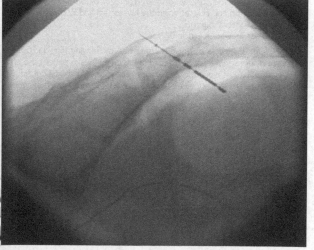

Fig. 11.30 Lateral x-ray of the sacrum. The SNS lead is located in the S3 foramina.

Technique

Stage 1

Peripheral nerve evaluation (PNE) to assess the feasibility of implantation and the benefits after a period a stimulation, the test stage. PNE is deemed successful if there is >50% reduction in incontinent episodes (80% of patients). Factors associated with successful PNE

- BMI <30
- Lead located in the S3 foramen
- Lower threshold to obtain a sensory/ motor response

Stage 2

Permanent SNS performed where PNE is successful. Factors associated with long-term SNS success

- Successful PNE
- Intact anal sphincter complex

Operative technique

Electrode insertion technique is the same for PNE and SNS. Under LA or GA with a short-acting muscle relaxant, the patient is positioned prone on an x-ray table. The landmarks are identified (Fig. 11.31) aided by fluoroscopy so that the medial border of the 3rd sacral foramina can be localized. The S3 foramina bilaterally are cannulated to determine the optimum sensory response or muscular contraction in response to the lowest electrical stimulus (aim <2mA). The typical muscular responses are

- S2—perineal muscle contraction, external leg rotation
- S3—contraction and relaxation of the levator ani and EAS, plantar flexion of ipsilateral big toe
- S4—circular EAS contraction only.

The optimum electrode position is confirmed by imaging (Fig. 11.32). For PNE the temporary electrode is taped and with an awake patient the electrode is stimulated to produce a sensory response, usually described as a tingling or pulsing sensation. The patient is provided with a portable stimulator which remains activated for the test period of 2 weeks.

For SNS the permanent electrode is tunnelled to the ipsilateral buttock where the pacemaker is secured on the gluteal fascia in a subcutaneous pocket.

Post-operative care

- The pacemaker is programmed to reproduce the sensation and continence effects of the PNE.

Complications

PNE
- Minor wound infection (<1%)
- Lead dislodgement (14–17%).

SNS
- Pain at insertion sites (4–26%)
- Wound infection (3–17%)
- Electrode migration or breakage (1–6%)
- Loss of effect (6–21%)
- Removal of the device (<5%).

Outcome of SNS
- >90% of patients report >50% continence improvement (both passive and urge)
- >50% of patients report full continence
- Improved quality of life scores in all studies.

References

Tjandra JJ, Lim JF, Matzel K. Sacral stimulation: an emerging treatment for faecal incontinence. *ANZ J Surg* 2004;**74**:1098–1106.

Matzel KE. Sacral nerve stimulation for fecal disorders; evolution, current status and future directions. *Acta Neurochir Suppl* 2007;**97**:351–357.

Related specialties

Endometriosis

Introduction

Endometriosis is defined as the presence of endometrial stroma or glands outside the uterine cavity. Cyclical stimulation of ectopic endometrial tissue may induce a chronic inflammatory reaction associated with symptoms including chronic pelvic pain and infertility. Endometriosis is unusual in being a non-malignant condition that demonstrates invasive characteristics. The condition can exhibit a wide range of diverse clinical manifestations. Clinical appearances often correlate poorly with symptom severity. Severe endometriosis may be encountered in the asymptomatic patient.

Aetiology

- Sampson's theory describes implantation of endometrial cells into the pelvic peritoneum 2° to retrograde menstruation along the fallopian tubes
- This theory fails to explain the long-term cure possible with surgery when 're-seeding' might be expected or the occasional occurrence of endometriosis at extraperitoneal sites, e.g. pleura
- Alternative theories suggest endometriosis may result from metaplasia of pelvic peritoneal cells or migration of endometrial cells as a result of blood-borne or lymphatic spread.

Prevalence

- Quoted incidence varies widely depending on indication for investigation, differing populations and criteria used for diagnosis
- Estimated prevalence in the general female population is 10–12%
- Higher incidences seen in women undergoing diagnostic procedures for investigation of pelvic pain or infertility.

Presentation

Symptoms associated with endometriosis include:

- Dysmenorrhoea
- Deep dyspareunia
- Chronic pelvic pain
- Ovulation pain ('mittelschmerz')
- Cyclical or perimenstrual GI/genitourinary symptoms
- Infertility
- Chronic fatigue.

Objective classification systems, such as the revised American Fertility Society (rAFS) classification, may be used to stage disease severity according to operative appearances but there is no correlation between these scores and the type or severity of symptoms. The location of the lesion is probably more important for the colorectal surgeon.

Presentations to the colorectal surgeon include:

- Rectal dissatisfaction, rectal bleeding, altered bowel habit, or tenesmus
- Pelvic mass with intestinal involvement or where aetiology of the mass is unclear
- Mimic or cause of acute appendicitis
- Abdominal pain, bloating, and small bowel obstruction from terminal ileal deposits which may be mistaken for CD
- Incidental finding at laparotomy/laparoscopy.

Appearances and localization

- Most affected sites include pelvic organs and peritoneum
- Occasionally encountered at distant sites, e.g. pleural cavity
- Typical appearances of superficial 'powder-burn' or 'gunshot' lesions seen on ovaries and pelvic peritoneal surface
- Large range of appearances range from petechial and haemorrhagic to polypoidal or vesicular
- Scarring and puckering of adjacent tissue are often observed
- Deep infiltrating disease may underlie what appears to be a superficial lesion and result in cystic areas of altered blood/large nodules
- Deep infiltrative disease is most frequently encountered originating from the uterosacral ligaments and may result in fibrotic obliteration of the rectovaginal space with infiltration into adjacent rectum and vagina
- Deep infiltrating disease on the uterovesical peritoneum may lead to bladder involvement
- Endometriomas are ovarian endometriotic retention cysts often containing thick deposits of altered blood ('chocolate cysts'). They are frequently associated with dense surrounding fibrosis resulting in adhesions to adjacent structures such as pelvic side wall, fallopian tubes, adjacent bowel, and the uterosacral ligaments.

Diagnosis and investigation

- Bimanual pelvic examination may reveal tenderness, a fixed retroverted uterus, an adnexal mass, and rectovaginal or uterosacral nodules
- Often clinical examination is unremarkable and further investigation is undertaken based on symptoms alone
- Visual inspection of the pelvis at laparoscopy is the 'gold standard'
- Histological confirmation is not usually required, although in cases of endometrioma/deeply infiltrating disease a biopsy should be obtained to exclude rare instances of malignancy
- Transvaginal ultrasonography (TVS) is useful for assessment of endometriomas and rectal endometriosis
- MRI may be useful to investigate symptoms of pain or where symptoms are suggestive of bowel or bladder involvement and infiltrating endometriosis is suspected
- CA125 should not be used to diagnose endometriosis as it is often raised and is not a sensitive or specific screening test. However, a raised CA125 does still merit further investigation as endometriosis is associated with an increased risk of clear cell and endometrioid ovarian cancer
- Colonoscopy may be useful for colonic symptoms where full-thickness bowel infiltration is suspected and may also be used to exclude alternative diagnoses.

Medical management

- In many cases patients presenting with symptoms suggestive of endometriosis can be treated without a definitive diagnosis
- Medical treatment may involve the use of analgesia or hormonal treatments, e.g. COC, progestogens, gonadotropin-releasing hormone (GnRH) agonists, Levonorgestrel releasing-IUD, Aromatase inhibitors or Danazol
- Most hormonal treatments act through suppression of ovulation and by inducing amenorrhoea
- Medical therapies have shown efficacy but do not modify underlying biological mechanisms
- Symptom recurrence is common following discontinuation and some women fail to respond at all.

Surgical management

The aim of surgical treatment should be to remove all visible endometriosis and restore anatomy by the division of adhesions. Ideally this should be performed at the time of diagnostic laparoscopy, providing that appropriate pre-operative consent has been given. Given the specialized nature of endometriosis surgery it is often appropriate for definitive surgery to be deferred and performed in a tertiary setting.

- Excisional and ablative laparoscopic surgery has been shown to be effective in treating endometriosis-related pain (↓ pain scores 63–80%)
- Excisional surgery is generally regarded as superior, as ablation may result in incomplete destruction of lesions due to difficulty distinguishing superficial from deeply infiltrative disease
- Radical excision requires removal of all visible peritoneal disease. Excision of deep disease may entail resection of the uterosacral ligaments, vaginal nodular endometriosis, and rectovaginal disease. Ureterolysis, partial cystectomy, and bowel resection may be necessary
- Intestinal involvement most commonly affects the rectovaginal septum and local excision (single lesion <3cm) or formal anterior resection may be required
- Surgical treatment of endometriomas includes oophrectomy or cyst drainage with ablative destruction/excision of the capsule. Capsule excision is more effective in treating symptoms
- Hysterectomy + BSO can be effective in women who have completed their families. It is important that all endometriotic deposits are excised and that adhesiolysis is performed as endometriosis-related pain can persist following surgical menopause.

Chronic pelvic pain

Chronic pelvic pain has various potential causes and symptoms suggestive of IBS or interstitial cystitis are often present in conjunction with those suggestive of endometriosis. A multidisciplinary approach is desirable and referral to a specialist pain clinic may be helpful for those women with symptoms refractory to treatment. Addressing psychological and social issues may also be important in resolving symptoms.

Pelvic inflammatory disease

Introduction

Pelvic inflammatory disease

Introduction

PID is inflammation of the genital tract and encompasses pathologies such as endometritis, salpingitis, parametritis, oophritis, tubo-ovarian abscess, and pelvic peritonitis. The most common mechanism is ascending infection from the lower genital tract. PID most frequently results from STIs but may also follow childbirth (puerperal sepsis) or abdominopelvic surgery.

- PID accounts for 1 in 60 primary care consultations for women <45yrs
- Causative organisms include *Neissseria gonorrhoea* and *Chlamydia trachomatis*. Other organisms commonly found in the lower genital tract, e.g. *Gardnerella vaginalis* and mycoplasmas such as mycoplasma genitalium, have been implicated
- Spectrum of severity ranges from asymptomatic disease to generalized peritonitis, septicaemia, and death
- Post-infective scarring following recovery can give rise to long-term sequelae such as chronic pelvic pain, ectopic pregnancy, and infertility.

Risk factors

- Young age (<25yrs)
- Multiple sexual partners or recent new sexual partner (<3 months)
- Past history of STI
- Termination of pregnancy
- Insertion of intrauterine contraceptive device in past 6 weeks
- Hysterosalpingography
- IVF treatment
- Post-partum endometritis.

Clinical features

- Bilateral lower abdominal tenderness (may radiate to legs or back)
- Abnormal vaginal or cervical discharge
- Fever (>38°C)
- Abnormal vaginal bleeding (intermenstrual/post-coital)
- Deep dyspareunia
- Cervical excitation on vaginal examination
- Adnexal tenderness on vaginal examination (± palpable mass).

Diagnosis

- Symptoms and signs lack sensitivity compared with laparoscopy with peritoneal swabbing. A low threshold for empiric treatment is recommended
- Both chlamydia and gonorrhoea can now be identified by molecular testing, the specimen of choice being a vaginal swab. Gonococci isolation by culture requires an endocervical swab
- Absence of infection in the lower genital tract does not exclude PID
- A pregnancy test should be performed for all women of child-bearing age with lower abdominal pain or vaginal bleeding
- TVS may be useful in identifying pelvic masses such as tubo-ovarian abscesses or pyosalpinx
- Limited evidence exists to support routine use of diagnostic CT/MRI
- Laparoscopy is not undertaken routinely

- Useful if diagnostic doubt or where the woman is unwell with no response to antibiotics within 72h
- Findings include inflammation of pelvic organs, free fluid/pus ± pelvic adhesions. The fallopian tubes may be grossly dilated indicating hydrosalpinx/pyosalpinx
- Characteristic perihepatic 'violin-string' adhesions of Fitz-Hugh–Curtis syndrome may be evident
- Laparoscopic findings are subjective and may miss intratubal inflammation where there is little visible serosal hyperaemia.

Differential diagnosis

- Ectopic pregnancy
- Threatened miscarriage
- Acute appendicitis
- Endometriosis
- IBS or other GI disorders
- Complicated ovarian cyst, e.g. rupture, torsion
- UTI
- Functional pain (pain of unknown physical origin).

Treatment

- Antibiotic treatment covering *N. gonorrhoea*, *C. trachomatis*, and anaerobes should be started, ideally <2 days from onset of symptoms
- Microbiological samples are taken prior to commencing treatment
- Mild cases may be treated with oral antibiotics on an outpatient basis
- Parenteral therapy is recommended when there is clinical evidence of severe disease, pelvic abscess, or when oral treatment has failed.

Recommended oral antibiotic protocol

- Ofloxacin 400mg bd + oral metronidazole 400mg bd for 14 days (this may not treat gonorrhoea adequately due to resistance)

  or

- IM ceftriaxone 1g single dose followed by oral doxycycline 100mg bd + metronidazole 400mg bd for 14 days.

Recommended IV antibiotic protocol

- Ceftriaxone 2g od + doxycycline 100mg bd

  or

- Clindamycin 900mg tid + gentamicin (2mg/kg loading dose followed by 1.5mg/kg tid)
- Review at 72h recommended. Failure to improve suggests need for further investigation, parenteral therapy ± surgical intervention
- Review 4 weeks after therapy is useful to ensure adequate response to treatment, compliance with antibiotics, screening and treatment of sexual contacts, and awareness of the significance of PID
- Patient education is important. Use of barrier contraceptives should be recommended, as should screening of sexual contacts to prevent re-infection
- Patient management should ideally be multidisciplinary, involving gynaecology and genitourinary medicine (GUM) services.

Ovarian cysts

Ovarian cysts are common and may occur at any stage of life. Symptomatic presentations include abdominal pain associated with cyst accidents and abdominal distension. Intervention may be offered if the cyst is associated with pain or where there is concern about a possible complication such as cyst torsion. In many cases the $1°$ objective is to exclude underlying malignancy. It is also important to avoid unnecessary intervention as complications of surgery, e.g. adhesions, may result in the future development of infertility or chronic pelvic pain.

- Functional follicular cysts common in women of reproductive age
- Incidence of malignancy rises following the menopause and with advancing age
- 90% of surgically managed cysts in pre-menopausal women are benign compared with 60% in the post-menopausal population.

Acute ovarian cyst complications

Rupture

- May result in irritation of the peritoneum which is particularly severe with dermoid cysts or endometriomas
- *Mittelschmerz* pain resulting from the rupture of a follicular cyst accompanying ovulation is a common, self-limiting phenomenon.

Haemorrhage

- May result in haemoperitoneum or severe pain if haemorrhage occurs within the cyst.

Ovarian torsion

- Infarction and ischaemia of the ovary and/or tube occurs usually in conjunction with severe pain
- Urgent operative de-torsion is required if ovary is to remain viable.

Classification

Epithelial ovarian tumours

- Epithelial tumours account for 95% of $1°$ ovarian malignancies
- May be benign, borderline, or malignant
- Account for 60–65% of all ovarian cysts and 90% of malignant cysts
- Serous cysts are the most common (75% of epithelial carcinomas)
- Mucinous tumours (10%) may be associated with pseudomyxoma peritonei
- >10% of endometrioid carcinomas are associated with co-existing endometrial carcinoma
- Histological subtypes include:
  - High grade serous
  - Low grade serous
  - Mucinous adenocarcinoma
  - Endometrioid carcinoma
  - Clear cell carcinoma
  - Carcinosarcoma
  - Transitional (Brenner)
  - Undifferentiated

- Many experts now believe that
  - High grade serous cancers arise from the fallopian tubes with a pre-malignant phase called serous tubal intraepithelial carcinomas (STIC)
  - Clear cell and endometroid ovarian carcinomas originate from endometriotic deposits
  - Müllerian inclusion cysts give rise to low grade serous and mucinous tumours.

Sex-cord stromal tumours
- Three main groups
  - Pure stromal—fibromas and thecomas
  - Pure sex cord—adult and juvenile granulosa cell tumours
  - Mixed sex cord stroma—Sertoli–Leydig
- Most pure stromal tumours are benign, Sertoli–Leydig can be benign or malignant, and granulosa tumours are the most prevalent malignant form
- Sex cord stromal tumours frequently possess endocrine function, most commonly oestrogenic or androgenic but may produce both.

Ovarian germ-cell tumours
- Most frequently observed in the first two decades of life
- Represent 30% of all ovarian tumours but account for only 5% of ovarian malignancies
- Dysgerminomas are the most common germ-cell malignancy
- In contrast to other ovarian malignancies, most present as stage I disease
- Histological subtypes include:
  - Benign teratoma (dermoid cyst)
  - Dysgerminoma
  - Immature teratoma (malignant)
  - Yolk sac tumour
  - Embryonal carcinoma
  - Choriocarcinoma
  - Mixed germ-cell tumours.

Evaluation of ovarian masses

Clinical examination may identify ovarian masses, but small lesions may escape detection and it can be difficult to distinguish pelvic masses of ovarian origin from other lesions, such as uterine fibroids.
- TVS provides detailed images of the ovaries and adnexal masses and is recommended as the preferred imaging modality for assessment
- Image resolution greatly exceeds that of abdominal US
- The role of other imaging modalities in distinguishing between benign and malignant lesions, e.g. MRI, CT, PET is not yet clearly established.

TVS sonomorphological features suggestive of ovarian malignancy
- Presence of septations (multiloculations)
- Evidence of solid areas
- Bilateral lesions
- Presence of ascites/fluid in the pouch of Douglas
- Evidence of metastases.

Biochemical markers
- CA125 usually elevated with epithelial ovarian cancer
- Elevated CA125 is not specific to ovarian malignancy and may remain low in early epithelial ovarian cancer or non-epithelial ovarian cancer
- Germ-cell tumours may secrete alpha fetoprotein (AFP) + β-human chorionic gonadotropin (β-hCG)
- CEA can be elevated in mucinous ovarian tumours and where a CA125:CEA ratio is less than 25:1 then a GI primary should be excluded.

Risk stratification

The 'risk of malignancy index' (RMI) combines the woman's menopausal status (pre- or post-menopausal) with a TVS morphology score and serum CA125 level to produce a score that corresponds to the woman's risk of malignancy (Fig. 12.1).

RMI score
- >250 corresponds to a high risk of >75% positive predictive value.

This score is commonly used to determine the type of surgery performed and whether this is in a general gynaecological unit, a cancer unit, or a tertiary cancer centre.

Management of ovarian cysts

- Management is defined by the nature of the presentation (incidental finding or a symptomatic cyst complication) and the perceived risk of malignancy
- Simple follicular cysts <5cm in younger patients are usually managed conservatively and will generally resolve spontaneously. If 5–7cm and asymptomatic then follow with US to ensure resolution is recommended
- Cyst complications leading to pain, hypovolaemic shock, or where ovarian viability is threatened will require prompt surgical intervention
- Where the risk of malignancy is low a laparoscopic approach is generally preferable
- Great caution should be taken to avoid the risk of upstaging an ovarian cancer where laparoscopic excision or cyst drainage has led to intraperitoneal spillage of cyst contents
- Where malignancy is suspected, a full staging laparotomy should be performed including careful evaluation of the entire peritoneal cavity, biopsy or excision of any suspicious lesions, peritoneal washings, and biopsies of common metastatic sites such as the greater omentum or the appendix.

Box 12.1 Risk of malignancy index
RMI = U × M × CA125
U = 0 (ultrasound score 0); **U** = 1 (score 1); **U** = 3 (score 2-5)
Ultrasound scores one point for each of multilocular cyst, solid areas, evidence of metastases, ascites and bilateral lesions
M = 1 for pre-menopausal and **M** = 3 for post menopausal women
CA125 serum measurement in U/ml

Ovarian malignancy

Ovarian malignancy

Epidemiology

There are 17,000 new cases of gynaecological cancer in the UK each year, leading to 7,500 deaths. Ovarian cancer is the second most common gynaecological cancer after endometrial cancer. It is the sixth most common cancer in females out of all cancer types (not just gynaecological cancers).

- There are ~7,400 new ovarian cancer cases in the UK each year
- Ovarian cancer is a major cause of mortality in women with ~4,100 deaths/yr in the UK, representing 6% of all female cancer-related deaths
- Incidence in UK is stable or falling slightly
- Most present in their 60s although more than a quarter of new cases are in females aged 75yrs and over.

Risk factors

- Factor associated with an increased risk include:
  - Increasing age
  - Obesity
  - Nulliparity/infertility
  - Endometriosis
  - Diabetes
  - Smoking
- 5–15% of ovarian cancers are hereditary, usually associated with a family history of ovarian or breast cancer but some are new mutations. Several genes have been shown to increase risk of ovarian cancer
  - General population: 1.3% lifetime risk
  - BRCA1 gene mutation: 65% lifetime risk
  - BRCA2 gene mutation: 35% lifetime risk
  - Lynch syndrome (HNPCC): 3–14% lifetime risk
- Factors associated with reduced risk include:
  - Previous pregnancy
  - History of breast feeding
  - Use of the oral contraceptive pill
  - Tubal ligation.

Screening

Large scale trials of screening have not produced any evidence to support the use of screening in high risk or low risk female populations.

Presentation

- Survival is poor as 60% present late with advanced disease
- Symptoms are often non-specific
- Typical symptoms include abdominal pain, distension or bloating, weight gain/loss, anorexia, and malaise
- Breathlessness may be related to pleural effusion or ascites
- Urinary symptoms or DVT may result from local pressure effects
- Abnormal vaginal bleeding may occur
- A fixed, irregular pelvic mass may be felt on abdominal, vaginal, and rectal exam
- Incidental adnexal mass may be seen on imaging for other indication.

Investigation

- Routine blood tests, serum CA125, CXR, and TA/TVS may be followed by CT/MRI of abdomen and pelvis
- CEA should be measured to identify primary GI tumours
- Upper/lower GI endoscopy may be useful if the 1° site is in doubt
- AFP and β-hCG should be measured in younger patients as germ cell tumours are the most common malignancy in those <20yrs
- Pathological classification of ovarian tumours has previously been outlined (➔ Ovarian cysts, discussed earlier in this chapter, p.612).

Staging

Staging is by laparotomy and involves assessment of anatomical spread. More detailed TNM can be used but FIGO staging is a common standard.

Stage I
- Disease confined to the ovaries (Ic: surface disease/ruptured ovarian capsule or malignant ascites/positive peritoneal washings).

Stage II
- Involvement of one/both ovaries + pelvic structures.

Stage III
- Stage I/II + peritoneal implants outside pelvis or +ve retroperitoneal LNs.

Stage IV
- Distant metastases (e.g. liver parenchyma/+ve pleural cytology).

Management

- Ovarian cancer commonly presents with advanced disease and curative surgical resection is uncommon for advanced disease. The overall 5yr survival is 46% and 10yr survival is 35%
- Surgery alone may be enough in low risk stage I disease
- For advanced stage disease the surgical aim should be complete cytoreduction at surgery with chemotherapy following surgery or, in some cases, chemotherapy with surgery midway through chemotherapy
- Combination carboplatin and paclitaxel are commonly used
- Surgery involves total hysterectomy and BSO, omentectomy, cytology for peritoneal washings, removal of diseased peritoneum and other areas where disease is present including bowel resection to achieve no residual disease
- Improved survival after resection is seen in patients with earlier stage disease and complete cytoreduction
- Germline BRCA mutated patients have a significant survival advantage if treated with PARP inhibitors
- PARP inhibitors may also be effective in platinum-sensitive patients and BRCA-mutated tumours
- Most women with advanced disease will relapse after initial treatment. Time between last platinum-based chemotherapy and relapse (platinum-free interval) is an important prognostic indicator
- Recurrent disease may be treated with second-line chemotherapy, secondary cytoreductive surgery, or palliative surgery (most frequently indicated for bowel obstruction)
- Multidisciplinary approach with colorectal input may be required for advanced disease with colonic involvement.

Endometrial cancer

Introduction

- Endometrial cancer is the commonest gynaecological malignancy and the fourth commonest cause of cancer in women
- High levels of oestrogens (particularly post-menopausal) are a recognized risk factor for endometrial cancer
- Causes include obesity (due to peripheral conversion of oestrogens to androgens in adipose tissue), oestrogen therapy unopposed with progestogens, tamoxifen therapy, late menopause, and polycystic ovarian syndrome (PCOS)
- Genetic factors also appear important and there is an established link to HNPCC
- Mortality approaches 2,300 deaths/year in the UK.

Presentation

- Endometrial cancer usually presents with vaginal bleeding in post-menopausal women
- Up to 10% of women with this presentation will have an underlying endometrial cancer
- Risk increases with age
- Screening is not useful for endometrial cancer where early investigation of symptoms, usually vaginal bleeding, is the most appropriate approach
- A high proportion of women are early stage at diagnosis.

Investigation

- TVS is the preferred first-line investigation for post-menopausal bleeding (PMB)
- If endometrial thickness is ≤3mm the probability of malignancy is reduced from 10% to <1%
- Endometrial tissue sampling can be performed as an outpatient
- Hysteroscopic examination with endometrial curettage should be performed where PMB is associated with tamoxifen use or where TVS is suspicious of malignant disease. Increasingly performed as an outpatient without the requirement for a GA
- The staging of endometrial cancer is based on surgical and subsequent pathological findings, although MRI may be used pre-operatively to assess myometrial invasion and the presence of nodal disease
- CT should be performed if there is a clinical suspicion of ureteric, bladder, or distal tumour involvement.

Pathology

- 95% are adenocarcinomas arising from the endometrium of which there are two subtypes:
  - Type I (endometrioid) endometrial adenocarcinoma. Account for 80% of uterine adenocarcinomas
  - Type II. Account for 20% endometrial adenocarcinomas. These include serous, clear cell, mucinous. The carcinomas are more aggressive and associated with up to 50% of relapses
- Uterine sarcomas account for around 5% of uterine tumours. They are derived from the myometrium and associated connective tissue. They have a poorer prognosis compared to uterine adenocarcinoma.

Staging

Stage I

• Tumour confined to corpus uteri.

Stage II

• Tumour confined to corpus and cervix.

Stage III

• Tumour spread beyond corpus but not outside pelvis; may include vagina, adnexa, and pelvic/para-aortic LNs.

Stage IV

• Bladder/rectal involvement or distant metastases.

Management

• Most endometrial cancers present at an early stage
• Overall 5yr survival rate is 75%
   • Stage I disease: 80–90%
   • Stage II 70–80%
   • Stage III/IV 20–60%
• Curative surgical resection is usually possible by hysterectomy and BSO ± pelvic and para-aortic node dissection. The procedure is now commonly performed via laparoscopic or robotic surgery
• Adjuvant RT may be offered to patients based on the stage and grade of disease
• Even considering co-morbidity and stage at presentation, older patients have a poorer prognosis compared to younger patients
• Progestogen therapy for women who have undergone surgery for early stage disease is not recommended as it does not improve overall survival
• Progestogen therapy may have a role in those unfit for surgery, to allow fertility options or with advanced disease
• Chemotherapy has a role for women with advanced or recurrent disease.

Cervical cancer

Introduction

- Cervical cancer is the 14th most common malignancy in females but the second most common in women <35yrs
- Annual incidence is 8.5 per 100,000 (i.e. 3,2000/year in UK)
- Peak incidence is between 30 and 34yrs
- The major risk factor for the development of cervical cancer is HPV infection
- Other risk factors include smoking, early age of onset of sexual activity, increasing number of sexual partners, and low socio-economic group
- Although there are more than 100 HPV subtypes and 40 that affect the genital area, types 16 and 18 account for more than 70% of cervical cancers in the UK.

Cervical screening

In the UK, the NHS Cervical Screening Programme (NHSCSP) was introduced in 1988. The screening has recently changed to HPV primary screening of the smear and a cytological assessment is only performed if high risk HPV is identified. Women aged 25–64 are screened by cervical smear sample. Cervical smears are not a diagnostic test and women with suspicious symptoms should be seen in colposcopy.

The programme has had a dramatic effect, halving the mortality of cervical cancer since introduction. In the UK, mortality rates have decreased by 75% since the early 1970s although the incidence has been stable over the last decade. The screening programme refers women with abnormal results for colposcopic assessment when appropriate. High grade, glandular, and invasive abnormalities should be seen urgently. In the vast majority cervical intraepithelial neoplasia (CIN) can be treated colposcopically.

HPV vaccine

- Vaccination has been offered to ♀ aged 12–13yrs in the UK since 2008/9 with catch-up programmes for those under 18yrs. The impact of vaccination on cervical cancer incidence will not be seen until well into the 2020s but the impact is already being seen for CIN
- Commencing 2019, all 12–13-year-olds (♂ and ♀) were offered the Gardasil® vaccine, effective against HPV types 6, 11, 16, and 18.
- HPV 16 and 18 account for more than 70% of cervical cancers in the UK and HPV 6 and 11 are responsible for 90% of genital warts
- Cervical screening is still important as vaccination does not protect against all types of HPV.

Presentation

- Frequently asymptomatic; early symptoms include post-coital bleeding, intermenstrual bleeding, or offensive vaginal discharge
- Invasive and pre-invasive disease may be identified through screening
- Advanced disease may present with back pain, dysuria, haematuria, renal failure, rectal bleeding, and lower limb lymphoedema.

Investigation

- Women with abnormal cervical screening should undergo colposcopy which involves high resolution visual assessment of the cervix using acetic acid and allows for biopsy/treatment of suspicious areas under direct vision
- 85% of cervical malignancies are squamous or adenosquamous carcinomas which are associated with more favourable prognosis than the less common adenocarcinoma
- Staging is based on clinical examination and MRI pelvis
- Stage 1B2 or greater should have a PET-CT scan.

Staging

Stage 0
- Pre-invasive disease (carcinoma in situ): CIN.

Stage I
- Tumour confined to the cervix.

Stage II
- Tumour extending into, but not beyond, upper 2/3 vagina or parametrium.

Stage III
- Tumour extending into lower 1/3 vagina or involving pelvic side wall and/or regional lymph nodes.

Stage IV
- Locally invasive disease involving bladder, rectum, or metastatic disease outside the pelvis.

Management

- In patients with Stage 0 disease or 1A (microinvasive disease only) (often asymptomatic and discovered through cervical screening), cone biopsy or loop diathermy excision may be all that is required
- For all other stages of disease, surgical resection by radical hysterectomy with pelvic lymphadenectomy or radical RT is indicated
- In some cases of small volume disease, in women wishing to conserve their fertility, loop diathermy and pelvic lymphadenectomy/ trachelectomy (radical excision of the cervix with uterine body preservation) and pelvic lymphadenectomy may be appropriate but require MDT approval
- Adjuvant pelvic RT is used in patients with positive pelvic nodes, large volume tumours, or where disease is found at excision margins
- Radical RT ± cisplatin-based chemotherapy is used for patients deemed unsuitable for surgery
- Further surgery, e.g. pelvic exenteration may offer cure in certain circumstances
- RT and cisplatin-based chemotherapy may be used as palliative therapies or in the treatment of recurrent disease
- Colorectal involvement may be required for the management of rectovaginal fistula in advanced disease or post-RT
- In the UK, 5year survival for all stages is 61%
- 5yr survival in women with microinvasive stage I disease approaches 100%. This falls to 70–85% for small volume stage I/II tumours, 50–70% for large volume stages I/II tumours, 30–50% for stage III, and 5–15% for stage IV disease.

Ectopic pregnancy

Ectopic pregnancy describes any embryonic implantation site outside the uterine cavity. Most ectopic pregnancies are tubal, but other sites are occasionally encountered. The thin wall of the tube is unable to withstand the trophoblast invasion of implantation and bleeding frequently occurs, either into the tubal lumen or as a result of tubal rupture which may result in sudden haemodynamic collapse.

Background

- Incidence has ↑ from 4.9 to 11.1/1,000 pregnancies in the last 30yrs
- Rate of increase closely follows ↑ incidence of PID, particularly chlamydia
- Ruptured ectopic pregnancy is a true surgical emergency
- Maternal mortality is 2 per 10,000 estimated ectopic pregnancies.

Sites of ectopic pregnancy

- Fallopian tube (98.3%)
- Abdominal (1.4%)
- Ovarian (0.15%)
- Cervical (0.15%).

Aetiology

- Any tubal injury, e.g. previous PID, tubal surgery, caesarian section, or previous ectopic pregnancy can result in obstruction of the fertilized oocyte's progress along the tube
- Ectopic pregnancy is associated with assisted conception techniques
- Pregnancy with IUCD *in situ*
- Incidence rises with maternal age
- Around 30% of women will have no known risk factors.

Diagnosis

- Early clinical diagnosis of an unruptured ectopic pregnancy remains a significant challenge and is often missed or delayed
- Symptoms and signs include amenorrhoea associated with lower abdominal pain, shoulder tip pain, vaginal bleeding, shock, tenderness/cervical excitation on vaginal examination, and signs of haemoperitoneum
- Collapse in early pregnancy should always be considered an ectopic pregnancy until an intrauterine pregnancy can be positively diagnosed
- Atypical presentations, e.g. vomiting + diarrhoea, have been repeatedly observed in cases resulting in maternal death, emphasizing the importance of a high index of suspicion
- Serum β-hCG + high resolution TVS enable earlier diagnosis
- The absence of an intrauterine pregnancy on TVS with a serum β-hCG level >1,000–1,500mIU/ml should prompt further investigation and definitive management
- Features suggesting ectopic pregnancy on TVS include an extrauterine sac, a complex adnexal mass, or free fluid in the pelvis
- TVS has a 90–99% sensitivity and a specificity of 95–99% for the diagnosis of ectopic pregnancy

- Initial TVS is non-diagnostic in 10–30%. In many cases of unruptured ectopic pregnancy the only finding will be the absence of an intrauterine pregnancy
- Although rare (1 in 3000 spontaneous and 1–3% of assisted conceptions), the possibility of a heterotopic pregnancy, where there are co-existing ectopic and intrauterine pregnancies, should always be considered, particularly following assisted conception.

Management options available for the treatment of ectopic pregnancy include laparotomy, operative laparoscopy, medical management, and occasionally observation alone. Management must be tailored to the clinical condition and the future fertility requirements of the woman.

Management

Management depends on the clinical presentations, findings on TVS, hCG level, and the patient's preference.

Medical treatment

- A single dose of methotrexate (folic acid antagonist which interferes with rapidly growing cells) is administered by IM injection in selected situations
  - No significant pain
  - Unruptured ectopic, no visible heartbeat and <35mm in size
  - No intrauterine pregnancy, confirmed in TVS
  - hCG <1,500 IU/L
  - Patient can return for follow-up
- Close follow-up required with monitoring of β-hCG. A 15% drop should be observed between days 4 and 7. If not, a repeat dose should be administered
- <10% of treated women will require surgical intervention. The tube is conserved and there is an 80% chance of tubal patency
- Tubal rupture occurs in 7% of women treated and it is imperative that immediate access to an early pregnancy/emergency gynaecology service is available in the event of complication.

Surgical management

- Surgery for ectopic pregnancy should be offered as first-line treatment in the following circumstances:
  - Ruptured ectopic with collapse or significant fluid on TVS
  - Significant pain
  - Adnexal mass >35mm
  - Ectopic with viable foetal heartbeat
  - Serum hCG >5,000 IU/L
- Surgical treatment may involve excision of the tube (salpingectomy), incision of the tube and removal of the ectopic pregnancy (salpingotomy), or extrusion of the ectopic pregnancy from the fimbrial end of the fallopian tube
- In the presence of a healthy contralateral tube, a salpingectomy should be performed in preference to a salpingotomy
- Conservation of the tube (e.g. salpingotomy) may be considered in women who have a history of fertility reducing factors (previous ectopic, PID, or contralateral tube damage)

- Salpingotomy associated with ↑ risk of post-operative tubal bleeding, persistent trophoblastic disease (5–10%), and recurrent ectopic pregnancy due to implantation at the site of tubal damage
- Future intrauterine pregnancy rates are similar for salpingectomy and conservative surgery.

Laparoscopic approach
- Preferable in haemodynamically stable patients as it is associated with shorter operation times, less intraoperative blood loss, shorter hospital stay, and lower analgesic requirement
- No significant difference in subsequent intrauterine pregnancy rate, rate of tubal patency, or incidence of recurrent ectopic pregnancy
- In the shocked patient the surgical procedure performed should be that which most quickly controls haemorrhage and in many cases a laparotomy will be required.

Expectant management
- NICE guidelines suggest expectant treatment should be *offered* if
    - Clinically stable and pain-free
    - Tubal ectopic pregnancy <35mm with no visible heartbeat on TVS
    - Serum hCG ≤1000 IU/L
    - Patient can return for follow-up
- It may be *considered* if the above apply but the serum hCG levels >1000 IU/L and <1500 IU/L
- hCG test should be repeated on days 2, 4, 7 after original test
- Continue conservative treatment if hCG falls by ≥15% of the preceding result until <20 IU/L
- If hCG does not fall as expected, early clinical review/reassessment should be performed
- There seems to be no difference in outcomes for expectant or medical management of women with ectopic pregnancy.

Reference

Ectopic pregnancy and miscarriage: diagnosis and initial management. NICE guideline [NG126] April 2019. Available at https://www.nice.org.uk/guidance/ng126

Sexually transmitted infections

STIs can cause several colorectal presentations. Because sex is not always discussed, these conditions can be missed.

Taking a sexual history

Receptive anal sex is reported by ~10% of heterosexual women in the UK. About 30% of MSM in the UK will have had unprotected anal sex in the last year with a casual partner.

If you suspect symptoms might be due to an STI:

- Explain your concerns and that you need to ask some more personal questions
- Do not ever assume gender of sexual partner: ask if this was a man or a woman
- Ask about recent and lifetime receptive anal sex and whether this was protected or not
- Ask whether they have ever had tests for STIs such as HIV
- If relevant to the presentation (e.g. rectal trauma) ask about use of sex toys, fisting, use of 'poppers' and other recreational drugs.

Colorectal surgery can significantly impact someone's sex life, indirectly (e.g. due to a stoma) or directly in the case of MSM who may be unable to have desired anal sex (e.g. following APER).

Ask:

- 'Have you had any problems with sex since your operation?'
- 'Has your surgery affected your sex life in any way?'

Human papilloma virus

- Ubiquitous: 20% carriage
- Genitoanal warts normally caused by HPV type 6 and 11 (Fig. 12.1)
- Transmitted by skin-to-skin contact
- Condoms not 100% protective
- Perianal warts can be seen in men and women with no history of receptive anal sex
- Intra-anal warts usually in MSM who have had receptive anal sex
- Oncogenic types (e.g. 16, 18) are the cause of AIN and anal cancer but tend not to cause visible warts
- Gardasil 9® vaccine covers nine strains of HPV (6, 11, 16, 18, 31, 33, 45, 52, and 58) which covers >90% of genital cancers and genital warts associated with HPV.

Investigations

- Usually clinical diagnosis
- Biopsy unusual or persistent lesions not responding to therapy.

Treatment

- Self-applied topical creams
  - Podophyllotoxin or imiquimod suitable for most
- Cryotherapy with liquid nitrogen
- Surgical debulking by excision or diathermy
  - May need follow-up to treat recurrences.

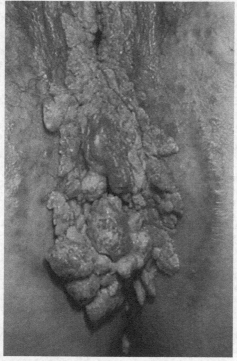

Fig. 12.1 Perianal warts.

Proctitis

Infectious causes

- *Neisseria gonorrhoeae* (gonococcus (GC))
- *Chlamydia trachomatis* (non-lymphogranuloma venereum (LGV))
- *Chlamydia trachomatis* (LGV type)
- *Treponema pallidum* (syphilis)
- Herpes simplex virus.

Investigations

- Culture for GC (+ Gram stain if available, e.g. in GUM clinic)
- Nucleic acid amplification test (NAAT) test for chlamydia and gonorrhoea
- PCR test for HSV (and *T. pallidum* in some centres)
- Biopsy (warn lab suspected LGV)
- Syphilis serology (NB: can be negative in very early infection).

Lymphogranuloma venereum

- Caused by *C. trachomatis* serovars L1–3 which are lymphotropic and invasive. Recent resurgence in MSM in cities in USA/Europe
- Causes significant tissue damage ('genitoanorectal syndrome')
- ~75% of UK LGV cases are HIV seropositive. 20% have hepatitis C
- National reference labs in the UK will test for LGV on chlamydia-positive rectal specimens in symptomatic proctitis
  - Non-LGV *C. trachomatis*, found in ~8% of all MSM, is usually asymptomatic.

Assume chlamydia-positive proctitis is due to LGV until proven otherwise; organize reference lab LGV testing of positive sample and give 3 weeks doxycycline 100mg bd PO.

HIV infection

Worldwide ~40 million are infected. In the UK, it is most common in MSM (prevalence 5–15%) and those from countries with established HIV epidemics.

HIV can present to the colorectal surgeon with
- Anal cancer. 30-fold ↑ risk (➔ Anal cancer, Chapter 7, p.384)
- Unexplained weight loss with bowel symptoms
- GI bleeding (e.g. due to Kaposi's sarcoma).

HIV is fully treatable. >90% of patients on HAART fully suppress viral load and have near-complete immune recovery. Unfortunately, this immune recovery has not greatly reduced rates of anal cancer or lymphoma.

Deaths and AIDS occur almost exclusively in late missed diagnoses.

Practice point: an HIV test should be part of the routine medical work-up for anal cancer or unexplained weight loss.

Herpes simplex

HSV types 1 and 2 (Fig. 12.2).
- Cause recurrent genitoanal ulceration (more frequent with type 2)
- Most shedding is asymptomatic
- Carriage of type 2 is ~8% in UK
- Acquired by skin-to-skin contact
- Condoms offer ~50% protection if consistent use
- Constellation of other symptoms common with recurrence, e.g. buttock or sciatic pain, flu-like illness, and fatigue.

Investigation
- PCR test (or less ideally, culture) on swab from ulcer sample
- Serology is not useful in acute ulceration but may help in specialist settings.

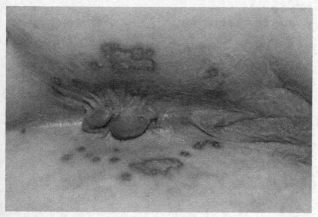

Fig. 12.2 Anorectal herpes.

Syphilis

Caused by *Treponema pallidum* sp. *pallidum*.

Primary stage

- Local 'chancre'
- Classically solitary ulcer but ~30% are multiple, painful, and can look like HSV ulcers
- Can be asymptomatic or hidden in anal canal (➔ Solitary rectal ulcer, Chapter 6, p.280)
- Can cause proctitis.

Secondary stage—dissemination

- General malaise, rash (especially affecting palms/soles), headache, 'the great pretender'
- Rapid progression in some HIV patients to neurosyphilis.
- *Latent stage* is then followed in ~30% untreated by *late syphilis*
- Gummata, neurosyphilis, cardiac syphilis.

Investigations

- Suspected chancre
  - Dark-ground microscopy and (if available) PCR testing
- Secondary stage
  - Serology is always positive
  - Screening enzyme immunoassay (EIA) is confirmed with venereal disease research laboratory (VDRL) test/rapid plasma reagin (RPR) and *Treponema pallidum* particle agglutination (TPPA) tests
  - EIA and TPPA usually stay positive for life
  - VDRL test and IgM fall after treatment.

Treatment
- Long-acting IM benzathine penicillin 2.4MU, 1–3 doses depending on stage
- If penicillin allergic, doxycycline 100mg bd for 2–4 weeks.

Case history: LGV proctitis

Shaun is a 23-year-old man. He has 7 days of increasing tenesmus, constipation, and anal pain. His GP suspected a fissure, but he is no better with simple treatment. Suspecting an STI, he attends his local GUM clinic. They establish that he has had recent unprotected sex in a London gay venue with a new partner. Proctoscopy shows boggy inflamed tissue with a purulent discharge which is negative for diplococci on Gram stain. Molecular testing demonstrates *Chlamydia trachomatis* and subsequent reference lab PCR confirms this as an LGV subtype. Shaun has already recovered with 3 weeks doxycycline 100mg bd. Unfortunately, he was seropositive for HIV at presentation and seropositive for hepatitis C at his follow-up visit, suggesting recent hepatitis C seroconversion.

Case history: early syphilis

Gerald, a 52-year-old man, was referred urgently to the local colorectal service with a rapidly expanding anal ulcer, thought to be malignant. After referral he had become generally unwell with fevers, lymphadenopathy, and a generalized though faint maculopapular rash. He had been having sex with a steady male partner for 6 months.

The ulcer was positive for *T. pallidum* on dark-ground microscopy and by PCR. Syphilis serology was positive by EIA with VDRL 1:64, TPPA >1:1,280, and a strongly positive IgM. He was seronegative for HIV. He made a full recovery with a single injection of benzathine penicillin 2.4MU.

Ureteric injury/reconstruction

Anatomy of the ureter

The ureter is frequently and inadvertently injured because of its close proximity to pelvic structures, the relatively long course in the retroperitoneum, and the tenuous blood supply.

Relationships

The ureter can be divided into three parts based on its association with the iliac vessels and pelvic brim (Fig. 12.3). The ureters descend in the retroperitoneum anterior to the psoas muscle and closely adherent to posterior peritoneum. The left ureter is crossed anteriorly by the left colic or inferior mesenteric and sigmoidal vessels. On the right the ureter is crossed by the right colic, ileocolic vessels, and the root of the mesentery containing the superior mesenteric vessels. Before entering the pelvis, the ureter passes under the gonadal vessels before crossing over the common iliac vessels.

In the pelvis the male ureter continues anterior and medial to the obturator vessels. Before entering the bladder, the ureter passes under the superior vesical vessels and the vas deferens.

The female ureter courses posteriorly to the infundibulo pelvic ligament containing the ovarian vessels. It continues anteromedial to the obturator structures, posterior to the superior vesical vessels, uterine artery, and the ovary. As the ureter turns medially towards the bladder it lies in the base of the broad ligament and ~2cm lateral to the cervix. The ureter is again crossed by the uterine artery before entering the bladder.

Blood supply

- Upper 2/3 receives blood supply medially from the renal artery and abdominal aorta
- The distal 1/3 receives blood supply from laterally placed iliac and superior vesical arteries.

Ureteric injury

- Iatrogenic injury (75%) is the most common mode of injury to the ureter
  - Gynaecological surgery (70–75%)
  - Urological (10–15%)
  - General surgical (10–15%)
  - It is also seen during vascular, pancreatic, and spinal surgery
- Overall incidence of iatrogenic ureteric injuries during colorectal surgery varies between 0.5 and 10%
- The injury is seen mostly in distal third (74%) of ureter compared with upper and middle third (13% each).

Mechanism of injury

Mechanisms of injury include ligation, kinking by a suture, complete/partial transection, avulsion, crush and ischaemic injury (delayed necrosis and stricture).

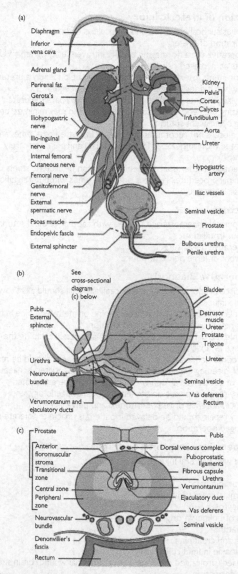

(a)

Diaphragm
Inferior vena cava
Adrenal gland
Perirenal fat
Gerota's fascia
Iliohypogastric nerve
Ilio-inguinal nerve
Internal femoral Cutaneous nerve
Femoral nerve
Genitofemoral nerve
External spermatic nerve
Psoas muscle
Endopelvic fascia
External sphincter

Kidney
Pelvis
Cortex
Calyces
Infundibulum
Aorta
Ureter
Hypogastric artery
Iliac vessels
Seminal vesicle
Prostate
Bulbous urethra
Penile urethra

(b)

See cross-sectional diagram (c) below
Pubis
External sphincter
Urethra
Neurovascular bundle
Verumontanum and ejaculatory ducts

Bladder
Detrusor muscle
Ureter
Prostate
Trigone
Ureter
Seminal vesicle
Vas deferens
Rectum

(c)

Prostate
Anterior floromuscular stroma
Transitional zone
Central zone
Peripheral zone
Neurovascular bundle
Denonvillier's fascia
Rectum

Pubis
Dorsal venous complex
Puboprostatic ligaments
Fibrous capsule
Urethra
Verumontanum
Ejaculatory duct
Vas deferens
Seminal vesicle

Fig. 12.3 Anatomy of the ureter.
Reproduced with permission from Morris, Peter J. and Wood, William C. (2000). *Oxford Textbook of Surgery*, 2nd edition. Oxford, UK: Oxford University Press.

Prevention of ureteric injury

- Generous surgical exposure and meticulous technique
- Identification of ureter
- Pre-operative ureteric imaging by CT/intravenous urogram (IVU) for patients at increased risk (see below)
- Ureteric stents inserted pre-operatively can help identify a ureteric injury when it does occur; they do not prevent injury
- Prophylactic stents can increase the ability to palpate the ureter, minimizing the need for ureteric dissection, and may minimize ureteric kinking by adjacent suturing
- Routine use is not recommended due to increased cost, time, and associated morbidity, i.e. UTI, haematuria, flank pain, and rarely ureteric injury
- Simultaneous rather than sequential insertion of ureteric stents during abdominal procedures reduces operative times without a significant increase in morbidity.

Risk factors

- Intraoperative haemorrhage treated with cautery or blind suturing
- Previous irradiation
- Re-operative pelvic surgery
- Recurrent or large pelvic tumours.

Intraoperative diagnosis

- Wall discoloration and absence of capillary refill should alert towards possible injury
- Intraoperative injection of indigo carmine or methylene blue in the ureter helps to confirm injury and location
- On-table retrograde ureterography can accurately establish the presence or absence of ureteric injury
- If site confirmed, careful evaluation of ureteral wall should be made. Lack of bleeding edge raises the suspicion of associated ischaemic injury
- Status of contralateral kidney or ureter should be established
- Primary repair depends on the length, location, aetiology, and presence/absence of retroperitoneal and pelvic infection
- Primary repair should be delayed if patient is unable to tolerate a prolonged operation.

Post-operative symptoms and signs

- Anuria with bilateral injury
- Ileus
- Flank or loin pain
- Abdominal mass (urinoma)
- Leucocytosis
- Sepsis of unknown origin
- Haematuria
- ↑ urea and creatinine
- ↑ creatinine in fluid collection
- Increased/prolonged drainage from abdominal wound/drain site
- Fistula formation
- Pathology report demonstrating a segment of ureter!
- Stricture and ipsilateral renal unit loss (long term).

Investigation of suspected ureteric injury

- US—hydronephrosis, ascites, and absent ureteric jets
- CT/IVU—contrast extravasation, ascites, hydronephrosis + urinoma
- Retrograde studies—in case of partial injury a double pigtail stent may be safely inserted
- X-ray—ground glass appearance, non-specific, and largely replaced by modern imaging techniques.

Treatment options

Initial percutaneous nephrostomy insertion can help treat sepsis and facilitate a later insertion of an antegrade stent. Favourable reports have been demonstrated with early repair of ureteric injury.

Principles of repair of partial injury

- If identified intraoperatively these should be managed with primary closure of the ureteral ends over a stent, with placement of an external, non-suction drain adjacent to the injury
- If identified post-operatively, a retrograde or antegrade stent is placed after retrograde ureteropyelogram or antegrade nephrostoureterogram. May reduce incidence of ureteric stricture.

Principles of repair of complete injury

- Debridement of ureteral ends to fresh tissue
- Spatulation of ureteral ends
- Placement of internal stent
- Watertight closure of reconstructed ureter with absorbable suture
- Placement of external, non-suction drain
- Isolation of injury within peritoneum or omental wrapping
- Type of reconstructive repair chosen by the surgeon depends on the nature and site of the injury.

According to the European Association of Urology guidelines (2009) the following are the treatment options for ureteric injury:

Upper third

- Ureteroureterostomy*
- Transureteroureterostomy (Fig. 12.4)
- Ureterocalycostomy.

Middle third

- Ureteroureterostomy*
- Transureteroureterostomy
- Boari flap and reimplantation* (Fig. 12.5).

Lower third

- Direct reimplantation
- Psoas hitch* (Fig. 12.6)
- Blandy cystoplasty.

Complete

- Ileal interposition
- Autotransplantation.

---

* denotes preferred techniques.

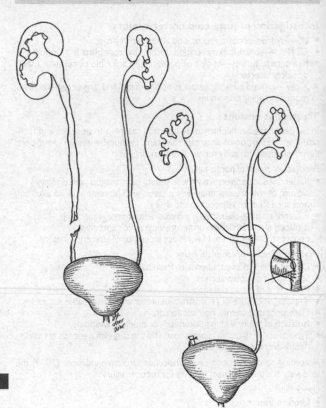

Fig. 12.4 Transureteroureterostomy.

Reproduced with permission from Presti, JC, Carroll, PR (1996). Ureteral and renal pelvic trauma: diagnosis and management. In McAninch, JW. *Traumatic and reconstructive urology.* Philadelphia, USA: W. B. Saunders.

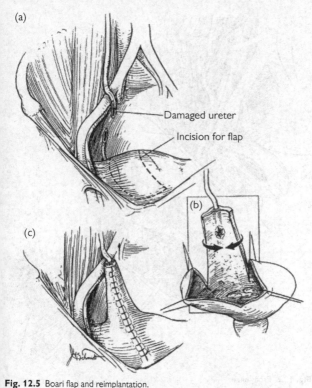

Fig. 12.5 Boari flap and reimplantation.

Reproduced with permission from Coburn M. (1996) Ureteral injuries from surgical trauma. In McAninch, JW. *Traumatic and reconstructive urology*. Philadelphia, USA: W. B. Saunders.

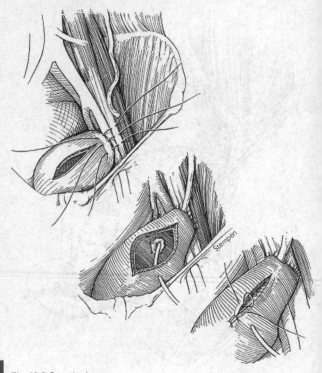

Fig. 12.6 Psoas hitch.

Reproduced with permission from Presti, JC, Carroll, PR (1996). Ureteral and renal pelvic trauma: diagnosis and management. In McAninch, JW. *Traumatic and reconstructive urology.* Philadelphia, USA: W. B. Saunders.

References

Dobrowolski Z, Kusionowicz J, Drewniak T et al. (2002) Renal and ureteric trauma: diagnosis and management in Poland. *BJU Int* **89**: 748–51.

Pokala N, Delaney CP, Kiran RP et al. (2006) A randomised controlled trial comparing simultaneous intra operative vs. sequential prophylactic ureteric catheter insertion in re-operative and complicated colorectal surgery. *Int J Colorectal Dis* **22**: 683–7.

Blandy JP, Badenoch DF, Fowler CG et al. (1991) Early repair of iatrogenic injury to the ureter and bladder after gynaecological surgery. *J Urol* **146**: 761–5.

Parpala ST, Paananen I, Santala M, Ohtonen P, Hellstrom P (2008) Increasing number of ureteric injuries after the introduction of laparoscopic surgery. *Scand J Urol Nephrol* **42**: 422–7.

Djakovic N, Plas E, Martinez-Pineiro L, Lynch TH, Mor Y, Santucci RA, Serafetinidis E, Turkeri LN, Hohenfellner M. *Guidelines on Urological Trauma.* European Association of Urology, 2009. https://uroweb.org/wp-content/uploads/EAU-Guidelines-Urological_Trauma-2012.pdf

Bladder reconstruction injury

Bladder resection/injury

Management of colorectal cancer invading the bladder

~10% of CRCs will involve surrounding structures, with most involving the urinary bladder. Adherence to bladder does not always mean invasion and attachment may represent inflammatory adhesion in 2/3 of cases. Pre-operative imaging is often suboptimal. *En bloc* resection should be the goal in localized disease, with 5yr survival for margin-negative resection between 40 and 72% in published series (Fig. 12.7).

- Tumours involving the dome can be managed with partial cystectomy
- Rectal tumours invade more caudally and may require total cystectomy
- Local invasion unilaterally near the ureteric insertion may still be managed by *en bloc* partial cystectomy combined with proximal transureteroureterostomy, direct re-implantation ± psoas hitch
- Partial cystectomy is sufficient to provide *en bloc* clearance in most cases and morbidity is significantly less than with enterocystoplasty or total cystectomy
- In older and unfit patients, urinary diversion with ileal conduit remains a popular option (Fig. 12.8)
- In younger patients with good life expectancy, a continent reservoir or neobladder may be constructed because these procedures improve patient's quality of life substantially.

Classification of bladder trauma

Intraperitoneal injury

- This should be repaired if identified, intra- or post-operatively
- Bladder drainage, e.g. urethral/suprapubic, is maintained post-operatively
- Cystogram may be used to assess repair post-operatively.

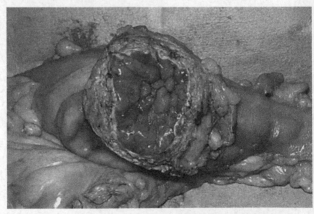

Fig. 12.7 *En bloc* resection of colon cancer involving partial cystectomy.

Extraperitoneal injury
- Any obvious injury to the bladder should be repaired intraoperatively
- If identified post-operatively can usually be managed with bladder drainage for 2 weeks followed by a cystogram to ensure that perforation has healed.

Laparoscopy and iatrogenic bladder/ureteric injuries

There have been reports of increased incidence compared with open surgery with the advent of laparoscopic colorectal procedures. Most of these injuries are not identified intraoperatively.
- Mostly caused by suprapubic trocar insertion or bladder dissection
- Injury, if suspected, can be confirmed by instilling the bladder with methylene blue
- It should be suspected with presence of gas in the Foley catheter
- If ureteric injury is identified, an attempted 1° closure over a double pigtail stent may be attempted, but in most instances, they require an open conversion
- Small injuries to bladder can be closed with 7–10 days' bladder drainage
- Injury can be prevented by catheterizing the bladder in complex pelvic surgery and avoiding directing the suprapubic trocar towards the space of Retzius.

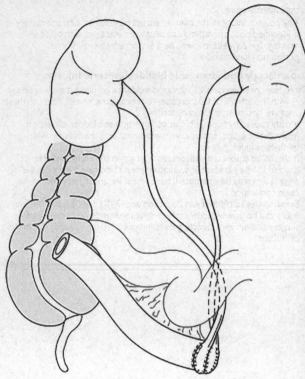

Fig. 12.8 Ileal conduit.

Index

Note: Tables, figures, and boxes are indicated by an italic *t*, *f*, and *b* following the page number.